Studies in Big Data

Volume 73

The series "Studies in Big Data" (SBD) publishes new developments and advances in the various areas of Big Data- quickly and with a high quality. The intent is to cover the theory, research, development, and applications of Big Data, as embedded in the fields of engineering, computer science, physics, economics and life sciences. The books of the series refer to the analysis and understanding of large, complex, and/or distributed data sets generated from recent digital sources coming from sensors or other physical instruments as well as simulations, crowd sourcing, social networks or other internet transactions, such as emails or video click streams and other. The series contains monographs, lecture notes and edited volumes in Big Data spanning the areas of computational intelligence including neural networks, evolutionary computation, soft computing, fuzzy systems, as well as artificial intelligence, data mining, modern statistics and Operations research, as well as self-organizing systems. Of particular value to both the contributors and the readership are the short publication timeframe and the world-wide distribution, which enable both wide and rapid dissemination of research output.

** Indexing: The books of this series are submitted to ISI Web of Science, DBLP, Ulrichs, MathSciNet, Current Mathematical Publications, Mathematical Reviews, Zentralblatt Math: MetaPress and Springerlink.

More information about this series at http://www.springer.com/series/11970

Chinmay Chakraborty · Amit Banerjee ·
Maheshkumar H. Kolekar · Lalit Garg ·
Basabi Chakraborty
Editors

Internet of Things for Healthcare Technologies

Springer

Editors
Chinmay Chakraborty
Department of Electronics
and Communication Engineering
Birla Institute of Technology, Mesra
Ranchi, India

Amit Banerjee
Department of Electrical
and Computer Engineering
National University of Singapore
Singapore, Singapore

Maheshkumar H. Kolekar
Department of Electrical Engineering
Indian Institute of Technology Patna
Patna, India

Lalit Garg
Department of Computer Information
Systems, Faculty of Information and
Communication Technology
University of Malta
Msida, Malta

Basabi Chakraborty
Faculty of Software and Information Science
Iwate Prefectural University
Takizawa, Japan

ISSN 2197-6503 ISSN 2197-6511 (electronic)
Studies in Big Data
ISBN 978-981-15-4111-7 ISBN 978-981-15-4112-4 (eBook)
https://doi.org/10.1007/978-981-15-4112-4

This Springer imprint is published by the registered company Springer Nature Singapore Pte Ltd.
The registered company address is: 152 Beach Road, #21-01/04 Gateway East, Singapore 189721, Singapore

Preface

The general interest in the Internet of things (IoT) for healthcare technologies has been increasing significantly because of its enormous and promising application prospects in the advancement of human civilization. Among literally thousands of different technologies related to the Internet of things for health care, there are some definite trends that have a high impact in the future health care and are focused on the current title, e.g., Advanced Medical Imaging, Biomedical Signal Processing, IoT with Different Biomedical Sensors, Biotechnological Advances, etc. This title focuses on the recent advances and different research issues in biomedical technology by seeking out for theoretical, methodological, well-established, and validated empirical work dealing with these different topics. This book volume deals with the emerging applications in Internet of things for healthcare technologies like IoT in smart healthcare system, IoT-based diseases prediction and diagnosis system for health care, methodology for improving efficiency in data transmission in healthcare systems, correlation of tension-type headache and diabetes; IoT perspective in health care, machine learning applications for a real-time monitoring of arrhythmia patients using IoT, human heart arrhythmia identification using ECG signals; an approach toward biomedical signal processing, deep learning and its applications in medical imaging, brain tumor classification using deep learning, early detection of dementia disease using data mining techniques, social, medical, and educational applications of IoT to assist visually impaired people, design of embedded system for remote monitoring of malnutrition for people living in rural areas, review on security and privacy concern in IoT health care, applications of Internet of things in medical area, and bigdata in the management of diabetes mellitus treatment. This title covers a very vast audience from basic science to engineering and technology experts and learners. This could eventually work as a textbook for engineering and biomedical students or science masters programs and for researchers. This title also serves the common public interest by presenting new methods to improve the quality of life in general, with better integration into society.

The title also covers various aspects of future healthcare technologies like medical imaging, which currently employs from simple 2-D X-rays, ultrasound, CT scans, MRI, and host of other technologies, but researchers are developing new and improved imaging options like various forms of EM imaging, terahertz or Infrared imagining, thermography, combined with medical virtual reality, which would provide more accuracy and better outcomes in image-guided surgery, improved cardiac and lung imaging, giving physicians real-time and accurate views. Artificial intelligence is to revolutionize all industries, but perhaps none so much as health care. Both biomedicine and machine learning could analyze data availed in national health databases to identify potential complications, as well as effective protocols, using the intelligence gained via data. A wave of wearable devices targeting the biomedical and healthcare applications far beyond tracking your steps each day emerged. These devices are capable of collecting detailed information about our health, while also serving as a smartwatch or simple attachment combined with our mobile phones. The data are collected and analyzed in standard protocols by machine intelligence looking for possible predictions of health-related issues. Beyond these, prosthetic technologies have already made significant strides in recent decades with the advances in materials and development. Chip-enabled prosthetics are on the horizon with more mobility and flexibility, or even auxiliary motors that can help provide additional strength and power, or additional robotic devices that will continue to blur the lines between therapeutic and assistive devices. The IoT enabled wireless ECG sensors to reduce healthcare costs and lead to improving the overall quality of cardio patients' life. The amount of data acquired by ECG sensors should be minimized for the efficient performance of the IoT healthcare systems. Various biomedical advances are extremely prominent and may transform the way we look at health care.

Ranchi, India

Dr. Chinmay Chakraborty
Assistant Professor
cchakrabarty@bitmesra.ac.in

Singapore

Dr. Amit Banerjee
Senior Scientist
amitbanerjeeiacseru@gmail.com

Patna, India

Dr. Maheshkumar H. Kolekar
Associate Professor
mahesh@iitp.ac.in

Msida, Malta

Dr. Lalit Garg
Senior Lecturer
lalit.garg@um.edu.mt

Takizawa, Japan

Dr. Basabi Chakraborty
Professor
basabi@iwate-pu.ac.jp

Contents

Editors and Contributors

About the Editors

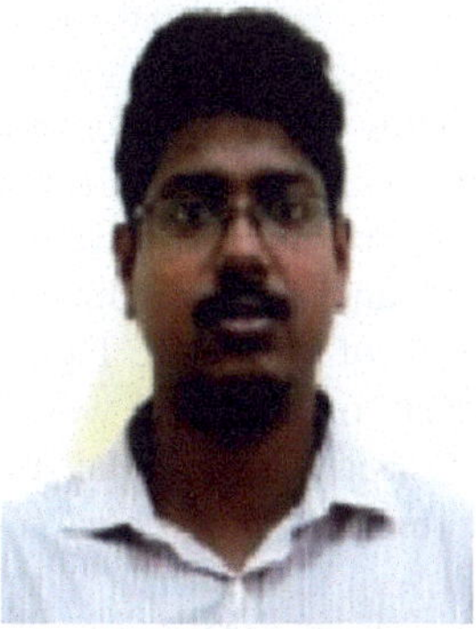

Dr. Chinmay Chakraborty is an Assistant Professor at the Department of Electronics and Communication Engineering, BIT Mesra. His primary areas of research include wireless body area networks, the Internet of Medical Things, energy-efficient wireless communications and networking, and point-of-care diagnosis. He received an Outstanding Researcher Award from TESFA in 2016, a Global Peer Review Award from Publons in 2018, and also a Young Faculty Award from VIFA in 2018. He is also the recipient of a Young Research Excellence Award, and a Global Peer-Review Award.

Address: Electronics and Communication Engineering, Birla Institute of Technology, Mesra, Jasidih, Deoghar, Jharkhand, Pin 814142, India

Phone: +91-9973871459
Email: cchakrabarty@bitmesra.ac.in
Business url: https://sites.google.com/view/dr-chinmay-chakraborty
LinkedIn: https://www.linkedin.com/in/dr-chinmay-c-35017310

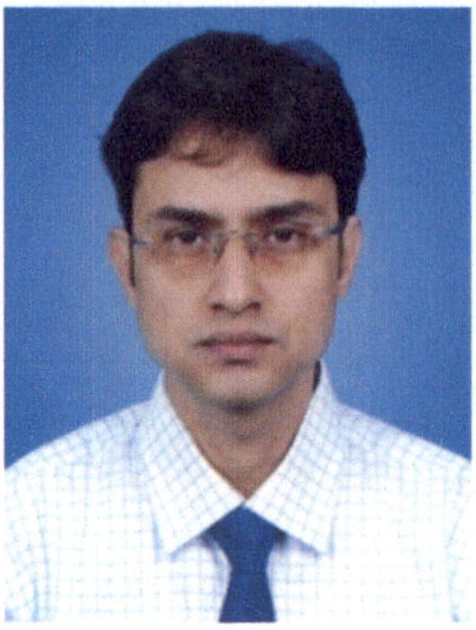

Dr. Amit Banerjee worked as a Scientific Researcher at the Research Institute of Electronics, Japan, from 2016, and became a Scientist at the Department of Electrical and Computer Engineering of the prestigious National University of Singapore in 2018. Amit has worked extensively on Terahertz devices for biomedical applications.

Scientist, Microelectronic Technologies & Devices, Department of Electrical and Computer Engineering, National University of Singapore, 21 Lower Kent Ridge Rd, 119077, Singapore

Email: eleami@nus.edu.sg
LinkedIn: https://www.linkedin.com/in/dr-amit-banerjee/
Web page: http://nfet.nshm.com/faculty/dr-amit-banerjee/

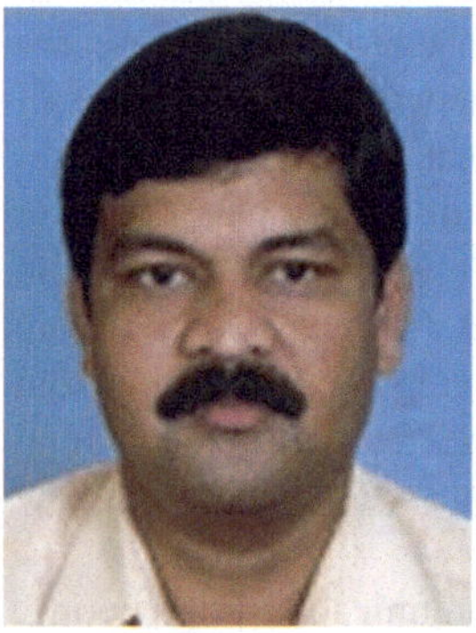

Dr. Maheshkumar H. Kolekar is an Associate Professor at the Indian Institute of Technology Patna. His research interests include digital image and video processing, video surveillance, and medical image processing. He was a recipient of the Best Paper Award from the Computer Society of India and was a DAAD fellow at TU Berlin, Germany, from May to July 2017, where he pursued research in the area of biomedical signal processing.

Associate Professor, Electrical Engineering Department, Indian Institute of Technology, Patna

Phone: +91-612-302 8043 (Off.)
Email: mahesh@iitp.ac.in
Web page: https://www.iitp.ac.in/index.php/departments/engineering/electrical-engineering/people/faculty/dr-maheshkumar-h-kolekar.html
LinkedIn: https://www.linkedin.com/in/maheshkumar-kolekar-68646a8/

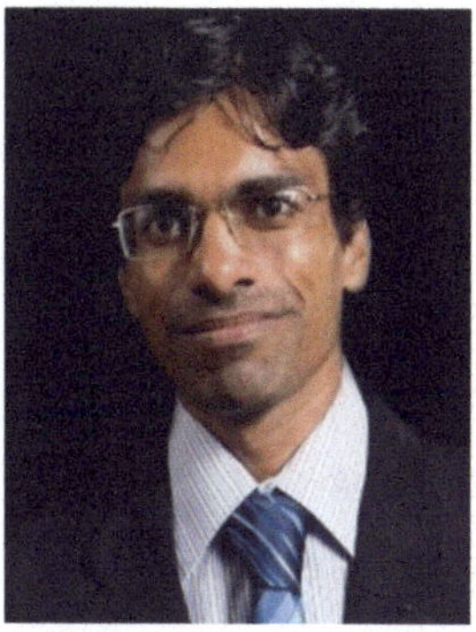

Dr. Lalit Garg is a Senior Lecturer in Computer Information Systems at the University of Malta, and an Honorary Lecturer at the University of Liverpool, UK. He has also worked as a researcher at Nanyang Technological University, Singapore, and at the University of Ulster, UK. His research interests include handling missing data, machine learning, data mining, mathematical and stochastic modeling, and operational research, and their applications, especially in the healthcare domain.

Assistant Professor, Faculty of Information and Communication Technology, University of Malta, MSD 2080, Malta

Phone: +356 7923 3327
Email: lalit.garg@um.edu.mt
Web page: https://www.um.edu.mt/profile/lalitgarg

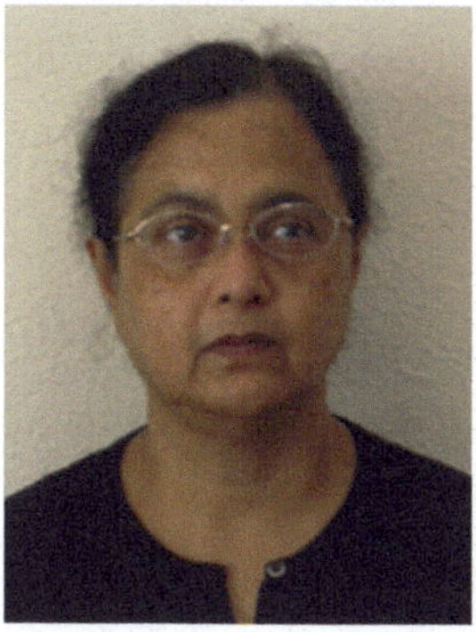

Dr. Basabi Chakraborty holds B.Tech., M.Tech., and Ph.D. degrees in Radio Physics and Electronics from Calcutta University, India, and worked at the Indian Statistical Institute, Calcutta, India, until 1990. From 1991 to 1993, she worked as a researcher at the Advanced Intelligent Communication Systems Laboratory in Sendai, Japan. Her main research interests include pattern recognition, machine learning, soft computing techniques, biometrics, data mining and social media data mining.

Professor, Faculty of Software and Information Science, Iwate Prefectural University, Japan

Email: basabi@iwate-pu.ac.jp
Web page: https://scholar.google.com/citations?user=qyqKH3cAAAAJ&hl=en

Contributors

Morteza Amirhosseini Allameh Tabataba'i University (ATU), Tehran, Iran

S. Ananda Kumar SCOPE, VIT-Vellore, Vellore, India

Rangel Arthur School of Electrical and Computer Engineering (FEEC), University of Campinas—UNICAMP, Campinas, SP, Brazil

Rajib Bag Supreme Knowledge Foundation Group of Institutions, Hooghly, India

Chinmay Chakraborty Department of Electronics and Communication Engineering, Birla Institute of Technology, Ranchi, Jharkhand, India

Joy Chatterjee Supreme Knowledge Foundation Group of Institutions, Hooghly, India

Devendra Kumar Chaturvedi Dayalbagh Educational Institute, Agra, India

Atanu Das Netaji Subhash Engineering College, Kolkata, India

Manab Kumar Das Supreme Knowledge Foundation Group of Institutions, Hooghly, India

Bikash Dey JIS College of Engineering, Kalyani, West Bengal, India

V. Dhanakoti Department of Computer Science and Engineering, SRM Valliammai Engineering College, Chennai, Tamil Nadu, India

Ravina Dnyaneshwar Edake MKSSS's Cummins College of Engineering for Women, Pune, Solapur, India

Reinaldo Padilha França School of Electrical and Computer Engineering (FEEC), University of Campinas—UNICAMP, Campinas, SP, Brazil

Sayon Ghosh Supreme Knowledge Foundation Group of Institutions, Hooghly, India

Mayank Gupta Tata Consultancy Services, Noida, India

Yuzo Iano School of Electrical and Computer Engineering (FEEC), University of Campinas—UNICAMP, Campinas, SP, Brazil

Maheshkumar H. Kolekar Department of Electrical Engineering, Indian Institute of Technology Patna, Patna, India

K. Lalitha Department of Information Technology, Kongu Engineering College, Erode, Tamil Nadu, India

G. Mahesh CSE, BMSIT&M-Bangalore, Bangalore, India

Farzaneh Mansouri Musolu Faculty of Management and Accounting, Department of Industrial Management, Allameh Tabataba'i University, Tehran, Iran

Ana Carolina Borges Monteiro School of Electrical and Computer Engineering (FEEC), University of Campinas—UNICAMP, Campinas, SP, Brazil

Iman Raeesi Vanani Faculty of Management and Accounting, Department of Industrial Management, Allameh Tabataba'i University, Tehran, Iran

Dhanaraj Rajesh Kumar School of Computing Science and Engineering, Galgotias University, Greater Noida, India

K. Rajkumar Department of Information Technology, Galgotias College of Engineering and Technology, Greater Noida, India

Rohit Rastogi ABES Engineering College Ghaziabad and Dayalbagh Educational Institute, Agra, India

Mamata Rath School of Management (Information Technology), Birla Global University, Bhubaneswar, Odisha, India

V. S. K. Reddy Department of Electronics and Communication Engineering, Malla Reddy College of Engineering and Technology, Hyderabad, India

Saeid Sadeghi Darvazeh Faculty of Management and Accounting, Department of Industrial Management, Allameh Tabataba'i University, Tehran, Iran

Soham Sharma Department of Computer Science, CHRIST (Deemed to be University), Bengaluru, India

Parul Singhal ABES Engineering College Ghaziabad and Dayalbagh Educational Institute, Agra, India

Rajendran Sree Ranjani RISE Lab, Department of Computer Science and Engineering, Indian Institute of Technology Madras, Chennai, India

S. Srinivasa Rao Department of Electronics and Communication Engineering, Malla Reddy College of Engineering and Technology, Hyderabad, India

M. Sucharitha Department of Electronics and Communication Engineering, Malla Reddy College of Engineering and Technology, Hyderabad, India

M. Umme Salma Department of Computer Science, CHRIST (Deemed to be University), Bengaluru, India

Vishal K. Waghmare Department of Electrical Engineering, Indian Institute of Technology Patna, Patna, India

Chapter 1
IoT in Smart Healthcare System

S. Ananda Kumar and G. Mahesh

Abstract Automation has taken over the world of the twenty-first century. Within every field, new ground-breaking technology has emerged that makes life easier, fast, and all the more efficient. A lot of changes can be wrought in the scope of medicine and pharmacy as well. One such instance is medication which has become an extremely common practice these days. Especially for the elderly, they have to consume multiple sets of medication every day. It becomes difficult to remember which to take and at what time. Monitoring the aged people for each and every second is a major issue which motivated us to take certain issues providing general solutions for healthcare systems using Internet of things (IoT). Due to the drastic increase in traffic and population with limited resources, the new technologies like IoT will be greatly useful in the field of healthcare monitoring and also used to take a decision before any critical event can occur.

Keywords Internet of things · Wearable devices · Healthcare system

1.1 Wearable Devices in IoT for Health care and Their Communication Models

1.1.1 Introduction

A wave of wearable devices targeting the biomedical and healthcare applications far beyond tracking your steps each day has emerged. These devices are capable of collecting detailed information about our health, while also serving as a smartwatch or simple attachment combined with our mobile phones. The data is collected and analyzed in standard protocols by machine intelligence looking for possible predictions

S. Ananda Kumar (✉)
SCOPE, VIT-Vellore, Vellore, India
e-mail: s.anandakumar@vit.ac.in

G. Mahesh
CSE, BMSIT&M-Bangalore, Bangalore, India

C. Chakraborty et al. (eds.), *Internet of Things for Healthcare Technologies*, Studies in Big Data 73, https://doi.org/10.1007/978-981-15-4112-4_1

of health-related issues. Beyond these, prosthetic technologies have already made significant strides in recent decades with the advances in materials and development. Chip-enabled prosthetics are on the horizon with more mobility and flexibility, or even auxiliary motors that can help provide additional strength and power, or additional robotic devices that will continue to blur the lines between therapeutic and assistive devices. The major goal of wearable devices is activity recognition and sensing what we are doing, in which location [1, 2].

1.1.2 Classification and Categories of Wearable Devices

The wearable devices are classified based on requirement and usage. Some devices are used based on doctors instruction because it may lead to serious issues in humans if not used with proper medical intervention, just for an example, ingestible sensors, wearable injectors, and wearable insulin pumps require proper medical intervention, with that experts can decide the proper dosage. On the other hand, some wearable sensors can be used without any intervention by experts for monitoring in various applications represented in Fig. 1.1 and Tables 1.1, 1.2, and 1.3 [3].

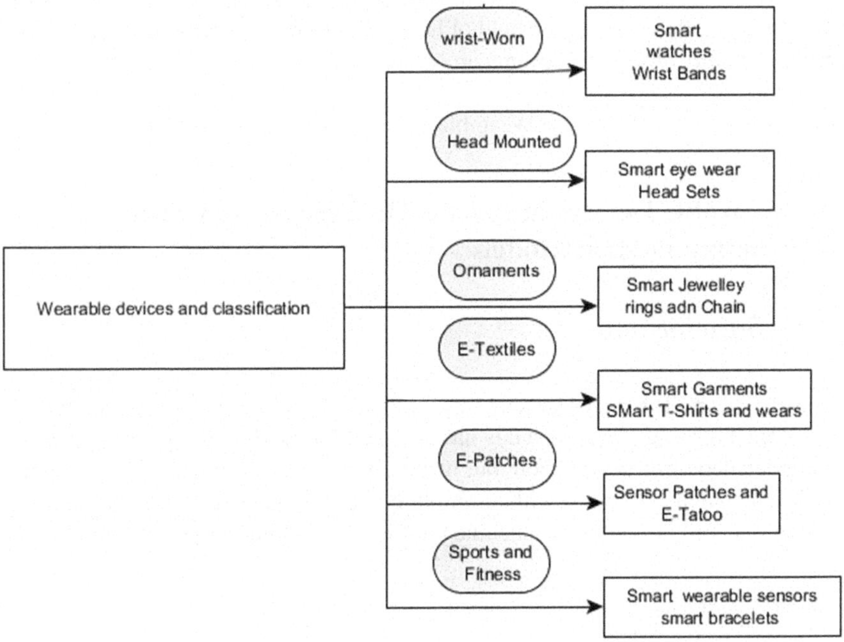

Fig. 1.1 Classification and categories of wearable devices

Table 1.1 Wearable devices categories [3]

Accessories		Description	Existing product	Research prototype
Wrist worns	Smartwatches	Wrist-worn devices with a touchscreen display	Apple iWatch Samsung Gear S2 Moto 360 Pebble Time	Smartwatch lifesaver Finger-writing with Smartwatch
	Wrist band	Wrist-worn devices with fitness tracking capabilities	UP by Jawbone Fitbit Flex MOOV NOW Nymi Band	Wrist-worn bioimpedance sensor Wrist-worn smoking gesture detector Ultrasonic-speaker-embedded wrist piece and neck piece
Head mounted device	Smart eyewear	Spectacles or contact lenses with sensing, wireless communications, or other capabilities	Microsoft HoloLens FUNI'KI Ambient Glasses Recon Jet	Google Glass Google Contact Lens Object modeling eyewear iShadow Mobile Gaze Tracker Indoor landmark identification supporting wearables Chroma
	Headsets and earbuds	Bluetooth-enabled headsets or ear plugs	Sony Xperia Ear Apple AirPods Bragi Dash Pro	–
Other accessories	Smart jewelry	Jewelry designed with features such as health monitoring and handless-control	Smarty Ring Kery Bellabeat Leaf	TypingRing Gesture detection ring
	Straps	Chest straps, belts, arm bands, or knee straps equipped with sensors for health tracking or other functionalities	MYO armband Zephyr Bioharness	Pneumatic armband BodyBeat
E-Textiles	Smart garments	Main clothing items that also serve as wearable such as shirts, pants, and undergarments	Athos Hug shirt Solar shirt Spinovo	Myovibe Dopplesleep
	Foot/hand-worn	Shoes, socks, insoles, or gloves embedded with sensors	Lechal Sensoria Fujitsu gesture-control Gloves	LookUp Gait analysis foot worns Foot-worn inertial sensors

(continued)

Table 1.1 (continued)

Accessories		Description	Existing product	Research prototype
E-Patch	Sensor patches	Sensor patches that can be adhered to the skin for either fitness tracking or haptic application	HealthPatch MD Thync UPRIGHT	DuoSkin Tattoo-based iontophoretic-biosensing system Smart tooth patch
	E-tatto/E-skin	Tattoos with flexible and stretchable electronic circuit to realize sensing and wireless data transmission	Motorola e-tattoo Wearable Interactive stamp platform	–

Table 1.2 Sub-categories of wearable devices [3]

E-textiles		
Sub-category	Product	Description
Smart garments and sports fitness	Hug shirt	Recreate the sensation of touch
	T Jacket	Designed for children with autism
	Solar shirt	Integrated with solar cells used to charge the smartphone and other smart devices
	Hovding	Helmet sense the cyclist movement
	Athos	For athletes and sports persons in training aids
	OMsignal	For fitness tracking made of special material
	Citizen sciences	Fitness tracking, tight fitting cloth with microsensors
	MYONTEC	Muscle sensing smart shorts monitor muscle load, hear rate, speed, and distance
	Ofseth	Monitor the respiratory movement
	Myovibe	Wearable MMG System, detect the activation of skeletal muscle

1.1.3 Communication Modes of Wearable Devices in IoT

Even though the devices are small in size and work with a small battery, they need to consume minimum power for operation. Also, each of the devices has its own constraints like processing, storing, computing power, and transmission power. Based

Table 1.3 Products of wearable devices [3]

Wrist-worns		
	Product	Descriptions
Smartwatches	Apple Watch Series 2 (aluminum case—38 mm)	A smartwatch with notifications and health tracking functionalities
	Motorola Moto 360 (42 mm)	A smartwatch with notifications and health tracking functionalities
	Samsung Gear S2	A smartwatch with notifications and health tracking functionalities
	Huawei Watch (42 mm)	A smartwatch with notifications and health tracking functionalities

on the distance coverage, there are three classifications very short distance, short distance, and long distance.

Very short distance—The technology adapted for very short distance communication is near-field communication (NFC), and it needs very low power consumption for shorter distance communication to transfer the tiny amount of data just by touching tow devices each other in 4 cm range, e.g., contactless payment system.

Short distance—Bluetooth is suitable for short-distance communication, with low cost and low power consumption, and the devices are powered by coin cell battery. These wearable devices can transfer limited data to the range up to 100 m theoretically. Maximum eight devices can pair in Bluetooth, one is acting as a master node and other seven nodes act as a slave node. Because of the limited data transfer, it is not suitable for multimedia communication. Some of the examples are calls through Bluetooth headset which is connected remotely to the cell phone.

ANT is another wireless network for short-distance communication technology for the application of sports and fitness to monitor the heart rate in cycling. Some of the ANT devices are SensRcore [3] (Fig. 1.2).

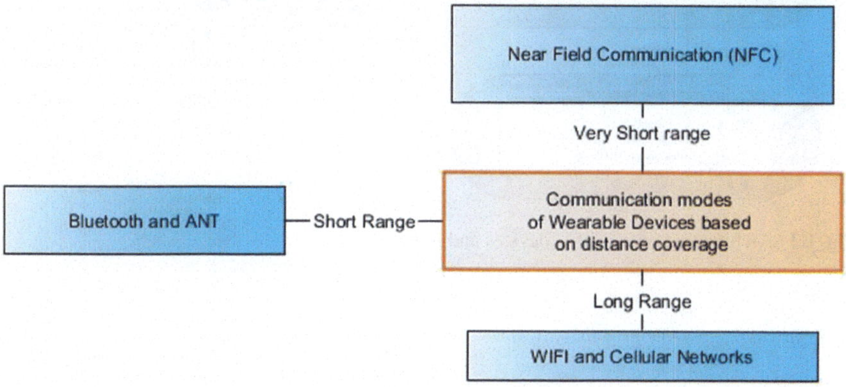

Fig. 1.2 Communication modes of wearable devices in IoT

Long-distance communication—If the application requires the data to transmit to longer distance with manageable delay, then Wi-Fi and cellular networks are the best available options. The device has more transmission power, processing power, and storage power than shorter communication models. These communication models transmit multimedia data like voice and video.

1.1.4 Working Principles of Wearable Devices in IoT

The working principles of wearable devices in IoT consist of three layers.

First layer—This layer contains the wearable sensors deployed in application for sensing data. As shown in Fig. 1.3, we considered the healthcare application, where the temperature and heartbeat are sensed and transmitted to the higher layer.

Second layer—The actual raw data from sensors is collected, processed in local network, and transmitted to cloud services for remote accessing with the help of various wireless communication technologies, like Bluetooth, Wi-Fi, ZigBee, and RFID.

Third layer or cloud service layer—The wearable sensors store data in the cloud, and this data is accessed from cloud service through communication technology. Also, the third layer is used for data analysis and monitoring the application in the remote system [4, 5].

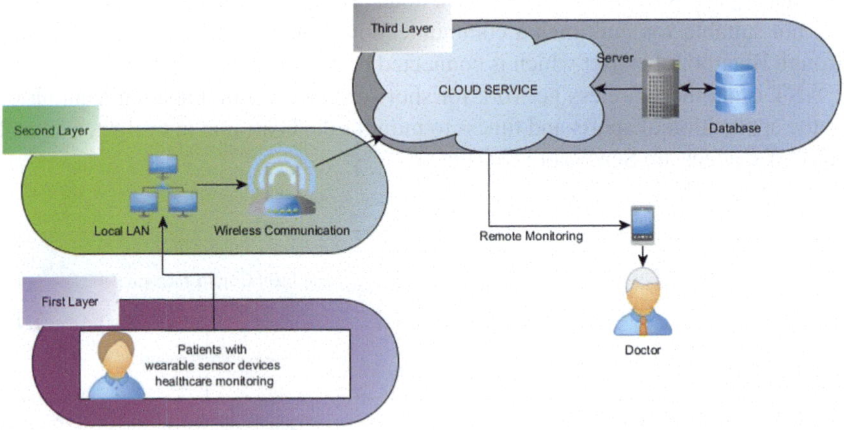

Fig. 1.3 Architecture of wearable devices and IoT

1.1.5 Applications of Wearable Devices in IoT

- Smartwatch-based wearable EEG system for driver drowsiness detection [6]. To avoid the major accidents in national highways due to drowsiness of drivers, a wireless EEG device contains sensory input unit (SIU) and sensory processing unit (SPU). The sensed data is converted to digital data transmitted to smartwatch through Bluetooth. The smartwatch contains vibrate sensor. If the driver had drowsiness, first it will give an early signal, and if the driver does not respond, it will vibrate and wake up the driver.
- Wearable IoT data stream traceability in a distributed health information system [7]. This technology is used to map the device data to the users in a heterogeneous environment.
- A wearable health monitoring system for post-traumatic stress disorder [8]. Post-traumatic stress disorder or PTSD is due to a shocking, traumatic event, and it commonly affects the veterans. With the help of wearable sensors, the patients are monitored for nightmare conditions. The existing collected data is used for training through machine learning techniques, and an optimized solution for patient monitoring and decision taking can then be designed.
- A model for predicting user intention to use wearable IoT devices at the workplace [9].
- A novel wearable device for continuous, non-invasion blood pressure measurement [10]. A wearable device which incorporates sensor is developed to measure the daily blood pressure; if any small volume of BP is detected, it will transmit the data and display on screen through Internet for remote patient monitoring. This data will go for further analysis and suggest medication, suggest the sports and diet to bring down the BP to a normal level.
- IoT-based intelligent fitness system [11].
- Virtual-blind-road following-based wearable navigation device for blind people [12].

1.1.6 Research Challenges and Open Issues

Apart from the challenges in constrained like size, power, and storage, wearable devices in IoT have some open challenges which are listed out [13].

- **Standards**: Several organizations maintain their own standards for communication, for example, ETSI maintains for machine to machine (M2M) and RFID. Some technologies are long-distance communication and some for short. 6LoWPAN is used for low-capacity devices. We have some diversity in standards. There is no common standard for IoT, and it is not integrated.

- **Scalability and adaptability**: Everyday adding a new type of wearable devices into the IoT application with that integration of devices in a heterogeneous environment is not a simple task [14].
- **Naming and addressing**: Due to scalability, the identification of devices in the application and real-time scenario is a great challenge, because we have a shortage of name and addressing. We already move from IPv4 to IPv6, in the near future; if 100 billion devices are joined for an application, then it will be a great challenge.
- **Traffic management**: The huge number of devices will generate a huge amount of data in terms of Gbps, managing those data is a crucial thing. Data identification and classification in healthcare application is a very challenging task, because at any point of time, the server is continuously receiving data [15].
- **Privacy**: Confidential data and health-related data are collected and shared without the knowledge of the concerned person. Validating the received data from the health care and other application is a challenging task.
- **HMI**: Human–machine interaction, interface for user to wearable devices, is still a challenging task.

1.2 IoT-Based Smart Pill Dispenser or Medicine Box

1.2.1 Introduction

The life span of human beings depends on the quality of life and every individual is prone to one or more disease during his/her lifetime. With aging, the probability of being diagnosed with a health issue is more, and medication is a common practice followed across the world for treating any illness. An important aspect of medication is that the individual needs to take the medicines as directed by a healthcare professional. The healthcare professional would have prescribed a particular medication regimen keeping in mind the history of the patient, and it would be effective only if the regimen is followed. However, adherence to the said routine of medication is a common issue, particularly among aged people.

Medication adherence can be defined as the behavior of the patient for the intake of medicines conforming to a routine, as specified by a healthcare professional. The routine includes the time at which the medicine needs to be taken and the dosage of medicine. The benefits of medication adherence include appropriate drug effect, proper treatment of the illness, and reduced healthcare cost.

Non-adherence could be because of missing a dose of medicine. Medication non-adherence can be defined as the incorrect taking of medication either in terms of quantity of medicine or the prescribed time. Medication non-adherence can be intentional or non-intentional. In intentional non-adherence, the patient deliberately misses a dose of medicine due to personal preference or lack of knowledge. In non-intentional adherence, the patient is not deliberately missing a dose but may forget to take medicine due to a complex medication regimen. Non-adherence to medication may lead to severe degradation of health, waste of medicines, and more healthcare cost.

Some of the reasons for medication non-adherence are

- **Forgetting**—One common reason is that patients forget to take some dose of medicine due to their busy schedule.
- **Confusion**—Patients may get confused to pick the right medicine from the medicine bag, when the number of medicines to be taken is more.
- **Ignorance after partial recovery**—Some patients stop taking medicines or will start their own regimen once they start feeling better. Worse sometimes, they may not take the medicines for the full duration specified.
- **Physical barriers**—In a few cases, there could be physical barriers, such as size of the tablet, as some patients find it difficult to swallow large tablets. The taste and odor of the medicine could also act as a barrier for non-adherence.
- **Early decision**—In some cases, the patients may feel that the medicines are not working for them in a short interval of time and may stop taking medicines.
- **Cost**—Some medicines might be costly and patients may skip doses or take less medicine than the prescribed dose to save money.

Medication adherence can be measured directly by any family member of the patient through observation or indirectly by counting the number of medicine units left in the medicine bag, in comparison with the number of units that should have been left, if the patient had followed the regimen correctly. With appropriate interventions, medical non-adherence can be reduced. The following are some of the ways that can be adapted to overcome medical non-adherence.

- Reminders in the form of a phone call or text may be sent to the patient who usually forgets to take medicines.
- Counseling the patient to bring in positive changes for medicine intake behavior.
- Family and peers intervention in providing a supportive environment can improve the medical non-adherence.

The advances in science and technology have enabled greater quality in healthcare systems, and as a result, the mortality and morbidity rate associated with a number of diseases is greatly reduced. After understanding the importance of medication adherence, monitoring it would result in better health and economic benefits. Medication adherence monitoring is the monitoring of the patient using some methods and analyzing whether the proper dose of medicines is taken on time. Traditional approaches of monitoring require a lot of efforts and attention toward the patient. Hence, it is preferred to take advantage of technology for monitoring medical adherence.

The vast network of devices connected to the Internet including smartphones, tablets, and related devices has a sensor on it. These “things” collect and exchange data. IoT in healthcare field referred to as Internet of Medical Things (IoMT). It is the purposeful connection of intelligent sensors, devices, and software to computer networking systems using Bluetooth, Wi-Fi, RFID, or M2M wireless technology in order to promote an interfunctionality that serves a greater purpose. In health care,

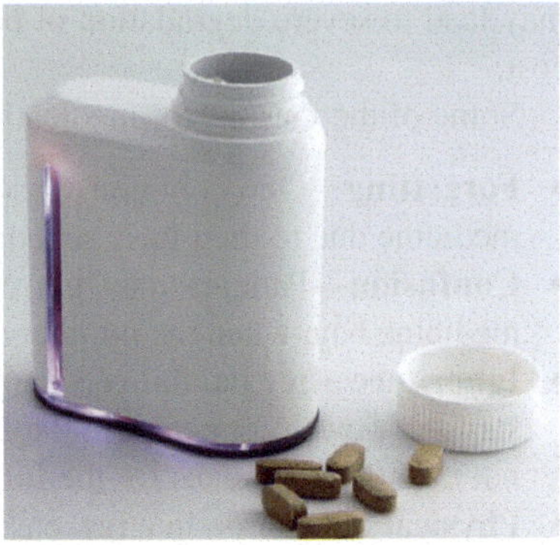

Fig. 1.4 AdhereTech's smart pill bottle [21]

that greater purpose is the achievement of cost-effective, information-driven, and efficient patient care system [16].

1.2.2 Smart Pill Boxes

A number of smart pill bottles are available in the market. The prominent ones among them are discussed in this section.

1.2.2.1 AdhereTech's Smart Pill Bottle

It is a plastic bottle with some circuitry, sensors, and software for detecting compliance with medications. The data flow starts with the bottle. Basically, the information about whether the medicine is taken by the patient or not is sent to the system. The system makes a comparison between the obtained information and the prescribed medication regimen of the patient. When a mismatch occurs, if it is the case of missing a simple dose of medicine, then the bottle will glow or a reminder by means of text or call is initiated by the system. If it is a serious non-adherence to medication like if multiple doses of medicine are missed, the system will initiate a call to the patient to know about the associated problems, or a call to a pharmacy or a healthcare professional is made to help out the patient (Fig. 1.4).

1.2.2.2 iMediPac

iMediPac is a pill dispenser in which pills are stored for each day of a week. The pill box has lights and alarms that will remind the patient to take the medicines as per the prescribed regimen. It can also remind the patient by means of a text message or a call. It also has an option of feeding data about the intake of medicine to an app,

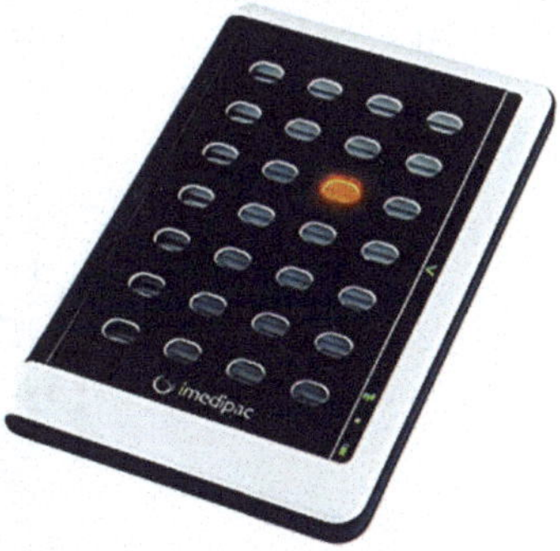

Fig. 1.5 IMediPac smart pill dispenser [22]

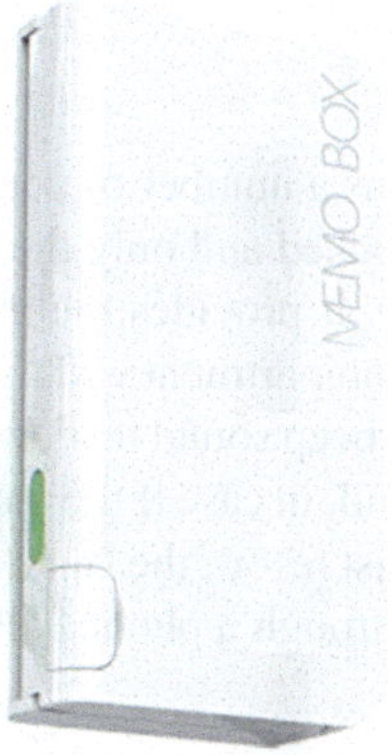

Fig. 1.6 MemoBox smart pill box [23]

using which the patient's family or the healthcare professional can get information about how well the patient is doing with medication adherence (Fig. 1.5).

1.2.2.3 MemoBox

MemoBox is a smart pill box with a compartment to store different pills to be taken at different time intervals. It reminds the patient about medication intake using audio and video alert as per the set time. It has a feature of double-dose alert for preventing the patient from overdose of medicines. It also has a feature of notifying the user when the box is left behind or misplaced (Fig. 1.6).

1.2.2.4 MedMinder

MedMinder smart pill box is a huge pill box that has its own built-in cellular connection. This eliminates the need for a separate phone line or Internet connection. It

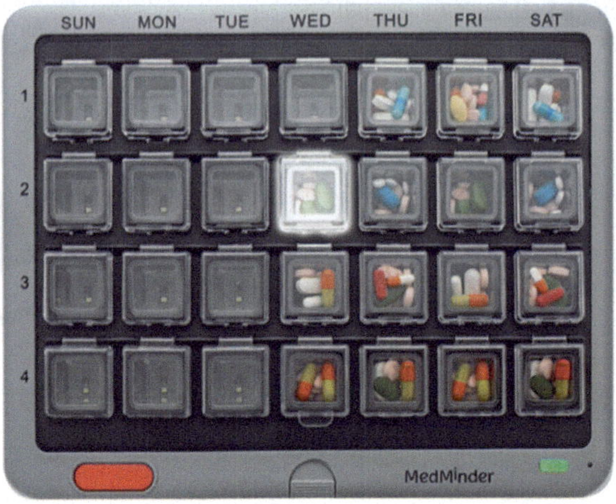

Fig. 1.7 MedMinder smart pill box [24]

has a number of compartments for storing the medicines. All the compartments are locked and only the right compartment is set to open at the right time (Fig. 1.7).

It provides the user with several different types of reminders. To start with, the compartment will flash if the medicine is not taken and then, the pill box will generate a beep sound to alert the patient. MedMinder will remind the patient through a phone call, in case if the patient fails to take the medicine even after the beep sound and as a last resort, the smart pill box notifies the family members or healthcare professionals through a phone call or text message.

1.2.2.5 uBox

uBox has a cylindrical structure with a number of compartments for storing the medicines. Each compartment can be used to store a dose of medicine. It has a reliable locking mechanism that ensures that the patient has access to the medicine, only at the time set. It provides an option for sharing information about the medicine intake, with the healthcare professionals and family members through notifications (Fig. 1.8).

1.2.2.6 Philips Medications Dispensing Service

This is a non-portable smart pill dispenser particularly helpful for aged people who stay at home. It can accommodate complex medication regimens with even six doses per day. It reminds the patient to take medicine by means of an audio alert, and with the press of a button, the medicine is dispensed. The dispenser is connected to a phone line, and when the patient misses a dose of medicine, the dispenser contacts the family members for their intervention to medication adherence (Fig. 1.9).

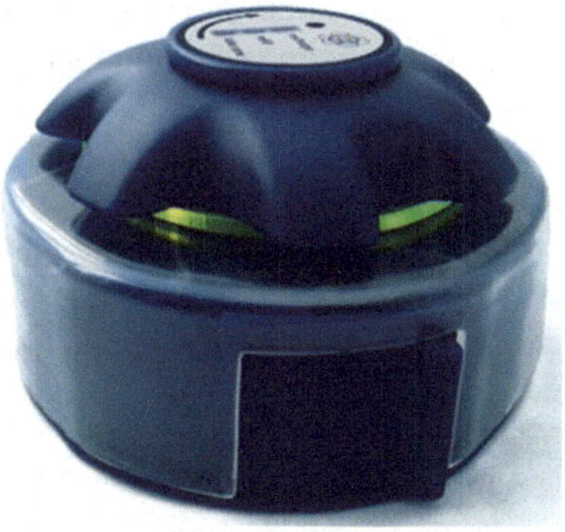

Fig. 1.8 uBox smart pill box [25]

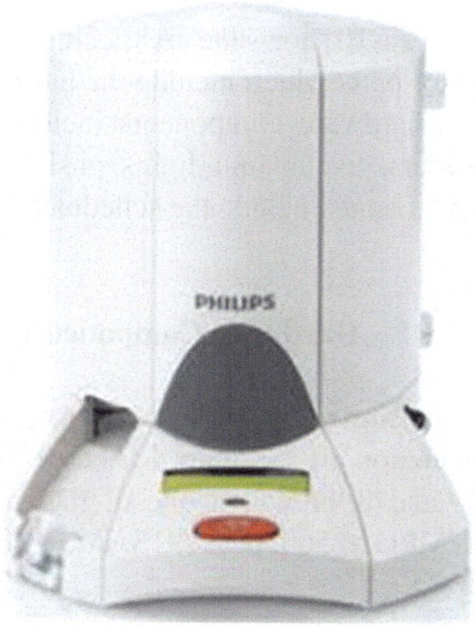

Fig. 1.9 Philips medication dispenser [26]

1.2.3 Desirable Characteristics of Smart Pill Boxes

Use of technology for medication adherence should help the users to adhere to the prescribed medication regimen without any kind of deviation. However, at the same time, the complexity and cost involved should not drive away the potential users from using it. After seeing the features of some prominent smart pill boxes, some of the desirable characteristics of smart pill boxes are as follows:

- **Ease of use**: It must be easy for the user to load medicines into the pill box, program the pill box as per the prescribed medication regimen, and dispense medicine from the pill box.
- **Capacity**: The pill box must be capable of holding the medicines required, for a given number of doses per day. Also, it should be capable of holding the required number of pills per dose.

- **Alerts**: The smart pill box must be able to alert the user in different ways including flashlight, beep sound, text and voice notifications.
- **Locking**: The pill box must provide a reliable locking service and must dispense the medicine only at the right time, as programmed by the user.
- **App interface**: The pill box must be interfaced with an application for remote monitoring of the patient by family members and healthcare professionals.
- **Cost**: The cost of the pill box must be reasonable, as high cost could drive away a number of users from using technology for medication adherence monitoring.

1.2.4 Smart Pill Dispenser Architecture

Figure 1.10 shows the architecture of a smart pill dispenser. The architecture has two major parts which include the hardware components and the software components. The hardware components include the microcontroller, GSM module, speakers, buzzers, display unit, lights, push-button, and containers with sensors. The software components include the scheduler, controller, and monitor modules.

1.2.4.1 Hardware Components

Microcontroller—The three prominent types of platform boards available for implementation are Arduino, Rasberry Pi, and the WiPy. Arduino comes in many models and is based on one of the microcontrollers ATMEGA328, ATMEGA32u4, ATMEGA2560, or AT91SAM3X8E. Arduino boards are capable of reading inputs

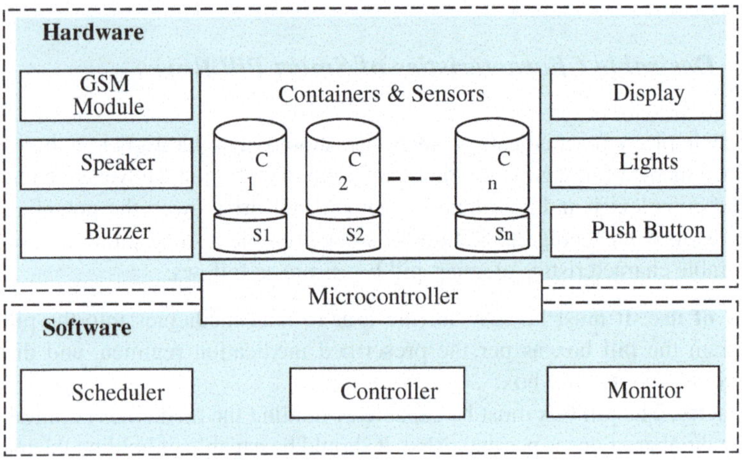

Fig. 1.10 Architecture of a smart pill dispenser

from different types of sensors both in analog and digital format and turn them into an appropriate output which includes rotating a motor, turning an LED on or off, connecting to the cloud and many other types of actions. The Rasberry Pi is a much bigger board than Arduino and has more processing capabilities which can include a complete operating system. It is like a small computer to which you can attach a keyboard, mouse, and a monitor. Because of its high power consumption and size, it may not be a suitable candidate for implementing the smart pill dispenser. The WiPy is an IoT development platform that runs MicroPython on a lightweight processor. It is very small, consumes less power, and has high processing capabilities which makes it suitable for implementing an IoT-based smart pill dispenser.

GSM module—This is used for establishing connectivity between the smart pill container and the mobile application.

Speakers, buzzers, display unit, and lights—These devices are used for reminding the user about the schedule for taking medicine or for locating a lost box. The reminder can be a simple one by means of switching on a LED light of a particular smart pill container or a sophisticated audio/video which uses the speakers and display unit of the smart pill dispenser. Typically, when the user is unable to find the smart pill box with the help of an application, on click of a button the buzzer can be turned on. The user on hearing the sound can then locate the smart pill box.

Push-button—The functionality of the push-button is to communicate to the controller upon two states: one for pressing the button and the other for releasing the button. This button must be activated only at the prescribed time for dispensing the medicines and in all other times, it must be inactive. It must also take care of dispensing duplicate/double dose of medicines.

Containers with sensors—Containers are designed for storing medicines of a single dose. The containers are closed with a magnetic lid, and a magnetic sensor placed beneath the container can be used to determine more information about the container and the lid. The containers can be fitted with infrared photo-interrupter to detect whether there are pills in the container. To improve the sensitivity, each container can be installed with three pairs of infrared emission LED and photo-detector receiver sensing circuits [17].

1.2.4.2 Software Components

Scheduler module—Initially, the user of the smart pill dispenser must configure the pill box, by specifying the events such as at what time the medicine must be taken, and in what container the medicine is stored. When the scheduled event occurs, the scheduler module will send notifications to the user reminding him/her to take medicine [18] and activate the push-button. The scheduler also sends information to the controller module, so that it can ensure that only the right container is opened at the scheduled time.

Controller module—The controller module upon receiving information from the scheduler module will unlock the container that needs to be opened. By using the relative locations of the magnetic lid and magnetic sensor, the controller can detect three states, viz. lid closed with no medicine, lid closed with medicine, and lid open [19, 20]. This information can be passed on to the monitor module for determining whether a patient has taken medicine in the prescribed time or not. For example, if the lid closed with medicine status is detected after the prescribed time for taking medicine, then it indicates that the patient has forgotten to take the medicine.

Monitor module—The monitor module upon receiving information from the controller module will take suitable actions based on the information received. If the patient has forgotten to take medicine, it will remind the patient by sending an audio or video reminder. If the patient has taken the medicine at the right time, then an entry about the same is made into the log file for further perusal by the patient's family members and the healthcare professional. Figure 1.11 shows the working of a smart pill dispenser.

1.2.5 Applications and Challenges

The smart pill dispenser would be helpful in terms of reminding to take medicine, ordering medicines, healthcare analysis, and monitoring. The following are some of the uses of smart pill dispensers.

- **Aged patients**: This would be helpful for aged people who tend to forget to take medicines at the prescribed time.
- **Patients with physical disabilities**: This would also be of great use to patients with certain diseases and physical disabilities who find it difficult to move or fold their hands and limbs.
- **Hospitals and pharmacy**: Customized smart pill dispensers can ease out the job of nursing staff at hospitals. The data logs obtained from it can be used for healthcare analysis. The pharmacist can receive orders for refilling the medicine as and when recommended by the healthcare professional or as required by the user.
- **Family members/Caretakers**: This would help the patient's family members or caretakers to monitor the health of their loved ones from a far-off distance.

The use of technology for health care comes with new promises, and however, a number of technological challenges exist which are to be addressed for these systems to make a greater impact on its users. The following are some of the challenges that need to be addressed.

- **Power consumption**: The smart pill box dispensers are typically battery-powered, and because of the small size of the box, there would not be enough room for using bigger batteries. Hence, power consumption is one big challenge that needs to be addressed. A battery monitoring system needs to be designed to keep track of the current battery usage of the pill box and notify the user when the battery level falls below a given threshold.

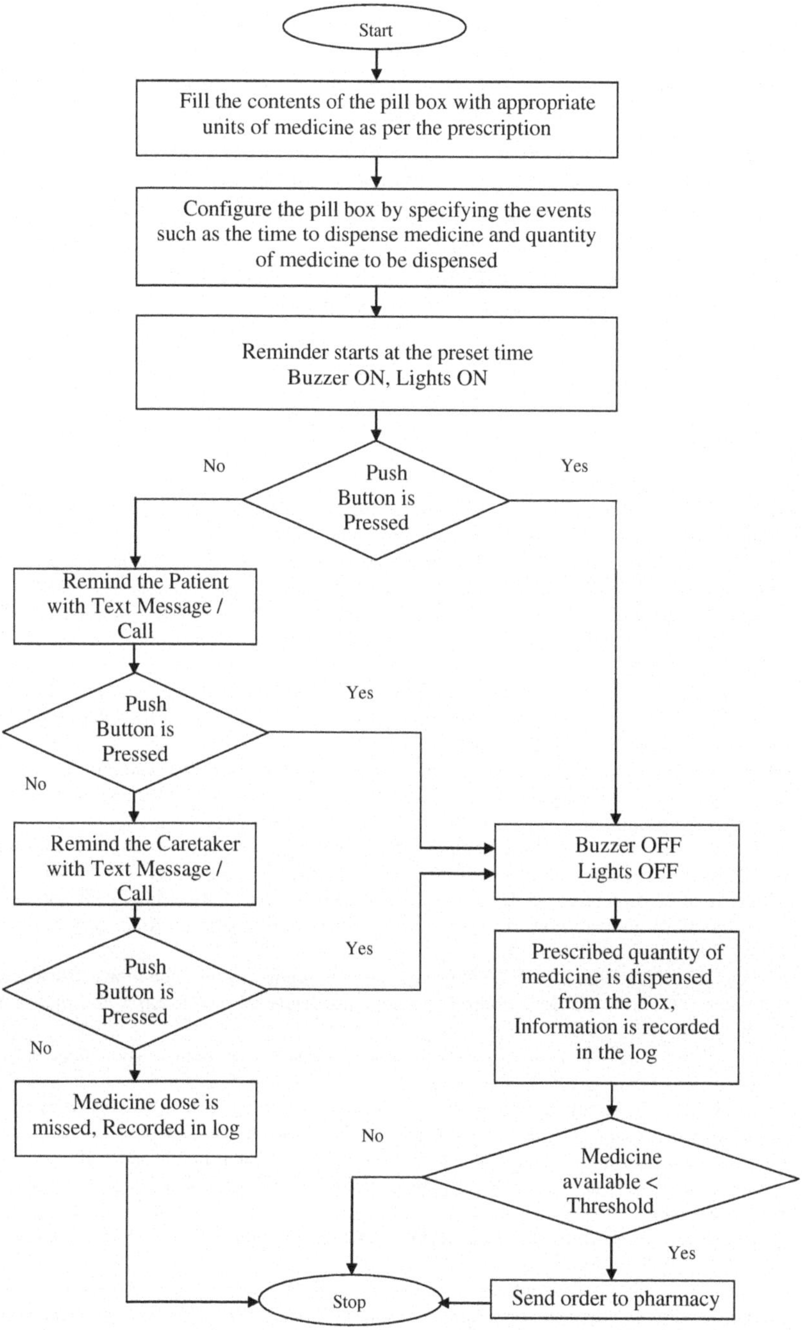

Fig. 1.11 Working of smart pill dispenser

- **Container design**: The pill containers need a creative design for making it capable of holding different types of pills which needs to be taken for one single dose.
- **Security**: The smart pill dispenser unlocks at the preset time and anybody in its vicinity will be able to access it making it highly insecure. Security for smart pill dispenser can be provided by means of a password, and this can be further enhanced by using biometrics of the patient or caretaker.
- **Additional hardware features**: Existing smart pill dispensers dispense medicine at the right time for the patient, and however, there are no means to find and confirm that the patient has taken the medicine. Some hardware in the form of a camera or sensor can be included with the smart pill dispenser to resolve this issue.

References

1. Martin, T., & Healey, J. (2007). 2006's wearable computing advances and fashions activity recognition. *Pervasive Computing Technology*, 2007–2009.
2. Avila, L., & Bailey, M. (2015). The wearable revolution. *IEEE Computer Graphics and Applications, 35*(2), 104.
3. Seneviratne, S., Hu, Y., Nguyen, T., Lan, G., Khalifa, S., Thilakarathna, K., et al. (2017). A survey of wearable devices and challenges. *IEEE Communications Surveys & Tutorials, 19*(4), 2573–2620.
4. Rodrigues, J. J. P. C., De Rezende Segundo, D. B., Junqueira, H. A., Sabino, M. H., Prince, R. M. I., Al-Muhtadi, J., et al. (2018, January). Enabling technologies for the internet of health things. *IEEE Access, 6*, 13129–13141.
5. http://www.infiniteinformationtechnology.com/iot-wearables-wearable-technology.
6. Li, G., Lee, B. L., & Chung, W. Y. (2015). Smartwatch-based wearable EEG system for driver drowsiness detection. *IEEE Sensors Journal, 15*(12), 7169–7180.
7. Lomotey, R. K., Pry, J., & Sriramoju, S. (2017). Wearable IoT data stream traceability in a distributed health information system. *Pervasive and Mobile Computing, 40,* 692–707.
8. Mcwhorter, J., Brown, L., & Khansa, L. (2017, September). A wearable health monitoring system for posttraumatic stress disorder. *Biologically Inspired Cognitive Architectures Journal, 22*, 44–50.
9. Yildirim, H., & Ali-Eldin, A. M. T. (2018). A model for predicting user intention to use wearable IoT devices at the workplace. *Journal of King Saud University—Computer and Information Sciences, 31*, 497–505.
10. Xin, Q., & Wu, J. (2017). A novel wearable device for continuous, non-invasion blood pressure measurement. *Future Generation Computer Systems, 69,* 134–137.
11. Yong, B., Xu, Z., Wang, X., Cheng, L., Li, X., Wu, X., et al. (2018). IoT-based intelligent fitness system. *Journal of Parallel and Distributed Computing, 118,* 14–21.
12. Bai, J., Lian, S., Liu, Z., Wang, K., & Liu, D. (2018). Virtual-blind-road following-based wearable navigation device for blind people. *IEEE Transactions on Consumer Electronics, 64*(1), 136–143.
13. Atzori, L., Iera, A., & Morabito, G. (2010, October). The Internet of Things: A survey. *Computer Networks, 54*(15), 2787–2805.
14. Pyattaev, A., Johnsson, K., Andreev, S., & Koucheryavy, Y. (2015). Communication challenges in high-density deployments of wearable wireless devices. *IEEE Wireless Communications, 22*(1), 12–18.
15. Pasluosta, F., Gassner, H., Winkler, J., Klucken, J., & Eskofier, B. M. (2015). An emerging era in the management of Parkinson's disease: Wearable technologies and the internet of things. *IEEE Journal of Biomedical and Health Informatics, 19*(6), 1873–1881.

16. Srinivas, M., Durgaprasadarao, P., & Raj, V. N. P. (2018). Intelligent medicine box for medication management using IoT. In *2018 2nd International Conference on Inventive Systems and Control (ICISC)*, Coimbatore (pp. 32–34).
17. Tsai, H., Tseng, C. H., Wang, L., & Juang, F. (2017). Bidirectional smart pill box monitored through internet and receiving reminding message from remote relatives. In *2017 IEEE International Conference on Consumer Electronics—Taiwan (ICCE-TW)*, Taipei (pp. 393–394).
18. Crema, C., Depari, A., Flammini, A., Lavarini, M., Sisinni, E., & Vezzoli, A. (2015). A smartphone-enhanced pill-dispenser providing patient identification and in-take recognition. In *2015 IEEE International Symposium on Medical Measurements and Applications (MeMeA) Proceedings*, Turin (pp. 484–489).
19. Chang, W.-W., Sung, T.-J., Huang, H.-W., Hsu, W.-C., Kuo, C.-W., Chang, J.-J., et al. (2011). A smart medication system using wireless sensor network technologies. *Sensors and Actuators, A: Physical, 172*(1), 315–321.
20. Hsu, W.-C., Kuo, C.-W., Chang, W.-W., Chang, J.-J., Hou, Y.-T., Lan, Y.-C., et al. (2010). A WSN smart medication system. *Procedia Engineering, 5*, 588–591.
21. https://adheretech.com/.
22. https://en.medissimo.fr/en/imedipac/.
23. https://pillbox.tinylogics.com/.
24. https://www.medminder.com/.
25. http://my-ubox.com/.
26. https://www.lifeline.philips.com/pill-dispenser/health-mdp.html.

Chapter 2
IoT-Based Diseases Prediction and Diagnosis System for Healthcare

Iman Raeesi Vanani and Morteza Amirhosseini

Abstract Nowadays, developments in high-tech have led to the emergence of Internet of Things (IoT) and Artificial Intelligence (AI) applications in the healthcare industry. IoT devices such as smart pills, wearable monitors, and sensors allow to collect data continuously, and AI systems can use this data for diseases detection. In this chapter, through introducing machine learning and relation between machine learning and disease detection, especially on IoT data, the authors discuss machine learning techniques. Machine learning can analyze the extensive amount of information available on IoT devices, streamline the diagnostic process. The literature focuses on applied machine learning techniques on health devices' data to diseases diagnosis and prediction. In this way, first of all, the authors mention the history of machine learning and some important and useful machine learning algorithms for healthcare usage; major objective of this chapter is describing machine learning methods and customized techniques on IoT data for disease detection. Then some real applied machine learning models in healthcare, are mentioned in this chapter. Future trends of machine learning using in disease detection are introduced through explaining a diagram about how IoT and AI work together to diseases diagnosis and prediction. Finally, the authors have summarized different sections of the chapter at the conclusion.

Keywords IoT · Machine learning · Disease diagnosis · Disease prediction · Healthcare

2.1 Introduction

The new advancements in disease prediction and diagnosis are used dataset from patient Electronic health records (EHR), Internet of Things (IoT) sensor devices, wearable and mobile devices, and social media. This new system applies Artificial Intelligence (AI) techniques to improve prediction and detection. Especially machine

---

I. Raeesi Vanani (✉) · M. Amirhosseini
Allameh Tabataba'i University (ATU), Tehran, Iran
e-mail: imanraeesi@atu.ac.ir

C. Chakraborty et al. (eds.), *Internet of Things for Healthcare Technologies*, Studies in Big Data 73, https://doi.org/10.1007/978-981-15-4112-4_2

learning techniques are used to develop analytic models. These models analyze the collected data from IoT to learn and identify patterns and conditions of the disease. Artificial Intelligence (AI) is changing our modern life and, in medicine, AI has two branches, virtual and physical [22].

The physical branch includes robotics, which can assist surgery and rehabilitation and the virtual branch includes informatics, which is expected to assist physicians in their clinical diagnosis and treatment decisions [35]. The recent progress of machine learning, with big data analysis, is contributing greatly, especially using big data collected by IoT devices.

Today, the role of Big Data and IoT proves that 90 percent of data currently available has been generated in the last couple of years, with rapid increases happening every day. The reason for this growth is increasing in communication through electronic devices, sensors, weblogs, global positioning system (GPS) data, mobile data, IoT, etc. [4].

The major objectives of medical data management are as follows: to improve patient care remotely with database support, to reduce health expenditure, and to give better consultancy by physicians [9], and one of the best ways to manage medical data is using IoT in healthcare.

Before talking about the IoT-based disease prediction and diagnosis, relationship with machine learning, Artificial Intelligence, and learning techniques is necessary to know. The easiest way to understand this relationship is by looking at the diagram in Fig. 2.1 [36].

Fig. 2.1 AI diagram

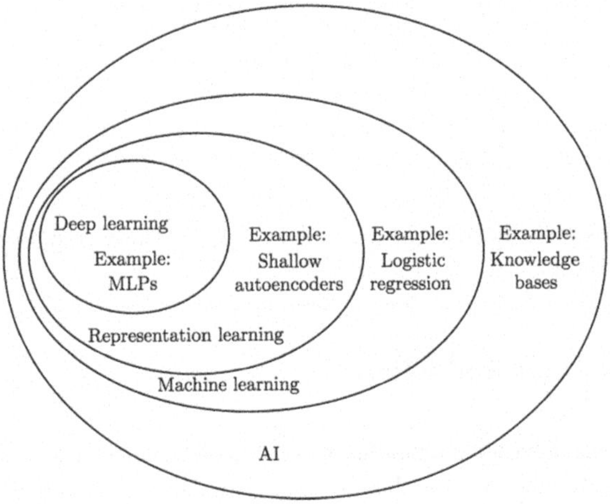

2.1.1 Artificial Intelligence

The term AI emerged in 1956 by John McCarthy, who is also referred to as Father of Artificial Intelligence [36]. The idea behind AI is fairly simple yet fascinating, which is to make intelligent machines that can take decisions on its own [36]. You may think it as science fantasy, but with respect to recent developments in technology and computing power, very idea seems to come closer to reality day by day.

Nowadays, computers have some intelligence power to all the programs that humans have created and which allow them to "do some intelligence things" that humans consider useful but there are many tasks which humans are able to do rather easily but stay out of reach of computers, at the beginning of the current century, many of these names under the label of Artificial Intelligence (AI). Researchers believe that we could create AI for some tasks because we do not know exactly how to do these tasks, even though our brain can do them and doing those tasks involve knowledge that is now implicit, but we have information about those tasks through data [36]. Fuzzy logic, neural networks, machine learning, evolutionary computations, pattern recognition are some of AI algorithms and methods that have been using as a solution for enabling computers to make a decision and allow them for learning [36].

2.1.2 Machine Learning

Now, that you are familiar with AI, let talk briefly about machine learning and understand what it means when researchers say that we're programming machines to learn. Let us begin with a very famous definition of machine learning:

> A computer Program find out from experience E with reference to some task T and a few performance measure P, if its performance on T, as measured by Performance, improves with experience [31].

So, if you want to do prediction, traffic patterns at a busy intersection (T), you can run it through a machine learning algorithm with data about past traffic patterns (E) [36]. Now, the accuracy of the prediction (performance measure P) will depend on the fact that whether the program has successfully learned from the dataset or not (experience E). Basically, machine learning refers to a type of Artificial Intelligence (AI) that provides computers with the ability to learn without being explicitly programmed by exposing them to the vast amount of data. The core principle behind machine learning is to learn from data sets and try to minimize errors or maximize the likelihood of their predictions being true [31].

Two main challenges in machine learning are as follows:

- Traditional ML algorithms are not useful while working with high-dimensional data that is where we have a large number of inputs and outputs. For example, in the case of disease recognition, we have a large amount of input where we will have different types of IoT devices with different types of diseases.

- The second major challenge is to tell the computer what features it should look for that will play an important role in predicting the outcome as well as to make better accuracy while doing so. This process refers to feature extraction.

Feeding raw data to the algorithm rarely ever works and this is the reason feature extraction is a critical part of the traditional machine learning workflow. Therefore, without feature extraction, the challenge for the programmer increases as the effectiveness of the algorithm very much depends on how insightful the programmer is [36].

2.1.3 Deep Learning

Deep learning is part of a broader family of machine learning methods based on learning data representations, as opposed to task-specific algorithms, learning can be supervised, partially supervised or unsupervised [5].

Deep learning is a class of machine learning algorithms that [13]:

- Use a cascade of multiple layers of nonlinear processing units for feature extraction and transformation [13]. Each successive layer uses the output from the previous layer as input.
- Learn in supervised (e.g., classification) and/or unsupervised (e.g., pattern analysis) manners [13].
- Learn multiple levels of representations that correspond to different levels of abstraction; the levels form a hierarchy of concepts.

Deep learning has various closely related definitions or high-level descriptions [13]. Deep learning is a sub-field within machine learning that is based on algorithms for learning multiple levels of representation in order to model complex relationships among data. Higher level features are defined in terms of lower level ones, and such a hierarchy of features is called a deep structure [36].

In recent years and after 2010 till now, several innovations, applied techniques and usages emerge in the world, some usages are in health, disease diagnosis, image recognition, natural language processing, drug discovery, customer relationship management, sentimental mining, text mining, bioinformatics, and mobile advertisement.

2.1.4 Machine Learning Algorithms

Recent successes of machine learning techniques in solving many complex tasks by learning from raw data and using various algorithms. The nature of this experience (E) in learning is typically considered for classifying machine learning algorithms into the following three categories: supervised, unsupervised, and reinforcement learning [7]. Nowadays, everyone could use some machine learning tools, and start to write code, but without knowing how those algorithms work, it is difficult. So is very important to understand be basics of learning algorithms and then study deep learning algorithm. One of the first concepts in machine learning is the difference between supervised, unsupervised, reinforcement, and deep learning.

In supervised learning, algorithms present with a dataset containing a collection of features. Additionally, labels or target values are provided for each sample. This mapping of features to the label of target values is where the knowledge is encoded. Once it has learned, the algorithm is expected to find the mapping from the features of unseen samples to their correct labels or target values. The purpose of unsupervised learning is to extract meaningful representations and explain key features of the data. No labels or target values are necessary in this case in order to learn from the data. In reinforcement learning algorithms, an AI agent interacts with a real or simulated environment. This interaction between the learning system and the interaction experience which is useful to improve performance in the task being learned. Finally, Deep learning (DL) techniques represent a huge step forward for machine learning. DL is based on the way the human brain process information and teaches [36]. It consists of a machine learning model composed of several levels of representation, in which every level uses the information from the previous level to train deeply [36]. Each level corresponds to a different area of the cortex, and every level abstracts more the information in the same way of the brain. Now each of these learning techniques explains to understand.

2.1.4.1 Supervised Learning Algorithms

Supervised learning algorithms learn how to associate an input with some output, given a training set of examples of inputs and outputs [20]. The following paragraphs cover the most relevant algorithms. Nowadays, in supervised learning: Feedforward Neural Networks, a popular variation of these called Convolutional Neural Networks (CNN), Recurrent Neural Networks (RNNs), and a variation of RNNs called Long Short-Term Memory (LSTM) models. Feedforward Neural Networks, also known as Multilayer Perceptions (MLPs), are the most common learning models. Their purpose is to work as function approximations. The approximated function is usually built by stacking together several hidden layers that are activated in the chain to get the desired output. The number of hidden layers is usually called the depth of the model, which explains the origin of the term deep learning: learning using models with several layers Convolutional Neural Networks (CNN). These models take their name from the mathematical linear operation of convolution which is always present in at least one of the layers of the network [7].

In contrast to MLPs, Recurrent Neural Networks (RNNs) are models during which the output may be a function of not only the present inputs but also of the sooner outputs, which encode into a hidden state. This suggests that RNNs have a memory of the previous outputs and may encode the knowledge present within the sequence itself, something that MLPs cannot do. As a result, this sort of model is extremely useful to find out from sequential data. RNNs are usually trained using Back Propagation Through Time (BPTT), an extension of backpropagation that takes under consideration temporality to compute the gradients. Using this method, with long temporal sequences can cause several issues. Gradients accumulated over an extended sequence can become immeasurably large or extremely small and these problems are mentioned exploding gradients and vanishing gradients, respectively [7].

Long STM (LSTM) models are a kind of RNN that successfully overcomes the matter of vanishing gradients by maintaining a more constant error, which effectively leaves continuous learning over a bigger number of your time steps [7]. Because it has been already stated, LSTM gated cells in RNN shave internal recurrence, besides the outer recurrence of RNNs. Cells store an indoor state, which may be written to and skim from them. There are gates control-ling how data enter and leave and are deleted from this cell state. Those gates act on the signals they receive, and, almost like a typical neural network, they block or expire information that supported its strength and importance using their own sets of weights. Those weights, because the weights that modulate input and hidden states, are adjusted via the recurrent network's learning process [7].

2.1.4.2 Unsupervised Learning Algorithms

Unsupervised learning aims towards the development of models that are capable of extracting meaningful and high-level representations from high-dimensional sensory unlabeled data. This functionality is inspired by the visual cortex which requires a very small amount of labeled data. Deep Generative Models such as Deep Belief Networks (DBNs) [23] allow the learning of several layers of nonlinear features in an unsupervised manner. DBNs are built by stacking several Restricted Boltzmann Machines (RBMs), resulting in a hybrid model in which the top two layers form an RBM and the bottom layers act as a directed graph constituting a Sigmoid Belief Network (SBN) [7].

Auto encoders are mainly composed of an "encoder" network, which transforms the input data into a low-dimensional code, and a "decoder" network, which reconstructs the data from the code. Training these deep models involves minimizing the error between the original data and its reconstruction. In this process, the weights initialization is critical to avoid reaching a bad local optimum; thus some authors have proposed a pertained stage based on stacked RBMs and a fine-tuning stage using back propagation [26].

The learning algorithm proposed in [23] is supposed to be one of the first efficient ways of learning DBNs by introducing greedy layer-by-layer training to get to a deep hierarchical model. In this greedy learning procedure, the hidden activity patterns obtained in the current layer are used as the "visible" data for training the RBM of the next layer. Once the stacked RBMs have been learned and combined to form a DBN, a fine-tuning procedure using a contrastive version of the wake-sleep algorithm is applied [7]. Deep neural networks can also be utilized for dimensionality reduction of the input data. For this purpose, deep "auto encoders" [38] have been shown to provide successful results in a wide variety of applications such as document retrieval and image retrieval [26]. An auto encoder is unsupervised neural networking in which the target values are set to be equal to the inputs.

2.1.4.3 Reinforcement Learning Algorithms

In reinforcement learning, an agent is defined to interact with an environment, seeking to find the best action for each state at any step in time. The agent must balance the exploration and exploitation of the state space in order to find the optimal policy that maximizes the accumulated reward from the interaction with the environment.

In this context, an agent modifies its behavior or policy with the awareness of the states, actions are taken, and rewards for every time step. Reinforcement learning composes an optimization process throughout the whole state space in order to maximize the accumulated reward. Robotic problems are often task-based with temporal structure. These types of problems are suitable to be solved by means of a reinforcement learning framework [25].

A general problem in real robotic applications is that the state and action spaces are often continuous spaces. A continuous state and/or action space can make the optimization problem intractable, due to the overwhelming set of different states and/or actions. As a general framework for representation, reinforcement learning methods are enhanced through deep learning to aid the design for feature representation, which is known as deep reinforcement learning. In this review, deep reinforcement learning methods are divided into two main categories: value function and policy search methods.

Value Function Methods allows simplifying more standard actor-critic style algorithms while preserving the benefits of nonlinear value function approximation [21]. NAF is valid for continuous control tasks and takes advantage of trained models to approximate the standard model-free value function. Policy search methods are policy-based reinforcement learning methods aim towards directly searching for the optimal policy, which provides a feasible framework for continuous control. Deep Deterministic Policy Gradient (DDPG) [27] is based on the actor-critic paradigm, with two neural networks to approximate a greedy deterministic policy (actor) and function.

2.1.4.4 Deep Learning Algorithms

Deep learning techniques are to get a deep neural network to train efficiently. They may also include latent variables organized layer-wise in deep generative models such as the nodes in Deep Belief Networks. Deep learning architectures such as deep neural networks, Deep Belief Networks, and recurrent neural networks have been applied to fields including computer vision, speech recognition, natural language processing, audio recognition, social network filtering, machine translation, bioinformatics, drug design, and opinion mining, where they have produced results comparable to and

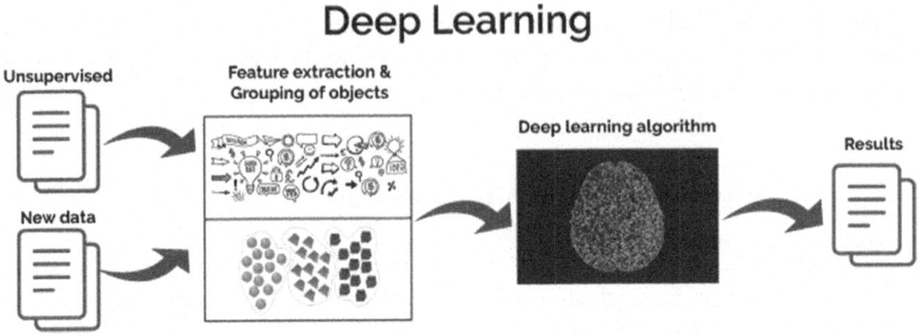

Fig. 2.2 An unsupervised deep learning process

in some cases superior to human experts [19]. In Fig. 2.2, an unsupervised deep learning is shown. Deep learning architectures are often constructed with a greedy layer-by-layer method. Deep learning helps to disentangle these abstractions and pick out which features are useful for improving performance [5]. For supervised learning tasks, deep learning methods obviate feature engineering, by translating the data into compact intermediate representations akin to principal components, and derive layered structures that remove redundancy in representation [13]. Deep learning algorithms can be applied to unsupervised learning tasks.

Deep learning includes many networks such as CNN (Convolutional Neural Networks), RNN (Recurrent Neural Networks), Recursive Neural Networks, DBN (Deep Belief Networks), and many more. CNNs have been used to perform a variety of natural language processing tasks, including part-of-speech tagging, named entity extraction, identification of semantic roles, and linking semantically similar words. More recently, CNNs have been used for end-to-end discriminative text classification tasks involving the identification of high-level concepts prevalent throughout an entire document. Additionally, a network with a single convolutional layer performed better than any traditional learner, such as Multinomial Naive Bayes and support vector machine (SVM), on their benchmarking datasets. CNNs have also been used to aid feature extraction from text [33]. The most famous example Socher has used is the Recursive Neural Network (RNN) for the representation of movie reviews from the website rottentomatoes.com [1].

2.2 Materials and Methods

First of all applying machine learning to IoT data will be reviewed. Machine learning has experienced a boost in popularity among industrial companies thanks to the Internet of Things (IoT). A lot of opportunities have begun to appear with the isotropy of AI and IoT. Since IoT will be the source of new data, data science will provide a considerable contribution to making IoT applications more intelligent. Data science is the combination of different scientific fields that uses data mining, machine learning, and other techniques to find patterns and new insights from data. These techniques include a range of algorithms applicable in different domain of experts. The process of applying data analytics methods to particular areas involves defining data types such as volume, variety, and velocity; data models such as neural networks, classification, and clustering methods, and applying efficient algorithms that match with the data characteristics [29].

2.2.1 ML Increases the Efficiency of IoT

There are some data models that implement data analytics, and these are often limited use when it comes to addressing rapidly changing and unstructured data. But when it comes to IoT, it is often necessary to identify the correlations between sensor inputs and various external variables that are producing millions of data records. We know that traditional data analysis needs a model that is built on past data and also an expert opinion to establish a relationship between different variables. When it comes to ML, it directly starts with the outcome factors and then automatically looks for different predictor variables and their interactions. Hence, ML is really valuable when we know what we want but do not know the important input variables to come to that decision. Different ML algorithms learn from the sets of data that are important in achieving that target. Machine learning helps to predict when a device connected to the IoT; this is incredibly valuable when it is used in healthcare.

Machine learning algorithms can learn from data to gain knowledge from experience and to make decisions and predictions. Health Informatics needs the effective use of probabilistic information for decision making. The combination of both has the greatest potential to rise the efficiency of treatment and care. This combination can call Health Artificial Intelligence Process that is shown in Fig. 2.3.

Leveraging Artificial Intelligence technology to build healthcare software products using cognitive technology has significant relevance in the healthcare IT industry. Integrating AI platforms for healthcare with your existing software and third-party applications can automate the workflow of healthcare systems. In healthcare, IoT

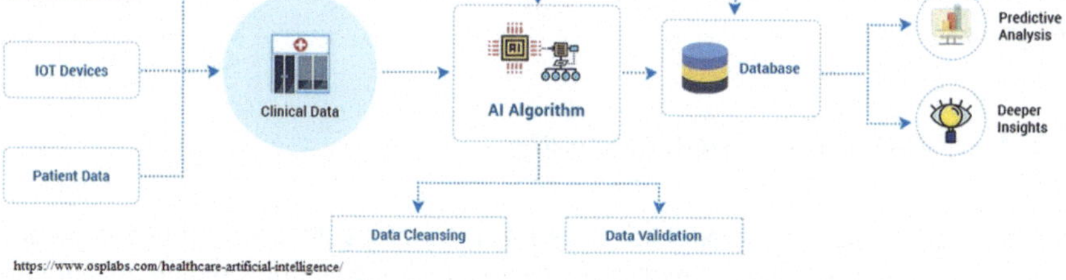

Fig. 2.3 Health Artificial Intelligence process

devices can gather different patient data and receive inputs from health practitioners and also Internet of Things Healthcare can greatly improve not only a patient's health and help in critical situations but also the productivity of health employees and hospital workflows. In IoT healthcare workflow first sensors collect data from a patient or a doctor/nurse inputs data then IoT device analyzes the collected data with the help of AI-driven algorithms like machine learning (ML), finally doctors, health practitioners, or even robots are enabled to make actionable and informed decisions based on the data provided by the IoT device.

IoT in the healthcare industry has many benefits. However, the most important is that treatment outcomes can be improved, as the data gathered by IoT devices are highly accurate, enabling decisions. Health facilities and practitioners will be capable of minimizing errors because all patient information can be measured quickly and sent to a doctor or a healthcare platform. AI-driven algorithms running on these IoT devices could also help make intelligible suggestions based on existing data. Another benefit of IoT in healthcare is reduced costs. With IoT in healthcare, some patients will be able to stay at home while various IoT devices monitor and send all important information to the health facility—meaning less hospital stays. With the information received from lots of IoT devices, health facilities will also be able to improve their disease management. IoT in the healthcare industry can improve components. It can also enhance healthcare applications, such as telemedicine, patient monitoring, medication management, imaging, and overall workflows in hospitals. It can also create new ways of treating different diseases. The Internet of Things for healthcare will not only be used by hospitals or facilities but also by research organizations, and even governmental institutions.

2.2.2 Applying ML in IoT Data to Disease Detection Model

This section explains the detail of disease prediction and diagnosis model based on the machine learning process. Figure 2.4 shows the conceptual model that consists of several modules such as data set (training and new data) as input, feature extraction, machine learning algorithms, disease detection, and the result.

The steps of the modeling process and the following subsections describe the details of each step. First of all, defining the problem and assembling a dataset is necessary. For example, diabetes disease diagnosis could be a problem and the needed dataset base on this problem must be defined and it is a process stat point of the process.

2.2.3 Dataset Types in Healthcare

The datasets used in this model has been taken from IoT devices and health record. The dataset is already partitioned into Test and Training samples which are suitable for machine learning models (Supervised and unsupervised). The quantity and quality

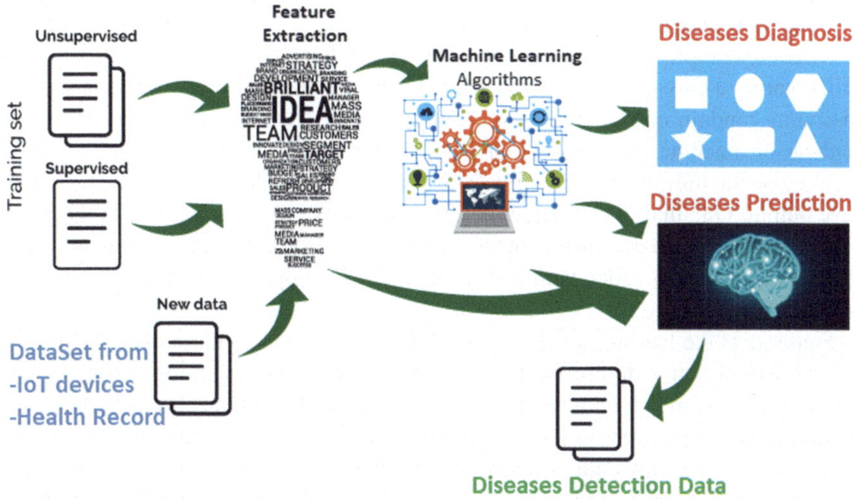

Fig. 2.4 Diseases detection process model

of your data dictate how accurate our model is The outcome of this step is generally a representation of data which will be used for training An analysis of the database is performed to attending to the nature of the variables: mean, standard deviation and extreme values are described for quantitative variables; absolute and relative frequencies for qualitative variables. The number of missing values is identified for each variable since for some of the algorithms to work it is anticipated that it may be necessary to eliminate observations with missing values. The missing values can be substituted using an appropriate imputation idea depending upon the type of column having missing values. Data Cleansing is very important that which may require it (remove duplicates, correct errors, deal with missing values, normalization, data type conversions, etc.) randomize data, which erases the effects of the particular order in which we collected and/or otherwise prepared our data. Visualize data to help detect relevant relationships between variables or class imbalances, or perform other exploratory analysis and finally split into training and evaluation sets.

2.2.4 Feature Extraction

The next step involves feature selection. It is essential to identify the chief features of the dataset which can contribute to a constructive model building for disease detection. Primary exploratory data analysis is performed based on which a set of features is selected, in order to assess the performance of various existing algorithms on datasets, we employ the following modeling approaches. Also, approaches are evaluated and compared to come up with the most optimal idea for the detection of diseases from real-time datasets.

Overfitting has many faces. What if the knowledge and data we have are not sufficient to completely determine the correct classifier? Then we run the risk of just hallucinating a classifier (or parts of it) that is not grounded in reality and is simply en-coding random quirks in the data. This problem is called overfitting and is the bugbear of machine learning. When your learner outputs a classifier that is 100% accurate on the training data but only 50% accurate on test data, when in fact it could have output. One that is 75% accurate on both, it has overfit. Everyone in machine learning knows about overfitting, but it comes in many forms that are not immediately obvious. One way to understand overfitting is by decomposing generalization error into bias and variance.

Some machine learning projects succeed and some fail. What makes the difference? Easily the most important factor is the features used. Learning is easy if you have many independent features that each correlate well with the class. On the other hand, if the class is a very complex function of the features, you may not be able to learn it. Often, the raw data is not in a form that is amenable to learning, but you can construct features from it that are amenable. This is typically where most of the effort in a machine learning project goes. It is often also one of the most interesting parts, where intuition, creativity and "black art" are as important as the technical stuff. First-timers are often surprised by how little time in a machine learning project is spent actually doing machine learning. But it makes sense if you consider how time-consuming it is to gather data, integrate it, clean it and preprocess it, and how much trial and error can go into feature design [15].

Also, machine learning is not a one-shot process of building a dataset and running a learner, but rather an iterative process of running the learner, analyzing the results, modifying the data and/or the learner, and repeating. Learning is often the quickest part of this, but that is because we have already mastered it pretty well! Feature engineering is more difficult because it is domain-specific, while learners can be largely general purpose. However, there is no sharp frontier between the two, and this is another reason the most useful learners are those that facilitate incorporating knowledge.

2.2.5 Model Evaluation

In this step, some performance evaluation and testing data are used for measuring the performance of the models. Uses some metric or combination of metrics to "measure" objective performance of model, test the model against previously unseen data. This unseen data is meant to be somewhat representative of model performance in the real world but still helps tune the model (as opposed to test data, which does not). Simple model hyperparameters may include number of training steps, learning rate, initialization values, and distribution, etc. In Fig. 2.5, a schema of a simple learning process and evaluation is shown.

The evaluation is most often based on prediction accuracy. There are some techniques that are used to calculate a model's accuracy. One technique is to split the

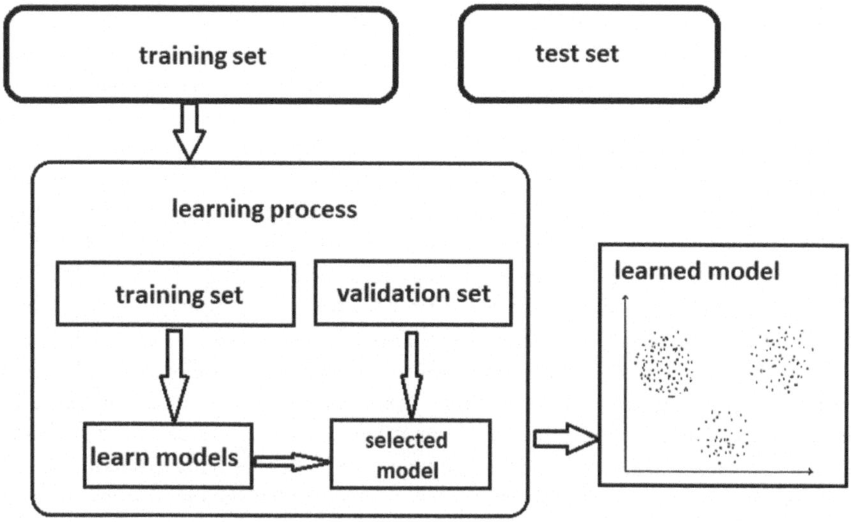

Fig. 2.5 learning process and evaluation

training set by using 66% for training and the other data for evaluating performance. In another technique, known as cross-validation, the training set is divided into mutually exclusive and equal-sized subsets and for each subset the model is trained on the union of all the other subsets. The average of error rate of each subset is, therefore, an estimate of the error rate of the model. Leave-one-out validation is special. All test subsets consist of a single instance. This type of validation is, of course, more expensive computationally, but useful when the most accurate estimate of a model's error rate is required.

2.2.6 *Model Selection*

A model is some relationships between the variables used to describe the system. Different algorithms are for different tasks; choose the right machine learning algorithm. The goal of training is to answer a question or make a prediction correctly as often as possible, for example, the linear regression algorithm would need to learn values for x and y (x is input, y is output) and each iteration of process is a training step. For predictions, using further (test set) data which have, until this point, been withheld from the model (and for which class labels are known), are used to test the model; a better approximation of how the model will perform in the real world. Classification is one of the most important aspects of supervised learning for disease diagnosis. Various classification algorithms like logistic regression, Naive Bayes, decision trees, random forests and many more can use as a machine learning algorithm. One of the principal responsibilities of a data scientist is to make reliable predictions based on data. When the amount of data available is enormous, it helps if some of the analysis can be automated. Machine learning is a way of identifying patterns in data and using them to automatically make predictions or decisions.

In this part, some of the popular algorithms describe as a good selectable algorithm. Decision Tree algorithms are used for both predictions as well as classification in machine learning. Using the decision tree with a given set of inputs, one can map the various outcomes that are a result of the consequences or decisions. In random forests, unlike a decision tree, where each node is split on the best feature that minimizes error, in random forests, we choose a random selection of features for constructing the best split. The reason for randomness is: even with bagging when decision trees choose the best feature to split on, they end up with a similar structure and correlated predictions. But bagging after splitting on a random subset of features means less correlation among predictions from subtrees. Linear regression predictions are continuous values (i.e., blood sugar level), logistic regression predictions are discrete values (i.e., whether a disease is detected) after applying a transformation function. Naive Bayes is an easy and quick way to predict the class of the dataset. Using this, one can perform a multi-class prediction. When the assumption of independence is valid, Naive Bayes is much more capable than the other algorithms like logistic regression. Furthermore, you will require less training data.

Learn many models, not just one in the early days of machine learning, everyone had a favorite learner, together with some a priori reasons to believe in its superiority. Most effort went into trying many variations of it and selecting the best one. Then systematic empirical comparisons showed that the best learner varies from application to application, and systems containing many different learners started to appear. Effort now went into trying many variations of many learners and still selecting just the best one. But then researchers noticed that, if instead of selecting the best variation found, we combine many variations, the results are better—often much better—and a little extra effort for the user [15].

2.3 Applications and Results

In this section and as a result, some successful applications of machine learning in the diseases diagnosis over IoT information are presented.

2.3.1 Diabetes and Hypertension

Early disease prediction plays an important role in improving healthcare quality and can help individuals avoid dangerous health situations before it is too late. Research proposed a disease prediction model (DPM) to provide an early prediction for type 2 diabetes and hypertension based on an individual's risk factors data. The proposed DPM consists of isolation forest-based outlier detection method to remove outlier data, synthetic minority oversampling technique to balance data distribution, and ensemble approach to predict the diseases. Four datasets (monitoring device, health records, personal information, and physician's experience) were utilized to build the model and extract the most significant risks factors. Some machine learning algorithms run over data and the results showed that the proposed DPM achieved the highest accuracy when compared to other models and previous studies. Also, a mobile application is developed to provide the practical application of the proposed DPM. The developed mobile application gathers risk factor data and sends it to a remote server so that an individual's current condition can be diagnosed with the proposed DPM. The prediction result is then sent back to the mobile application; thus, immediate and appropriate action can be taken to reduce and prevent individual risks once unexpected health situations occur (i.e., type 2 diabetes and/or hypertension) at early stages [18].

2.3.2 *Kidney Disease*

New predictive model for diabetic kidney diseases (DKD) using AI is constructed, processing natural language and longitudinal data with big data machine learning, based on the electronic medical records (EMR) of 64,059 diabetes patients. AI extracted raw features from the previous 6 months as the reference period and selected 24 factors to find time series patterns relating to 6-month DKD aggravation, using a convolutional autoencoder. AI constructed the predictive model with 3073 features, including time series data using logistic regression analysis. AI could predict DKD aggravation with 71% accuracy. Furthermore, the group with DKD aggravation had a significantly higher incidence of hemodialysis than the non-aggravation group, over 10 years ($N = 2900$). The new predictive model by AI could detect the progression of DKD and may contribute to more effective and accurate intervention to reduce hemodialysis [30].

2.3.3 *Cardiovascular Disease*

Cardiovascular disease (CVD) continues to be one of the most common causes of death in both men and women worldwide. American Heart Association reported in 2017, coronary heart disease (CHD) was an underlying cause of death in about 1 of every 7 deaths in the United States in 2014. The total CHD prevalence was 6.3% in adults $\geq$20 years of age and was 7.4% for males and 5.3% for females. In Hungary, for 10,000 residents the incidence of myocardial infarction (MI) in the capital city was 28.6 in males and 16.2 in females [24].

With constructing and validating prediction models on mortality, it becomes possible to separate patients who have high risk of death from those who are at low risk. In terms of knowledge-based systems: based on the knowledge base coming from historical data (the dataset), the system is aimed to reason and solve complex questions. With training and validating regression, decision tree, and neural network models, new knowledge can be derived—which can be used by physicians in the process of treatment. Predicting mortality risk helps physicians make better decisions during the treatment. Such models help them separate patients into groups of high and low risk of death. While the formers can receive specialized treatment and closer follow-up after leaving the institute; the latter may leave the hospital sooner. In addition to personal advantages, healthcare institutions can operate with better performance [32].

2.3.4 Risk of Coronary Heart Disease

In another study, the utility of several supervised machine learning (ML) algorithms for predicting clinical events in terms of their internal validity and accuracy is done. The results, which were obtained using two statistical software platforms, were also compared. The data used in this research come from the open database of the Framingham Heart Study, which originated in 1948 in Framingham, Massachusetts as a prospective study of risk factors for cardiovascular disease. Through data mining processes, three data models were elaborated and a comparative methodological study between the different machine learning algorithms—decision tree, random forest, support vector machines, neural networks, and logistic regression—was carried out. The global selection criteria for choosing the right set of hyperparameters and the type of data manipulation was the area under a curve (AUC). The Framingham study open database contains 4240 observations. The algorithm that yielded the greatest AUC when analyzing the data in R-Studio was neural network applied to a model that excluded all observations in which there was at least one missing value (AUC = 0.71); when analyzing the data and applying the same model, the best algorithm was support vector machines (AUC = 0.75) [6].

2.3.5 Predictors of In-Hospital Length

The In-hospital length of stay (LOS) is expected to increase as cardiovascular disease complexity increases and the population ages. This will affect healthcare systems especially with the current situation of decreased bed capacity and increasing costs. Therefore, accurately predicting LOS would have a positive impact on healthcare metrics. The aim of this study is to develop a machine learning-based model approach for predicting in-hospital LOS for cardiac patients. Using electronic medical records, retrospectively extracted all records of patients' visits that were admitted under adult cardiology service. Admission diagnosis and primary treating physician were reviewed to verify selection criteria. A predictive machine learning-based model approach was applied to incorporate simple baseline health data at admission time to predict LOS. Patients were divided into three groups based on their LOS: short (b3 days), intermediate (3–5 days) and long (N5 days). Information gain algorithm was utilized to select the most relevant attributes. Only attributes with information gain of more than zero were used in model building. Four different machine learning techniques were evaluated and their diagnostic accuracy measures were compared. The dataset of this study included adult patients who were admitted between 2008 and 2016 in King Abdul-Aziz Cardiac Center (KACC). Participants (dataset): A total of 16,414 consecutive inpatient visits for 12,769 unique patients (mean age of 58.8 ± 16 years of which 68.2% were males) between 2008 and 2016 were included. The study cohort had a high prevalence of cardiovascular risk factors (hypertension 56%, diabetes 56%, dyslipidemia 52%, obesity 33%, and smoking 24%). The most common admitting diagnosis was acute coronary syndrome (36%). The variables with the highest impact on the prediction of in-hospital LOS were on admission heart rate, on admission systolic and diastolic blood pressure, age, and insurance status (eligibility). Using machine learning models; Random Forest (RF) model outperformed among all other models [sensitivity (0.80), accuracy (0.80), and AUROC (0.94)] [12].

2.3.6 Prediction of Diseases with Pathological Characteristics

With a colossal development of data in the field of social insurance, there has been a noteworthy improvement made in foreseeing infections with the use of machine learning calculations. From the forecast of plague episode and different illnesses to giving better methods for putting away and verifying human services data, usage of machine learning in the field of social insurance guarantees exact outcomes. The principle center is around to utilize machine learning in social insurance to enhance tolerant consideration for better outcomes. Machine learning has been made less demanding to distinguish diverse illnesses and determine them accurately. Prescient analysis with the assistance of proficient different machine learning calculations predicts the illness all the more effectively and helps treat patients. Gathering therapeutic data of people utilizing IoT and assessing and examining them to foresee the illness has given a proficient system to a coordinated machine learning and IoT arrangement in human services. The study, for the most part, expects to give aggregate components that would execute machine learning advancements to yield exact outcomes. The anticipated infections and the manifestation were coordinating up to 70% of exactness. This motivation behind this study is to ponder streamlined machine learning calculations for their usage in different illness forecast [10].

2.3.7 Blood Diseases Detection

Blood has many secrets that affect human life. The growth in age should be reflected in blood. Depending on several attributes like age, gender, symptoms, and any health conditions, the physician can choose the specific blood tests for diagnosing the disease. Many blood tests are standard and essential for everyone to get. Blood tests are widespread because of that most of the blood tests do not need special conditions like fasting for 8–12 h before the test or preventing some kinds of medicine. By testing the fluid, different parameters in the blood can be measured. The results help to identify health problems in the early stages or nay predictable diseases. Physicians cannot diagnose diseases and health problems with blood tests alone. However, they can use them as a factor to confirm a diagnosis. These factors may include some signs and symptoms, which could be integrated with other vital signs for diagnosing the diseases. The disease is diagnosing, and the prediction process is a necessary process that is based on the quality of data and the physician's experience. Applying modern technological tools for helping physicians to improve the accuracy of disease diagnosing, become one of the hot topics of research, especially IoT and machine learning algorithms. Using classical machine learning algorithms are applied on 668 records that belong to four different classes as get by blood test devices. One of the essential disease detectors is the blood analysis; as it contains many parameters with different values that indicate definite proof for the existence of the disease. The machine learning algorithm accuracy depends mainly on the quality of the dataset; for this reason, a high-quality dataset is collected and verified from expert physicians and blood testing devices. This dataset is used for training the classifiers for obtaining high accuracy. In one study several classifiers are tested and achieved accuracy up to 98.16% which realize the research objective, which is helping the physicians to predict the blood diseases according to general blood test [2].

2.3.8 Cardiac Arrhythmia Diagnosis

Cardiac arrhythmia is a life-threatening disease that causes severe health problems in patients. A timely diagnosis of arrhythmia diseases will be useful to save their lives. Internet of Things (IoT) assures to modernize the healthcare sector through continuous, remote and noninvasive monitoring of cardiac arrhythmia diseases. An IoT platform for the prediction of cardiovascular disease using an IoT-enabled ECG telemetry system acquires the ECG signal, processes the ECG signal and alerts physicians for an emergency. It is helpful for the physician to analyze heart disease as early and accurate. This study is developed an IoT-enabled ECG monitoring system to analyze the ECG signal. The statistical features of raw ECG signals are calculated. The ECG signal is analyzed using Pan Tompkins QRS detection algorithm for obtaining the dynamic features of the ECG signal. The system is used to find the RR intervals from the ECG signal to capture heart rate variability features. The statistical and dynamic features are then applied to the classification process to classify cardiac arrhythmia disease. People can check their cardiac condition by the acquisition of ECG signal even in their home. The size of the system is small, and it requires less maintenance and operational cost. It is helpful for the physician to analyze heart disease as easily and accurately [14].

2.3.9 Chronic Wound Tissue Characterization

The output of the processed chronic wound image by an automated model is evaluated and validated by the expert clinician. He has to validate the results of naked-eye observation and automated machine learning-based observation in terms of the percentage of tissue characterization. Proper validation and verification are required before their use in clinical testing for providing useful service to clinicians and patients. According to the doctor's observation, the machine learning process provides a more accurate percentage of different tissues when comparing these two methods. The results are easily monitored using a smartphone, and the outcome can be predicted more easily, accurately, and rapidly. The research work on chronic wound tissue characterization using different machine learning approaches gave a very accurate assessment of ulcer stages. The digital medical chronic wound image and percentage of necrotic, sloughing, and granulation tissue, is better than manually determined, naked-eye assessment of the ulcer. This can provide an accurate assessment of the chronic wound from a distance to the treating clinician, and he/she can monitor the progress of wound healing [11].

2.4 Discussion

One of the essential parts of life is healthcare. Healthcare is the improvement of health via prediction and diagnosis of diseases. In recent years, technological development is at its top due to which several wearable health devices and gadgets are available. Even expert doctors figure out it as challenging to estimate the health from the symptoms observed from the diseased. Using this kind of technology and tools such as Internet of Things (IoT) and machine learning along with big data makes the job of physicians much easier in digging out the cause of disease and predicting its seriousness by using modern algorithms. The Internet of Things (IoT) is a potential solution to help the pressures on healthcare systems by providing many useful data with various devices. On the other hand, machine learning gains recognition as that of big data (collected by IoT devices) by analyzing and simplifying the task of data scientists in an automated process. Expansive scale informational collections are gathered and examined in the health area. Automating nonstop monitoring of health parameters through IoT is a novel solution and it is very important to monitor various medical parameters continuously. The performance of various machine learning algorithms depends on the nature of the dataset. The latest trend in healthcare technological methods is using IoT and machine learning techniques. Internet of things serves as a data provider for healthcare and plays a main role in a wide range of healthcare applications. Today, intelligent, assisted living environments for healthcare for patients are very essential. The environment combines the patient's clinical history and electronic data with the ability to monitor the disease conditions using IoT technologies. Thus the Internet of Things (IoT) and machine learning algorithms, when combined together, the following result is appeared. The resultant integrated healthcare framework can support significant improvement in general health. Machine learning algorithms, techniques, and machinery are already present in the market to implement reasonable disease diagnosis and prediction processes. So, this technology is sometimes described as supervised or predictive machine learning. As a discussion, authors must clarify that model selection and trustable data are two main factors of accuracy. Table 2.1 shows a comparison between different machine learning approaches used in healthcare [34].

From Table 2.1, we can find that the ML approach is used in many s-Health applications such as glaucoma diagnosis, Alzheimer's disease, bacterial sepsis diagnoses, ICU readmissions, and cataract detection. The ANN, SVM algorithm, and deep learning models, especially CNN, are the most commonly used machine learning approaches where they proved to get high evaluation performance in most cases [34].

Growth in IoT is good but how much of the data collected by IoT devices is actually useful, is the key question. To answer that, efficient data analytics software and technologies should be used. Machine learning and IoT should work towards creating a better technology, which will ensure efficiency and productivity for all healthcare sectors.

It is going to be the collaboration between humans and machines that is going to play a vital role in healthcare. Overall, most articles in the Diagnosis and Treatment category indicate that technologies such as IoT and AI provide patients and doctors with clear benefits. In this chapter, the impacts of technologies such as IoT and machine learning in healthcare disease prediction and diagnosis will be discussed and also will highlight key insights for the top application categories, which include wearable and connectivity, disease detection.

2.5 Conclusion and Future Trends

In this chapter, we understand that IoT plays a significant role in collecting and monitoring data, whereas AI is responsible for analyzing the growing amounts of data and taking action based on what it learns from the data. These useful technologies need to understand the variety of ML algorithms and how they can choose and use the right algorithm on trustable data (collected on IoT devices and health record data) to gain the best result on disease diagnosis and disease prediction.

Table 2.1 Machine learning approaches in health

Authors	Objective	Data set	Feature extraction	Machine learning and evaluation
Chai et al. [8]	Glaucoma diagnosis	Data collected from Beijing Tongren Hospital	Scale-Invariant Feature Transform (SIFT) features	Logistic regression Accuracy = 60.84%
			Local Binary Patterns (LBP) features	Logistic regression Accuracy = 62.67%
			Whole image	One-branch CNN (5-conv layers) Accuracy = 71.36%
			Extracted image	One-branch CNN (5-conv layers) Accuracy = 74.95%
				Two-branch CNN (6-conv layers) Accuracy = 74.89%
				Two-branch CNN (5-conv layers) Accuracy = 81.69%
Zhang et al. [39]	Prediction of the MMSE scores in Alzheimer's disease	ADNI database	Level 1	Linear regression, AUC = 0.318
				Ridge regression, AUC = 0.530
				Lasso regression, AUC = 0.520
				Elastic-net, AUC = 0.527

(continued)

Table 2.1 (continued)

Authors	Objective	Data set	Feature extraction	Machine learning and evaluation
Zhang et al. [39]	Prediction of the MMSE scores in Alzheimer's disease	ADNI database	Level 2	Linear regression, AUC = 0.453
				Ridge regression, AUC = 0.542
				Lasso regression, AUC = 0.550
				Elastic-net, AUC = 0.5441
			Level 3	Linear regression, AUC = 0.388
				Ridge regression, AUC = 0.427
				Lasso regression, AUC = 0.419
				Elastic-net, AUC = 0.424
			Level 4	Linear regression, AUC = 0.309
				Ridge regression, AUC = 0.318
				Lasso regression, AUC = 0.324
				Elastic-net, AUC = 0.322

(continued)

Table 2.1 (continued)

Authors	Objective	Data set	Feature extraction	Machine learning and evaluation
			Level 5	Linear regression, AUC = 0.266
				Ridge regression, AUC = 0.273
				Lasso regression, AUC = 0.262
				Elastic-net, AUC = 0.268
Liu and Choi [28]	Diagnose bacterial sepsis	Data Collected from the General Hospital of Guangzhou, China		Procalcitonin (PCT) (cutoff = 3.40) Accuracy = 78.4%
				PCT (cutoff = 8.56) Accuracy = 82.2%
				SVM Accuracy = 88.6%
				Random Forest (RF) Accuracy = 89.2%
Viegas et al. [37]	Prediction of ICU readmissions	MIMIC II	Area under the Sensitivity and specificity curves	Average ensemble decision criteria AUC = 0.77 ± 0.02
				Maximum distance ensemble decision criteria AUC = 0.77 ± 0.02
				Weighted distance ensemble decision criteria AUC = 0.77±0.02

(continued)

Table 2.1 (continued)

Authors	Objective	Data set	Feature extraction	Machine learning and evaluation
			Sensitivity and specificity at the intersection threshold	Average ensemble decision criteria AUC = 0.76 ± 0.02
				Maximum distance ensemble decision criteria AUC = 0.75 ± 0.02
				Weighted distance ensemble decision criteria AUC = 0.76 ± 0.02
			Sensitivity and specificity close to the intersection threshold	Average ensemble decision criteria AUC = 0.75 ± 0.02
				Maximum distance ensemble decision criteria AUC = 0.74 ± 0.02
				Weighted distance ensemble decision criteria AUC = 0.75 ± 0.02

(continued)

Table 2.1 (continued)

Authors	Objective	Data set	Feature extraction	Machine learning and evaluation
Dong et al. [16]	Cataract detection	Data was collected from different sources	Wavelet features	SVM Accuracy = 81.81%
			Texture features	Staking algorithm Accuracy = 84%
Zheng et al. [40]	The risk prediction of hospital readmissions	Data was collected from different hospitals		Radial Basis Function Accuracy = 56.1%
				Neural network Accuracy = 83.8%
Zheng et al. [40]	The risk prediction of hospital readmissions	Data was collected from different hospitals		Linear SVM Accuracy = 50.6%
				Polynomial SVM Accuracy = 52.7%
				RBF-based SVM Accuracy = 69.5%
Fialho et al. [17]	Predict ICU readmission	MIMIC II	Data missing for an intentional Reason was deleted. Data missing for unintentional reason was given the last available value was used	Sequential forward selection Accuracy = 71 ± 3%
				Intelligent tool titled: Acute Physiology And Chronic Health Evaluation (APACHE) version II Accuracy = 61 ± 2%
				APACHE version III Modified tool Accuracy = 65 ± 2%

Today, physicians can detect and remedy much more diseases than in the past. However, even after years of practice, they can still struggle to make the correct diagnosis efficiently. This is where technologies such as IoT and AI can play a key role in providing reliable support for determining a diagnosis and the best course of treatment. AI technologies such as machine learning can quickly analyze the extensive amount of information available to physicians, in the way of the diagnostic process, and help avoid mistakes by integrating both historical data and specific patient information [3].

IoT in the healthcare industry does not stand alone. All IoT devices and their networks need to be combined with other technologies to help healthcare facilities transformation. As mentioned before, IoT will revolutionize the healthcare industry but it also needs data, high-speed communication, and proper security and compliance. AI-driven solutions will make sense of the data lakes from a collection of devices.

Also, in this chapter, the impacts of technologies such as IoT and machine learning in healthcare disease prediction and diagnosis have been discussed and also highlighted key insights for the top application categories, which include wearable and connectivity, disease detection.

ML on IoT for healthcare is expected such trend to continue with more and better model designs. Researchers expect to see more AI applications over IoT information by healthcare as an assistant to physicians being ones. Researchers also expect to see more research on other bots to more disease detection and advising patients remedy. Finally, the authors expect to see more and more surveys and applications on this topic.

References

1. Ain, Q. T., Ali, M., Riaz, A., Noureen, A., Kamran, M., Hayat, B., et al. (2017). Sentiment analysis using deep learning techniques: A review. *International Journal of Advanced Computer Science and Applications, 8*(6), 424.
2. Alsheref, F. K., & Gomaa, W. H. (2019). Blood diseases detection using classical machine learning algorithms. *International Journal of Advanced Computer Science and Applications (IJACSA), 10*(7).
3. Amato, F., López, A., Peña-Méndez, E. M., Vaňhara, P., Hampl, A., & Havel, J. (2013). Artificial neural networks in medical diagnosis. *Journal of Applied Biomedicine (De Gruyter Open), 11*(2), 45–58.
4. Amit, B., Chinmay, C., Anand, K., & Debabrata, B. (2019). Emerging trends in IoT and big data analytics for biomedical and health care technologies. *Handbook of data science approaches for biomedical engineering* (Ch. 5, pp. 121–152). Elsevier. ISBN: 9780128183182.
5. Bengio, Y., LeCun, Y., & Hinton, G. (2015). Deep learning. *Nature, 521*(7553), 436–444. https://doi.org/10.1038/nature14539. PMID: 26017442.
6. Beunza, J.-J., Puertas, E., García-Ovejero, E., Villalba, G., Condes, E., Koleva, G., et al. (2019). *Comparison of machine learning algorithms for clinical event prediction*. Elsevier. https://doi.org/10.1016/j.jbi.2019.10325.

7. Carrio, A., Sampedro, C., Rodriguez-Ramos, A., & Campoy, P. (2017). A review of deep learning methods and applications for unmanned aerial vehicles. *Hindawi Journal of Sensors*. https://doi.org/10.1155/2017/329687463.
8. Chai, Y., He, L., Mei, Q., Liu, H., & Xu, L. (2017). Deep learning through two-branch convolutional neuron network for glaucoma diagnosis. In *Proceedings of International Conference on Smart Health* (pp. 191–201). Springer.
9. Chakraborty, C., Gupta, B., & Ghosh, S. K. (2013). A review on telemedicine-based WBAN framework for patient monitoring. *International Journal of Telemedicine and e-Health, 19*(8), 619–626.
10. Chandra kala, V., Venkateswarakiran, L., & Siva Prasad, P. (2019). Prediction of diseases with pathological characteristics classification using data mining. In *International Conference on Vision Towards Emerging Trends in Communication and Networking (ViTECoN)*, Vellore, India (pp. 1–5).
11. Chinmay, C. (2019). Computational approach for chronic wound tissue characterization. *Informatics in Medicine Unlocked, 17*, 1–10.
12. Daghistani, T. A., Elshawi, R., Sakr, S., Ahmed, A. M., Al-Thwayee, A., & Al-Mallah, M. H. (2019). Predictors of in-hospital length of stay among cardiac patients: A machine learning approach. *International Journal of Cardiology*. https://doi.org/10.1016/j.ijcard.2019.01.046.
13. Deng, L., & Yu, D. (2014). Deep learning: Methods and applications. *Foundations and Trends in Signal Processing, 7*(3–4), 197–387. https://doi.org/10.1561/2000000039.
14. Devi, R. L., & Kalaivani, V. (2019). Machine learning and IoT-based cardiac arrhythmia diagnosis using statistical and dynamic features of ECG. *Journal of Supercomputing*. https://doi.org/10.1007/s11227-019-02873-y.
15. Domingos, P. (2012). A few useful things to know about machine learning. *Communications of the ACM*. https://doi.org/10.1145/2347736.2347755.
16. Dong, Y., Wang, Q., Zhang, Q., & Yang, J. (2016). Classification of cataract fundus image based on retinal vascular information. In *Proceedings of International Conference on Smart Health* (pp. 166–173). Springer.
17. Fialho, A. S., Cismondi, F., Vieira, S. M., Reti, S. R., Sousa, J. M., & Finkelstein, S. N. (2012). Data mining using clinical physiology at discharge to predict ICU readmissions. *Expert Systems with Applications, 39*(18), 13158–13165.
18. Fitriyani, N. L. (2019). Development of DPM based on ensemble learning approach for diabetes and hypertension. *IEEE Access*. Special section on data-enabled intelligence for digital health. https://doi.org/10.1109/ACCESS.2019.2945129.
19. Ghasemi, F., Mehridehnavi, A. R., Fassihi, A., & Perez-Sanchez, H. (2017). Deep neural network in biological activity prediction using deep belief network. *Applied Soft Computing, 62*, 251.
20. Goodfellow, I., Bengio, Y., & Courville, A. (2016). *Deep learning*. Cambridge, MA: MIT Press.
21. Guo, Y. (2016). Deep learning for visual understanding. *Neurocomputing, 187*(26), 27–48.
22. Hamet, P., & Tremblay, J. (2017). Artificial intelligence in medicine. *Metabolism, 69*, S36–S40.
23. Hinton, G. E., Osindero, S., & Teh, Y.-W. (2006). A fast learning algorithm for deep belief nets. *Neural Computation, 18*(7), 1527–1554. https://doi.org/10.1162/neco.2006.18.7.1527. PMID: 16764513.
24. Jánosi, A., Ofner, P., Branyickiné Géczy, G., & Polgár, P. (2013) Incidence of myocardial infarction in Hungary. Population study in five districts of Budapest and Szabolcs–Szatmar–Bereg County. *Orvosi Hetilap, 154*(28), 1106–1110.
25. Kober, J., Bagnell, J. A., & Peters, J. (2013). Reinforcement learning in robotics: A survey. *The International Journal of Robotics Research, 32*(11), 1238–1274. https://doi.org/10.1177/0278364913495721.
26. Krizhevsky, A., & Hinton, G. E. (2011). Using very deep auto encoders for content based image retrieval. In *19th European Symposium on Artificial Neural Networks (ESANN'11)*, Bruges, Belgium.

27. Lillicrap, T. P., Hunt, J. J., & Pritzel, A. (2015). *Continuous control with deep reinforcement learning*. Cornel University Library. https://arxiv.org/abs/1509.02971.
28. Liu, Y., & Choi, K. S. (2017). Using machine learning to diagnose bacterial sepsis in the critically ill patients. In *Proceedings of International Conference on Smart Health* (pp. 223–233). Springer.
29. Mahdavinejad, M. S., Rezvan, M., Barekatain, M., Adibi, P., Barnaghi, P., & Sheth, A. P. (2018, August). Machine learning for internet of things data analysis: a survey. *Digital Communications and Networks, 4*(3), 161–175. https://doi.org/10.1016/j.dcan.2017.10.002.
30. Makino, M., et al. (2019). Artificial intelligence predicts the progression of diabetic kidney disease using big data machine learning. *Scientific Reports*. https://doi.org/10.1038/s41598-019-48263-5.
31. Mitchell, T. (1997). *Machine learning* (p. 2). New York, NY: McGraw Hill. ISBN: 978-0-07-042807-2.
32. Piros, P., Ferenci, T., Fleiner, R., Andréka, P., Fujita, H., Főző, L., et al. (2019). Comparing machine learning and regression models for mortality prediction based on the Hungarian Myocardial Infarction Registry. Knowledge-Based Systems. https://doi.org/10.1016/j.knosys.2019.04.027.
33. Prusa, J. D., & Khoshgoftaar, T. M. (2017). Improving deep neural network design with new text data representations. *Big Data, 4*(1), 7. https://doi.org/10.1186/s40537-017-0065-8.
34. Rayan, Z., Alfonse, M., & Salem, A.-B. M. (2019). Machine learning approaches in smart health. In *8th International Congress of Information and Communication Technology, ICICT 2019*. Elsevier.
35. Urban, G. (2018). Deep learning localizes and identifies polyps in real time with 96% accuracy in screening colonoscopy. *Gastroenterology, 155,* 1069–1078.e8.
36. Vanani, I. R., & Amirhosseini, M. (2019). Deep learning for opinion mining. *Extracting knowledge from opinion mining* (pp. 40–65). Hershey, PA: IGI Global.
37. Viegas, R., Salgado, C. M., Curto, S., Carvalho, J. P., Vieira, S. M., & Finkelstein, S. N. (2017). Daily prediction of ICU readmissions using feature engineering and ensemble fuzzy modeling. *Expert Systems with Applications, 79,* 244–253.
38. Vincent, P., Larochelle, H., Lajoie, I., & Manzagol, P. (2010). Stacked de noising auto encoders: Learning useful representations in deep network with a local de noising criterion. *Journal of Machine Learning Research, 11,* 3371–3408.
39. Zhang, J., Luo, Y., Jiang, Z., & Tang, X. (2017). Regression analysis and prediction of mini-mental state examination score in Alzheimer's disease using multi-granularity whole-brain segmentations. In *Proceedings of International Conference on Smart Health* (pp. 202–213). Springer.
40. Zheng, B., Zhang, J., Yoon, S. W., Lam, S. S., Khasawneh, M., & Poranki, S. (2015). Predictive modeling of hospital readmissions using met heuristics and data mining. *Expert Systems with Applications, 42*(20), 7110–7120.

Chapter 3
A Methodology for Improving Efficiency in Data Transmission in Healthcare Systems

Reinaldo Padilha França, Yuzo Iano, Ana Carolina Borges Monteiro, and Rangel Arthur

Abstract Given the numerous technological advances in communication reaching the health sector, the accelerated growth of telemedicine can be observed. This medical practice can be defined by the use of telecommunication means to provide care, health promotion, treatment, information exchange between doctors and researchers, and also for various health research. However, there are still many methodologies that present a large consumption of computational memory as well as slowness in sending medical data. And with that focus, the present research aims to implement discrete event modeling, called CBEDE (Coding of Bits for Entities by Discrete Events) to improve the transmission of medical data by specifying the wide spectrum of health-related themes. The modeling was performed using the MATLAB Simulink environment, where AWGN communication channel models with DQPSK (Differential Quadrature Phase Shift Keying) modulation were developed and analyzed in relation to information consumption medical data in MB (megabytes). The proposal directs a different approach with respect to signal transmission, employing in the discrete domain the effect of discrete entities' technique in the bit generation step, aiming to increase the information capacity transmission in healthcare systems, showing better memory consumption utilization regards improvement of 95.86%. Since diagnostic health interaction offered by e-health enables digital solutions for faster and better-quality health care, enabling the optimization of healthcare services, generating greater interaction between physician and patient, as well as all agents in system health care, where CBEDE methodology may enable faster and

R. P. França (✉) · Y. Iano · A. C. B. Monteiro · R. Arthur
School of Electrical and Computer Engineering (FEEC), University of Campinas—UNICAMP, Av. Albert Einstein—400, Barão Geraldo, Campinas, SP, Brazil
e-mail: reinaldopadilha@live.com; padilha@decom.fee.unicamp.br

Y. Iano
e-mail: yuzo@decom.fee.unicamp.br

A. C. B. Monteiro
e-mail: monteiro@decom.fee.unicamp.br

R. Arthur
e-mail: rangel@ft.unicamp.br

C. Chakraborty et al. (eds.), *Internet of Things for Healthcare Technologies*, Studies in Big Data 73, https://doi.org/10.1007/978-981-15-4112-4_3

more efficient scheduling of consultations, transmission devices monitoring data from patients, presenting great potential for the transmission of medical data.

Keywords Discrete events · Simulation · Precoding · Modulation · CBEDE · Healthcare

3.1 Introduction

In recent years, with the advancement of technology and its new discoveries, diagnostic medicine has evolved greatly favoring both patients and physicians, as tests, procedures, and results have become simpler, faster, and safer. Due to the evolution of technology in medicine over the years, it is remarkable for both professionals and patients, where health care has been changing and the way doctors relate to patients. Where in the present world scenario are the automation of procedures, strengthened with the arrival of the Internet of Things (IoT), big data, and artificial intelligence (AI), deeply influencing in the way medicine is employed [1].

When talking about technology and medicine, it is natural to think of robotic surgery, telemedicine, and stem cell use, very modern and current topics, and however, the relationship between medicine and technology is dated a long time. Taking a brief look back, in the Middle Ages, the period between the fifth and fifteenth centuries, some medicines for the treatment of diseases have already been developed in Europe. One was a type of anesthetic made from a mixture of hemlock juice, garlic juice, opium, vinegar, and wine that was given to the patient prior to a surgical procedure, and it is also dangerous and can lead to death if the mixture does not follow the right dose of each ingredient [1, 2].

At that time, surgeries were not safe procedures, and they were only performed in case of life-threatening, largely due to lack of hygiene, infrastructure, and knowledge. At the end of the fifteenth century, increased investments in universities, enhancing the study of sciences such as anatomy, physics, biology, and chemistry, wherefrom the scientific knowledge that experts developed new ways to harness discoveries and technologies for the improvement of medicine. The use of X-ray equipment spurred an unprecedented technological revolution in the medical field, so doctors have since been able to examine anatomical structures without the need for invasive procedures [3, 4].

At the beginning of the twentieth century, scientists have been able to develop different ways to study and record the functioning of the heart muscle, and from these initial studies, created the electrocardiogram machine. Conducting research on magnetism about electromagnetic radiation, addressing ions or charged particles, there was also a contribution to the production of the magnetic resonance apparatus. In addition to the diagnostics that innovations through technology that have impacted various medical specialties, the technologies used in communication are also important for advances in medicine [3–5].

These advances culminated in the emergence of specialties such as telemedicine, which employs Information and Communication Technologies to provide distance reports, becoming evident, especially from the nineteenth century, with the support of telegraphy, where doctors began transmitting reports of radiographic examinations with colleagues from distant locations. In the late nineteenth century, with the invention of the telephone, there was a leap forward with this communication gaining the possibility of sharing by voice. The Morse code was also employed for sending medical information [3–5].

And in the twentieth century, the invention and popularization of the Internet allowed the development of chats, applications, and other technologies that facilitated communication in medicine, boosting telemedicine, initially in European countries, to be applied in public health, where its use in fields beyond telediagnosis, such as tele-education, health management, and second medical opinion, has generated the current concept of telehealth. Telehealth can be defined as the provision of distance health services through information and communication technologies, where more recently digital health or e-health has also emerged—a unification of patient information such as medicines, consultations, and examinations, integrating software and devices through technology in medicine [3–5].

Innovations will be responsible for bringing many opportunities for doctors with the acquisition of knowledge and new skills and can improve their current practices and rely on this great ally in preventing and fighting disease. Being one of the trends in this field are the applications that assist in the collection of health information. Regarding the union between Internet and mobile should give more autonomy for patients, who can help their doctors with routine information, facilitating assertive diagnoses [6].

A great example of the use of technology in health is the electronic medical record, which has been gaining more and more adherence in the daily routine of a clinic, gathering all the information in one place, being one of the main advantages of an electronic medical record. Where coupled with a cloud system, this information can be accessed from anywhere, which is of great relevance when treating an emergency patient by having access to the Internet. Other features present in an electronic medical record are the customization according to the specialty and needs of the place, attach exams, and photographs, with the advantage of not occupying physical space, while considering that using an electronic medical record ensures the security of your data and makes the easier and more efficient services [1, 6].

Through Information Technology, management systems have helped doctors to manage their offices and offer better-quality care to their patients because this type of system offers more peace and transparency to the healthcare professional, as it organizes and optimizes all administrative tasks within the clinic or office, where these systems organize appointment scheduling, electronic medical records, and even clinic financial management, providing many benefits to the healthcare professional and his staff in the day-to-day tasks of medical practice [7, 8].

The digital revolution has brought about an adaptation in the way information is annotated and accessed, so keeping information on paper gradually ceases to be part of our reality, just as using patient records and records risks to maintaining this information due to time action, theft and poor communication between employees about information and processes. To solve this scenario, software purchased and installed on the computer for a long time was the only option [6–8].

However, just like paper, there is a risk of theft or problems with the computer, such as burning the board, circuitry, or formatting, which leads to the loss of this information and there is no support to help recover it. So, with cloud systems, data is stored on more than one server. Where in the event that any server has a problem such as power outages or accidents, the other servers will take action to meet the needs of users [8, 9].

Telemedicine is a means of communication and patient care that develops more and more. It is a form of assistance to remote patients, being initially used to reach distant places, and nowadays, it relies on the use of artificial intelligence until it reaches the operating tables. Being a reality and its use is increasingly frequent, having examples of its applications videoconferences, teleconsultations, tele-assistances, reports, and surgeries with the help of robots. Since its inception, this medical specialty has made significant strides in making health accessible anytime, anywhere, whether for interpretation of exams and issuing reports at a distance, this is decisive support, contributing to the prevention, diagnosis, monitoring, and treatment of diseases, injuries, and other medical conditions [1, 10].

Distance reports are already a reality in many countries, including Brazil, thanks to a combination of Internet, telemedicine platforms, trained professionals and specialists, nursing or radiology technicians, or health professionals can perform examinations that record pixel images (digital), where they are stored and shared online on secure systems. Thus, an expert can view the information of any device with Internet access, through login and password. Therefore, telemedicine is considered a significant advance of technology in world medicine [11–13].

All these advances also enable the empowerment of patients, making them responsible for their health status and engaged with the treatment prescribed by the health professional, where gradually there is an improvement in the lives of patients and family, reducing the delay with results, treatments, hospitalizations and, mainly, in the cure of several diseases. Wherever it is a simple message sent to patients confirming the consultation, interaction through social networks or even the computerization of all clinic data and processes is sure to make a difference for the patient [1, 14, 15].

Advances in health technology are not only restricted to electronic devices and digital applications, but also include alternative technologies designed to improve people's lives, wherein healthcare institutions the use of technology combined with communication is also a reality. Since in many hospitals already use communication solutions that alert and notify the emergency room doctors about each new result of rectified and critical examination that was updated in the system and also makes available by application the schedule of updated appointments for their doctors, so the hospital ensures clinical safety and agility and improves medical communication, where this interaction and follow-up between appointments can be of great value to the patient [15, 16].

From the above technologies, the predictions for the future of medicine are encouraging, since we are facing a perspective ranging from the end of transplantation queues, changes in DNA that can eliminate disease to new technological options to combat great ills. Since technology is an element of sustainability throughout the chain, since it generates greater service efficiency and cost reduction, as well as being a vector of economic development. Thus, telemedicine, as well as medical devices and healthcare applications, should also progress further, increasing access to services such as online reports, second opinion, and distance learning [15–17].

3.2 Telecommunications Channels

Telecommunications systems comprise a set of devices and techniques employed for the instantaneous transmission of long-distance information, operating and differing from each other especially in the type of information manipulated and the medium used to transmit it, be it voices, graphic signals (images), medical data, images, television signals, among others. These can be exemplified as telegraphy, telephony, radio, television, and computerized medical data networks, having as essential means of transmission radio communication, cable transmission, and artificial satellites [18].

Four fundamental elements comprise the general process of transmission by means of a communication system being a message, a transmitter (or sender), the means or channel of transmission, and the receiver being general principles of telecommunications. Where the transmission of the message from a sender to a receiver is usually by two channels the air (or vacuum) and the conductors of electricity [18, 19].

Being the used model quite due to its long-acting spectrum and a large set of physical channels is the Additive White Gaussian Noise (AWGN) channel model, featuring characteristic of introducing a statistically modeled noise into the transmitted signals, as the name itself leads being the white Gaussian additive process. Also said that this model mathematically considers imperfections in the communication channel as the existence of disturbances/noise in the channel (free space/atmosphere/copper line) being of multiple causes, so in this context, there is also the wireless mobile channel, referring to communication that is based on radio frequencies, being the communication path is mobile at both ends [18, 20].

Airborne transmission is based on the duality of electric and magnetic fields, which move together in space, or vacuum, in the form of an electromagnetic wave of physical magnitudes related to the intensity of the fields. Where variations in the received signal are observed on a large scale, and when the signals travel long distances or long periods of time, it is called large scale variation; which in turn the variation determined by loss in the course directly related to the distance and the frequency of its propagation presenting a linear variation [19, 21].

Likewise, in a system propagation can be done by means of electrical currents through conductive wires (cable transmission), taking advantage directly of the electrical character of electromagnetic fields (such as coaxial cables, extended wire pairs on poles, or buried under shallow, underground or submarine), widely used in the communication of sounds, telegraph signals, and low-speed data sets, this system uses several types of conducting lines [18, 22, 23].

Rician fading is also a useful model of real-world phenomena in wireless communications, used to describe the received signal level (affected by a flat fading channel) as a function of temporal variation, or the amplitude of individual multipath components, being a stochastic model for the radio signal propagation anomaly, caused by the partial cancelation of a radio signal by itself, that is, when the dominant component of the received signal is stationary, a condition normally found in channels with line of sight (LOS). The signal reaches the receiver exhibiting multipath interference, being fast, associated with terminal movement and multipath. Thus, communication networks are based on a sender sending a communication message to a particular receiver or to several via a channel, that is, a means for conveying the message to be communicated. Both types of channels can be employed for the transmission of medical data between hospitals, hospitals and patients, and physicians and patients [15, 24, 25].

3.3 Discrete Events

Systems are usually considered as sets of elements, between which a relationship can be defined and which operate as an organized structure. As well as the discrete event system can be outlined as a system whose dynamic evolution hangs on the occurrence of events. These so-called discrete events can be classified as a responsible occurrence for changing the state of this system and are commonly classified into three types, intentional, spontaneously controlled occurrence, or verification of a condition. Thus, it is necessary that there are actions taking place, which in turn generate events, where the system will change state only when it occurs, otherwise the system will remain in the same state [26–28].

If this system depends on variables that assume discrete values, i.e., be in a domain of finite or enumerable values such as the integer set. The goal of discrete event modeling is to reproduce the activities of the entities that make up the system, the state change being determined by the occurrence of an event at a deterministic or stochastic time, and from there, knowing the system behavior and performance, where it is necessary to define the system state and the activities that drive the system from state to state [26–28].

Discrete events evolve as system states are changed and easily identified, entities are discrete items of interest in a discrete event system, where the meaning of the entity depends on what is being modeled and the type of system, where the concepts entities and events are different. Thus, one or more phenomena of interest change their value, or state, at discrete points in time [26–28].

The occurrence of these events changes the state of the system at any given moment, where they are instantaneous discrete incidents that can change the state variable/output/occurrence from another event, which also means that an entity is relatively dependent on what is being modeled and the type of system [26–28].

The state of the event is represented by variables representing the properties of the system to be studied, an event is a conceptual notation that a state changes in a system, and may indicate an accident/earthquake/fault/control/person/heartbeat, or another desirable concept within a system, as well as the generation of a bit in a communication system. Wherefrom the point of view of simulation time is divided into small slices and the state of the system is updated according to the activities that occur in each slice of time [26–28].

3.4 Scientific Grounding

In 2009, Petri Net (PN) framework was studied, in the context of fault detection problem for discrete event systems, considering the previous knowledge that structure of the PN model and initial marking, still reflecting that faults are modeled by unobservable transitions, being such modeling employed by an algorithm computation grounded on the determination and establishment of some integer linear programming issues establishing whether the system behavior displays some possible faults or has normal behavior [29].

In 2010, the trend in the industrial area of communication network technologies was researched. Among these trends, the Controller Area Network (CAN) protocol was approached as a solution in distributed control systems. However, the effect of network communication delays on control system performance was seen as the biggest challenge in the development of distributed systems based on industrial networks. In this context, a model with colored Petri Nets for simulating these CAN-based systems using discrete events was presented [30].

In 2011, a discrete event-based packet transmission mechanism was implemented and applied to simulation environments. This implementation was performed for routing protocols in wireless networks, aiming at mapping and tracking their path in each node of the network. Events were used for the purpose of updating and tracking packages [31].

In 2012, it was studied the real-world problems related to impreciseness, subjectivity, and vagueness, taking into account fuzzy discrete event systems. Thus, in this context, the supervisor was designed as a controlled system, with a bisimilar specification, presenting the achievement that the supervisor exists over a certain finite fuzzy state space, through modeling of a theorem [32].

Also, in 2012, cloud computing combined with the IoT concept was studied as the trend with respect to the efficient processing, transmission, and management of data in relation to online sensors. Since, in turn, healthcare applications that use networks of body sensors generating volumes of data that need to be transmitted, stored, and managed for further processing. In this focus, the research presented a platform based on cloud computing related to the management of portable and mobile IoT health sensors, demonstrating how the IoT technology can be applied to health in a comprehensive way [33].

In 2013, it was studied that network coding can greatly influence the performance of flow control schemes. In this work, the processing of an end-to-end (SR) selective repetition (ARQ) automatic repeat request from an intermediate communication link was investigated. These studies were based on the network coding technique (NC). Simulink's SimEvents tool was employed in the available band where the channel was working. The results showed that throughput performance was sensitive to a series of node inbound links and width [34].

Still, in 2013, it was studied that IoT is the best way to collect information on a personal and public level, and along with its advent of connectivity, it gained the ability to cover related aspects in the physical field, since public health is important for governments and people, and the management, transmission of data and organization of this information can help improve social health, enabling the creation of an infrastructure focused on achieving a healthy society. In this sense, the research described how IoT can be applied in public health with governments helping citizens [35].

In 2014, the use of discrete event simulation for call centers was seen that many researchers as a tool that optimizes services and improves resource planning. In this sense, it was investigated in a more complex system, the use of discrete event simulation taking into account the multi-stage information technology service (ITC) center. Sales orders have gone through several processes involving different types and levels of service [36].

Also in 2014, it was studied that RFID tags in the medical context allow an accurate and quick identification of each intelligent entity, which allows data transmission and quick and ubiquitous access to Personal Health Records through IoT, as well as using the simple architecture from IoT combined with smart objects and mobile communications, the possibility of remote care of patients' well-being was seen, establishing a m-health service prototype, establishing a use-case scenario with respect to the proposed architecture assessment [37].

In 2015, it was studied process optimization focused on quality, productivity improvement, and cost reduction tools has excelled in industrial environments based on the results obtained by several companies, where research aimed at discrete events simulation as decision-making tools and the application of value stream mapping (VSM) directing among the available scenarios generated by simulation system as best option with respect to the management invest [38].

Also, in 2015, the variety of applications enabled by IoT with respect to intelligent health care was analyzed, since networked sensors enable the collection of rich information, captured continuously, aggregated and extracted, bringing a positive transformative change in the healthcare scenario, which indicates people's physical and mental health. The research highlights the challenges and opportunities of IoT in achieving this future vision of health care. Particularly, together the availability of data in time scales with a new generation of intelligent processing algorithms, and longitudes contribute to facilitating evolution in the practice of medicine, based on the current reactive diagnosis paradigm and post facto treatment, for the prognosis of diseases in an incipient stage, considering prevention, cure, and management; as well as (b) management permission directed especially to the individual's specific circumstances and needs as well as the customization of treatment options; and (c) helping to reduce the cost of health care together with improving outcomes [39].

In 2016, a discrete event simulation model was presented to analyze the processing of an email server. The sending and receiving of messages were analyzed, taking into account their lead time period [40].

Also, in 2016, a mobile health system (m-health) was described within the IoT context, taking into account issues related to security which is essential for the health system addressing issues of privacy and security, confidentiality in the context of an m- health insurance. Reflecting on the essential characteristics of m-health devices with relation to low power consumption, IP connectivity, security, and compactness, and discussing aspects regarding the acquisition of mobile health data through wearables and medical devices. As well as the application of data in the monitoring of various health aspects, such as blood pressure, asthma, ECG, blood sugar level, among others. In this way, several measures were listed regarding the protection of information contained in the m-health system about patients, as well as it was assessed that a general mobile health system has the capacity to significantly reduce the costs of unnecessary hospitalizations and medical assistance [41].

In 2017, it was found that exhaustive testing of wireless protocols on prototypic hardware is expensive and time-consuming. Thus, a discrete event simulator was presented allowing direct simulation of the existing code for wireless prototypes with a focus on the lower layers of the communication stack, since it was analyzed that an alternative approach is network simulation [42].

Also, in 2017, the integration of cloud computing with IoT technology was studied in order to obtain a better solution for a secure, continuous, uninterrupted, and ubiquitous structure, still considering aspects of processing, accessibility, storage, security, service sharing, and components, making the convergence suitable for the advancement of mobile technologies reflecting on the level of flexibility of this solution. In this sense, the health field is one of the locations that benefit from IoT-cloud technology, with respect to the restrictions of physical movement of patients and at the same time as the shortage of specialized professionals, as well as other factors. With this focus, the research discussed solutions for the voice pathology monitoring that afflicts people, through a voice pathology detection system using the IoT cloud, with the use of an extreme learning machine classifier and a local binary standard in a representation of the voice signal in the Mel spectrum and with the intention of detecting this type of pathology, still considering the easy use of this monitoring structure, which can still achieve high accuracy in detection [43].

In 2018, it was studied the difficulty of identifying risk and opportunities to quantify them and propose mitigation plans that minimize the impact of risk in manufacturing projects, and developed a model representative of a manufacturing plant and manufacturing strategy [44].

Also in 2018, the advancement of IoT in the health field was studied, the integrity and security of medical data became major challenges for healthcare services applications, which led to the development of a hybrid security model, through the integration of technique level 1 2D steganography with respect to the 2D discrete wavelet transform (2D-DWT-2L) or the 2D discrete wavelet transform (2D-DWT-1L) with a hybrid encryption scheme using a combination of the Rivest, Shamir algorithms, Advanced Encryption Standard, and Adleman, to protect this text diagnostic data with respect to medical images. The performance of the system is evaluated according to six statistical parameters; mean square error (MSE), bit error rate (BER), peak signal-to-noise ratio (PSNR), structural similarity (SSIM), correlation and structural content (SC), proving the ability to hide confidential data from patient by the proposed method [45].

In 2019, the importance of monitoring in the healing of chronic wounds was studied, which implemented a compression technique with qualification for use in a smartphone present in a telewinding network (TWN) system. Taking into account the need for bandwidth and memory savings for processing clinical data, images of wounds were then captured using a smartphone via a metadata application page, being reduced, followed by an improvement in the accuracy and sensitivity of the segmentation, which were compressed and sent to the hub telemedical according to partitioning configured in the hierarchical tree compaction algorithm (SPIHT), considering that a better healing treatment depends on the accuracy of the segmentation and classification of these images. Since the use of the SPIHT compression technique aided by YDbDr-fuzzy, c-means clustering significantly reduced the execution time (105 s), improving segmentation accuracy (98.39%), saving memory (18 kB), and producing better results even without using SPIHT. The proposal was evaluated in terms of compression rate, peak signal/noise rate, bit rates per pixel, transmission time, quality of diagnosis in the telemedicine structure, and mean square error. In this sense, the results showed the potential of this type of proposal to be implemented in the future in the field of chronic wound management and clinical evaluation [46].

Or even in the same year, trends were shown regarding data analytics for biomedical and healthcare technologies in the context of IoT and big, and WBAN framework for patient monitoring [47, 48].

3.5 Proposal and Objectives

The objective of discrete event modeling is to improve process performance based on the formulation of mathematical models already in use but which can be optimized, since the developed and validated simulation model can be used as a tool to predict the effects of a change, analyzing the performance obtained in the system, as well as helping in the implementation of future projects.

The importance of computer simulation is the result of the increase in the processing capacity of personal computers, which has favored greater access to computer simulation software, thus reducing costs of evaluation without the need for a physical experimental setup, allowing the increase of the performance of computers processes through newly developed approaches, ensuring that new processes are tested and validated, thus achieving a higher level of resource optimization. Through researches, it is clear that the technique of discrete events was employed in the transport layer in telecommunications systems.

Discrete events are a technique that can help in greater applicability and performance in telecommunications systems, such as the development of the methodology CBEDE, which employs the technique in the step of generation of bits (physical layer), is responsible for its conversion into discrete entities, where these are transmitted on a signal in an Additive White Gaussian Noise (AWGN) channel. The result of this process acting at a lower level of application at the physical layer reduces the consumption of computing resources, as memory consumption, being a fundamental parameter to meet the requirements of an exponentially technological world.

In this context, the medical data are related to the personal data of patients in the health context considered, in a broad sense, as all information that is identified or allows to identify individuals related to health, sexual life, family history, description and evolution of symptoms, and exams, in addition to indications and treatments and prescriptions, genetic or even biometric data; or even clinical medical data such as the digitalization of tests or the creation of electronic medical records of patients such as laboratory tests, images, anamnesis, pressure values, weight, heart rate, clinical reports, medications, and diagnoses, among many others.

Within this ambit, it is essential to develop new communication approaches based on discrete events that aim to transmit medical data with greater accuracy and speed, having positive impacts on the delivery of clinical information to the partners of the service chain, as well as the interaction facilities among all its members, making the same information available to the decision-making doctors of this chain; monitoring patients who need constant supervision, having devices attached sending medical data about heartbeat, pressure and other parameters to the doctor's computer; assisting hospitals and health institutions that already use technology for treatments, improving the exchange of information between systems. Since there must be synchrony between the old and the new, where technology and new proposals developed should add, not limit.

3.6 Methodology

This study employs the technique of discrete events in the stage of the generation of the signal, i.e., the discrete events are punctually employed to the process of creation of the bits, through a precoding process of bits dealing with discrete events in the signal before of the modulation process, for transmission in an AWGN channel, its use is responsible for giving rise to the methodology named by CBEDE, along with advanced modulation format DQPSK and fading Rician for multipath.

The modeling of the CBEDE was done through the Simulink simulation environment of MATLAB software, in its 64-bit version (2014a), and was chosen because it was consolidated in the scientific environment and has already tested and validated blocks, where the libraries were used: communications System, the DSP System, Simulink, and the SimEvents.

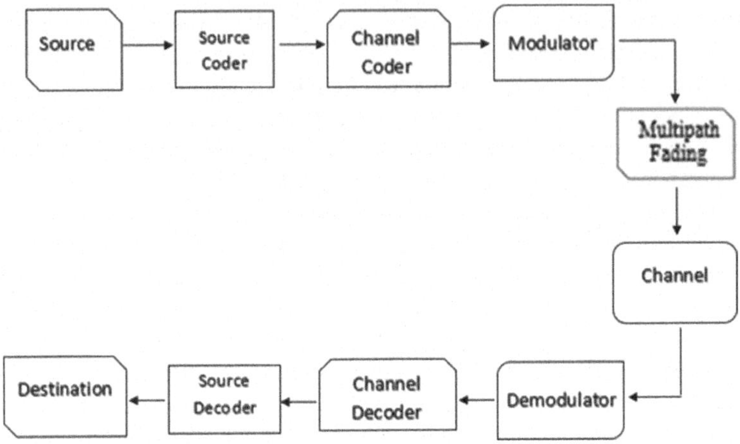

Fig. 3.1 Traditional telecommunication system modeling

In the proposed model (Fig. 3.1), the signals corresponding to the bits 0 and 1 are generated and modulated with the advanced modulation format DQPSK, which uses the phase shift, coming from the modulation format itself; passing through a multipath Rician fading channel with Jakes model with Doppler shift defined at 0.01 Hz, as also inserted a block with a math function $1/u$, required to track the channel time variability where the receiver implementation ordinarily incorporates an automatic gain control (AGC); then proceeding to an AWGN channel (parameters shown in Table 3.1); where this signal is then demodulated to perform the Bit Error Rate (BER) calculation of the channel, having these values obtained are sent to the MATLAB workspace, for verification of equality and generation of the BER signal.

Table 3.1 Parameters channel AWGN DQPSK

AWGN DQPSK	
Sample time	1 s
Simulation time	1000–10,000 s
Signal-to-noise ratio (SNR)	0–15 dB
Symbol period	1 s
Input signal power	1 W
Initial seed in the generator	37
Initial seed on the channel	67

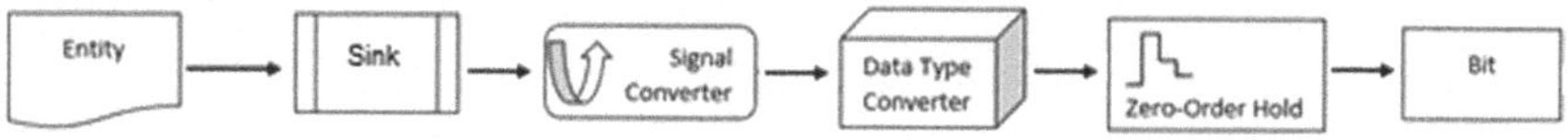

Fig. 3.2 Proposed bit precoding

3.6.1 Bit Treatment

The modeling according to the proposal implemented with discrete events is similar presented in the previous session, differentiating in the addition of the process of discrete events called precoding, being implemented through the discrete event methodology, where it is understood as the discrete event methodology in the step of generating signal bits (information) to make it more appropriate for a specific application.

The event-based signal is the signal susceptible to treatment by the SimEvents library, and is converted to the specific format required for manipulation by the Simulink library, being (both time-based signals and event-based signals are in the time domain) treatment has the emphasis on bits 1 and 0, which are generated as a discrete entity (parameters as shown in Table 3.1). Then, Entity Sink is used to represent the end of the modeling of discrete events by the library SimEvents, responsible for highlighting the specific point where the event-based signal conversion will be performed for a time-based signal.

This time-based signal is converted to a specific type that will follow the desired output data parameter (integer = the bit), By means of the Real World Value (RWV) function, and the current value of the input signal is preserved after then, rounding is performed with the "floor" function, responsible for rounding the values to the nearest smallest integer. Performing after a Zero-Order Hold (ZOH), responsible for defining sampling in a practical sense, used for discrete samples at regular intervals, which describes the effect of converting a signal to the time domain, causing its reconstruction and maintaining each sample value for a specific time interval. The treatment logic on bit 1 is presented in Fig. 3.2.

After this processing, the signal is modulated within DQPSK and inserted into the AWGN channel and thereafter demodulated for purposes of calculating the BER of the signal to verify equality and generate the BER graph of the signal, as represented in Fig. 3.3.

The models shown in Figs. 3.1 and 3.3 are executed with 10,000 s of simulation respecting the configuration defined according to Table 3.1.

3.6.2 Signal Validation

The verification of equality of the signals is performed through the "size" and "is equal" functions of the MATLAB by analyzing the DQPSK modulation through its constellation, by means of the "compass" function (where *n* is the number of elements

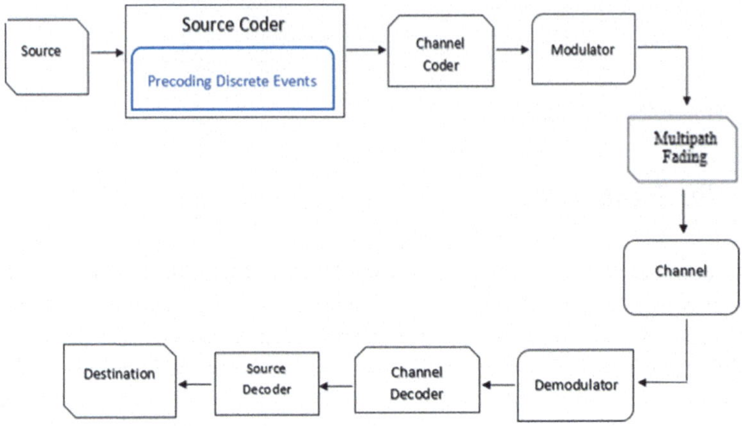

Fig. 3.3 Proposal applied to telecommunication system

in Z) which displays a compass graph with n arrows, and how the constellations will be PSKs, their representations of points are radial, as well as through the bit error rate (BER), being responsible for the mathematical comparison proving that the signals have the same Size Thus, together with the BER verification, it states that the same amount of information is transmitted (bits) in both the proposed methodology (CBDE) and the conventional methodology, flowing through the AWGN channel, where if the signals are of the same size, the logical value 1 (true) is returned and the same volume of medical data is transmitted, indicating that the equality of the signals is true, otherwise the value will be 0 (false), showing that the proposal does not add or remove information to the originally transmitted signal. And to the same end will be used the diagram of constellation [26, 27].

The DQPSK constellation has four possible states 0, π, $+\pi/2$, $-\pi/2$, where each symbol represents two bits of information, its division of the binary pattern is equal to QPSK, except when a bit string is shifted to about $\pi/4$ or $\pi/2$, meaning that there are a total of 8 status positions. Figure 3.4 shows the constellation diagram DPQSK

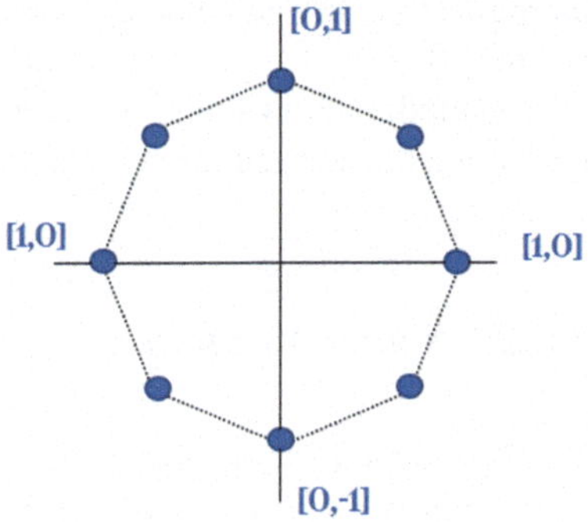

Fig. 3.4 Theoretical DQPSK constellation

for the offset version $\pi/4$, where this modulation format is widely used in several airborne systems [26, 27].

3.7 Results

In this section are presented the results of this research showing an AWGN transmission channel modeled with DQPSK modulation through MATLAB Simulink. Through the model shown in Fig. 3.5 are the traditional method (left) and the proposed innovation of this chapter (right), addressing signal transmission flow (bits 0 and 1), is generated and then modulated in DQPSK, and Fig. 3.6 is presented the constellations for proposed (left) and the traditional methods (right).

The models were investigated from the perspective of memory consumption evaluation, from the first simulation of both models because it is in it where all the

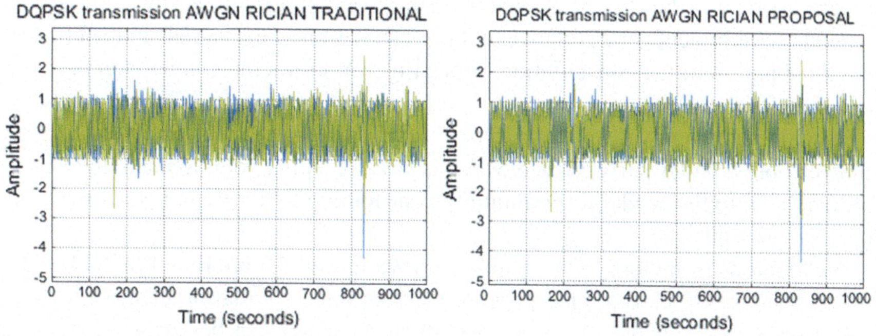

Fig. 3.5 Transmission flow DQPSK Rician

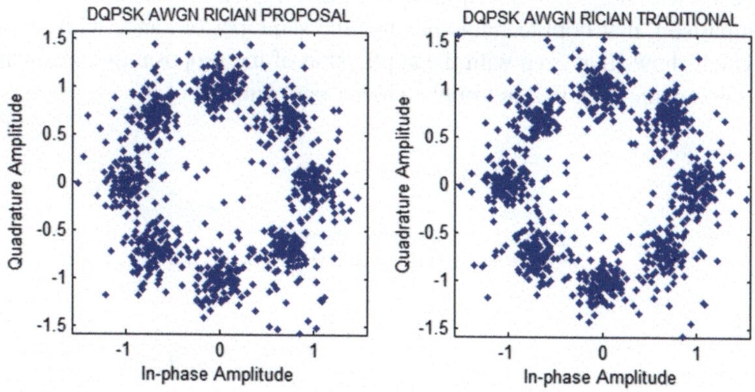

Fig. 3.6 Simulated DQPSK Rician constellations

variables of the model are allocated, it is in the first simulation that the construction of the model in a virtual environment is performed from scratch, as well as the memory of the operating system in which the MATLAB is running is reserved for the execution of the model and the results of this model.

With respect to memory calculation, the "sldiagnostics" function was used, where the "TotalMemory" variable receives the sum of all the memory consumption processes used by the "ProcessMemUsage" parameter, counting the amount of memory used in each process, throughout the simulation, returning the total in MB (megabyte). For this was used a computer with hardware configuration is an Intel Core i3 processor, containing two color processing, Intel Hyper-Threading Technology, and 4 GB RAM, relating the proposal to the dynamics of the real and modern world, stating its efficiency and applicability, being carried out through four simulations of each model, as shown in Fig. 3.7.

The DQPSK modulation was analyzed through its constellation, by "compass" function, displaying a compass graph with n arrows, and how the constellations will be PSKs, their representations of points will be radial, with the location of the base of each arrow will be its origin, where each arrow is determined by the real and imaginary components of Z, relative to the constellation of the signal, and confirmed with the diagram of the constellation. Thus, Fig. 3.8 shows the comparison between the methodologies.

Developing an innovative methodology for improving the transmission of a signal achieves both a better performance which is already a plus point to make the know-how available to the academic community contributing to the area of study theme is important as well.

The amounts of memory consumption shown in Fig. 3.7 are found in Table 3.2.

The relationship between the proposed x traditional simulation methodology as well as its impact on the physical layer of the channel can be analyzed through BER, where scripts were made in the MATLAB for processing the graph, where their results are shown in Fig. 3.9 with respect to performance of models during transmission with noise ranging from 0 to 25 dB. Where it is possible to see through this comparison, that both technologies had the same performance with respect to BER, which shows that even with the application of the proposal in a medical data transmission channel, it will not imply a lower performance of it.

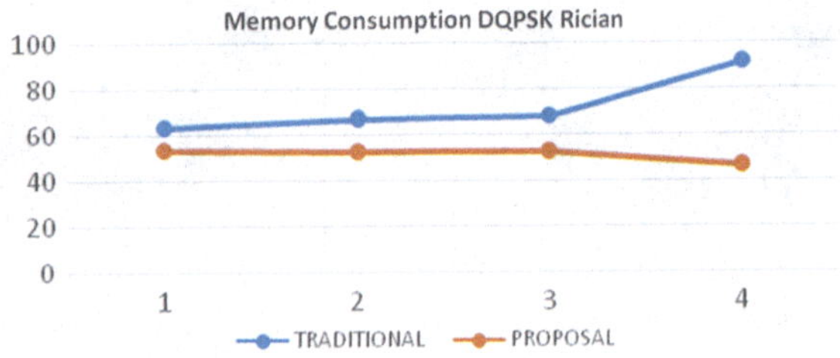

Fig. 3.7 Simulations (memory) DQPSK Rician

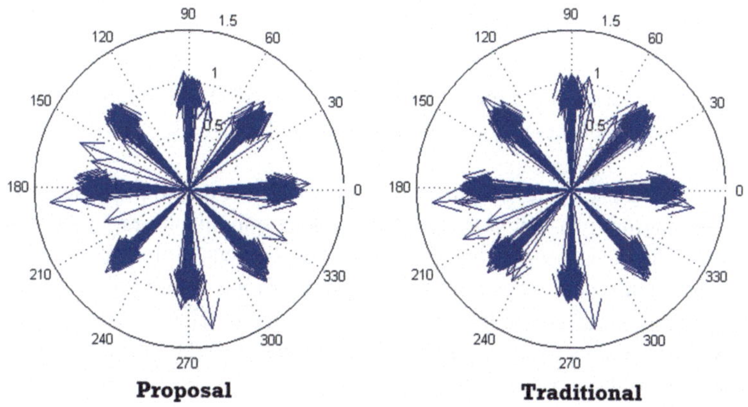

Fig. 3.8 Simulations (memory) DQPSK Rician

Table 3.2 Amounts of memory consumption

	Traditional	Proposal
Simulation		
1	63.2109	53.2539
2	66.8281	52.7422
3	67.9648	52.5508
4	91.0820	46.5039

Fig. 3.9 BER between the model DQPSK Rician

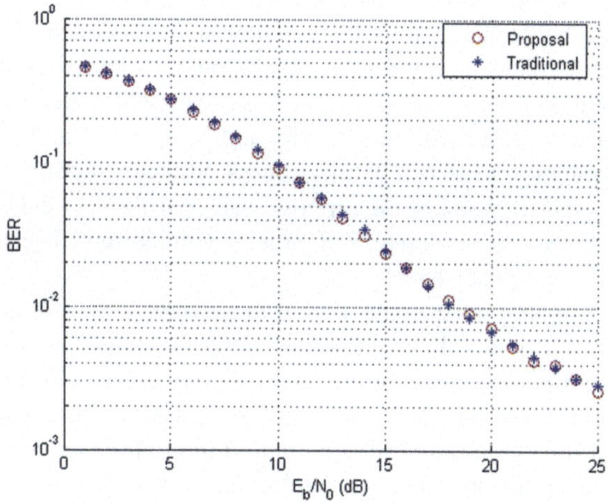

As already discussed, this proposal brings a new approach to signal transmission, which is performed in the discrete domain with the implementation of discrete entities in the bit generation process, providing optimal computational performance.

3.8 Discussion

The comparison between the methodologies showed results reaching up to 95.86% in the improvement of memory consumption through of the proposed methodology (CBEDE).

The increasing use of devices that allow medical data transmission at speed and quantity unimaginably a few years ago has made communication as a whole intensified, where the near-absolute presence of mobile devices in the hands of doctors, patients, and health workers enables transmission of images and voice, today being a reality. Telemedicine, e-health is one of the news that impacted the health universe positively, where the fact is how much technology has added to this area filling gaps that directly impact the patient's life.

Health systems around the world, public or private, face a constant tension between the need to serve patients well and budgets that are often in short supply, wherein this context CBEDE methodology demonstrates its great potential for employment in healthcare devices, emerging as a tool that allows agility and improvement in medical data transmission and efficiency in computational consumption.

Since one of the e-health's core values is not to fill that entire time interval between appointments, exams, speeding up urgent processes, shortening distances, optimizing time, and improving information communication, ensuring patient well-being where it will always return. The proposed proposal (CBEDE) can assist with patient data and images in Internet traffic with infrastructure that ensures better handling, information integrity, provided that the proposal demonstrates great potential for interconnected hospitals, physicians and patients to find in less time, the necessary medical services.

Based on these characteristics, e-health is not only an exclusively medical activity, but is the result of the union of health and technology professionals, forming an important synergy for the development of activities aimed at promoting the health and well-being of health professionals, where the correct application of this practice, together with the security and better medical data transmission throughout the system is what will define success. Still considering the low memory consumption, a positive point of the proposal can contribute to the transmission of large amounts of medical data streams of patients with chronic diseases, be seen as a crucial factor for emergency care.

In the same context of transmission and communication, videoconferencing broadcasting allows important hospital centers to connect with each other through high-performance online telemedicine, where CBEDE can contribute in this context. I also take into consideration that each center can cover the basic health units of its region (increasing its range) through more efficient telemedicine, organizing the healthcare process according to complexity.

Where beyond the technological aspects, e-health is an effective application of technology solutions for the purpose of optimizing education, care, logistics planning, and implementing methods that provide multicenter research reaching the entire health chain, providing and better generating management strategies resulting in sustainability in a new e-health model focused on better patient care.

Thus, the proposal presented in this chapter uses an effective technique that reaches the wide variety of healthcare issues, where conceptually discrete events have been used in the modeling of concepts with a high level of abstraction as patients, nurses, doctors, in the exchange of emails on a clinical server, transmission of medical data packets between devices in a hospital network, queuing concept to manage patient data, to an extent of a healthcare system, where different from the proposal through the implementation of discrete entities in the bit generation process, increasing the transmission capacity information for healthcare systems.

3.9 Future Scope of Research

As can be seen the potential of the proposal in the transmission of medical data, in future research it will be directed to Orthogonal Frequency-Division Multiplexing (OFDM) system since this modern scheme concerns modulation allowing the simultaneous transmission of multiple data streams in carrier frequencies orthogonal, that is, mutually perpendicular, still reflecting on the transmission distribution of the stream with a high bit rate, considering multiple slow flows, allowing the operation in channels with the occurrence of the multipath phenomenon, overcoming this type of problem, as long as the data transmitted are divided into subcarriers, each of which carries a piece of information.

Being applied in m-health, referring to tools and practices carried out on wireless mobile devices, dealing with medical practice acting from prevention work, monitoring even diagnosis of diseases, related to electronic health, through technological tools and solutions developed to improve people's quality of life.

As well as the future development of the proposal with support and focused on mobile devices such as smartphones, personal digital assistants (PDAs), or patient monitoring devices, other wireless devices, which facilitate not only the patient's life, concerning monitoring treatments and medication consumption, as well as for optimization of hospital services in laboratories and clinics.

3.10 Conclusions

This chapter introduces a new approach for signal transmission, implementing discrete entities in the bit generation process in the discrete domain, aiming at increasing the information transmission capacity in healthcare systems, since it is in the use of discrete events applied to the bit itself (physical layer of a transmission medium) related to low-level of abstraction, showing better computational performance with regard to memory utilization related to compression of information, reaching up to 95.86%, which is a major contribution to the area.

The proposal of this research also assists and contributes to e-health in any application that uses the Internet as well as internal medical data transmission networks, as well as being used in conjunction with other information technologies, focused on providing better conditions for clinical processes, patient care, and better costing conditions to the health system.

As well as providing a better optimization of time, helping to reduce operating costs, and likewise providing the doctor's approach with the patient, ensuring health care, greater speed of care, due to the systematization of the process.

References

1. Cruz-Cunha, M. M. (Ed.). (2016). *Encyclopedia of E-health and telemedicine*. Hershey, PA: IGI Global.
2. Zebroski, B. (2015). *A brief history of pharmacy: Humanity's search for wellness*. New York: Routledge.
3. Castiglioni, A. (2019). *A history of medicine*. New York: Routledge.
4. Ackerknecht, E. H., & Haushofer, L. (2016). *A short history of medicine*. Baltimore: JHU Press.
5. Magner, L. N., & Kim, O. J. (2017). *A history of medicine*. Boca Raton, FL: CRC Press.
6. Darcy, A. M., Louie, A. K., & Roberts, L. W. (2016). Machine learning and the profession of medicine. *JAMA, 315*(6), 551–552.
7. Hamet, P., & Tremblay, J. (2017). Artificial intelligence in medicine. *Metabolism, 69,* S36–S40.
8. Shapiro, J. S., et al. (2016). Health information exchange in emergency medicine. *Annals of Emergency Medicine, 67*(2), 216–226.
9. Lo'ai, A. T., et al. (2016). Mobile cloud computing model and big data analysis for healthcare applications. *IEEE Access, 4*, 6171–6180.
10. LeRouge, C. M., Tulu, B., & Wood, S. (2016). Project initiation for telemedicine services. *E-health and telemedicine: Concepts, methodologies, tools, and applications* (pp. 1–24). Hershey, PA: IGI Global.
11. Harzheim, E., et al. (2016). Telehealth in Rio Grande do Sul, Brazil: Bridging the gaps. *Telemedicine and e-Health, 22*(11), 938–944.
12. Pedrosa, F., et al. (2017). The impact of prospective telemedicine implementation in the management of childhood acute lymphoblastic leukemia in Recife, Brazil. *Telemedicine and e-Health, 23*(10), 863–867.
13. Mattos, S. d. S., et al. (2018). Impact of a telemedicine network on neonatal mortality in a state in northeast Brazil. *Population Health Management, 21*(6), 517.
14. Pandian, P. S. (2016). An overview of telemedicine technologies for healthcare applications. *International Journal of Biomedical and Clinical Engineering (IJBCE), 5*(2), 29–52.
15. Nelson, R., & Staggers, N. (2016). *Health informatics—E-book: An interprofessional approach*. Elsevier Health Sciences.
16. Celi, L. A. G., et al. (Eds.). (2017). *Global health informatics: Principles of eHealth and mHealth to improve quality of care*. Cambridge, MA: MIT Press.
17. Lau, F., & Kuziemsky, C. (2016). *Handbook of eHealth evaluation: An evidence-based approach.*
18. Morreale, P. A., & Terplan, K. (2018). *CRC handbook of modern telecommunications*. Boca Raton, FL: CRC Press.
19. Iannone, E. (2016). *Telecommunication networks*. Boca Raton, FL: CRC Press.
20. Omer, A. E. (2015). Review of spectrum sensing techniques in cognitive radio networks. In *2015 International Conference on Computing, Control, Networking, Electronics and Embedded Systems Engineering (ICCNEEE)*. IEEE.
21. Shavit, R. (2018). *Radome electromagnetic theory and design*. Hoboken, NJ: Wiley.
22. Butt, S. J., et al. (2015). Micro propagation in advanced vegetable production: A review. *Advancements in Life Sciences* 2(2), 48–57.

23. Van Regemortel, M., Sels, D., & Wouters, M. (2016). Information propagation and equilibration in long-range Kitaev chains. *Physical Review A, 93*(3), 032311.
24. Singh, R., & Tiwana, S. S. (2016). *Review paper on generalized Rician Fading.*
25. Le, K. N. (2019). A review of selection combining receivers over correlated Rician fading. *Digital Signal Processing.*
26. Padilha, R., Martins, B. I., & Moschim, E. (2016). Discrete event simulation and dynamical systems: a study of art.
27. Padilha, R. F. (2018) Proposta de um método complementar de compressão de dados por meio da metodologia de eventos discretos aplicada em um baixo nível de abstração [Proposal of a complementary method of data compression by discrete event methodology applied at a low level of abstraction].
28. Kogler, C., & Rauch, P. (2018). Discrete event simulation of multimodal and unimodal transportation in the wood supply chain: A literature review. *Silva Fenn, 52.*
29. Dotoli, M., et al. (2009). On-line fault detection in discrete event systems by Petri nets and integer linear programming. *Automatica, 45*(11), 2665–2672.
30. Godoy, E. P., Lopes, W. C., Sousa, R. V., & Porto, A. J. V. (2010). Modelagem E Simulação De Redes De Comunicação Baseadas No Protocolo Can—Controller Area Network. *Revista SBA: Controle & Automação, 21*(4).
31. Narra, H., Cheng, Y., Çetinkaya, K. E., Rohrer, P. J., & Sterbenz, G. P. J. (2011). The OMNeT++ discrete event simulation system. In *SIMUTools '11 Proceedings of the 4th International ICST Conference on Simulation Tools and Techniques* (pp. 439–446), Barcelona, Spain, March 21–25, 2011.
32. Xing, H., Zhang, Q., & Huang, K. (2012). Analysis and control of fuzzy discrete event systems using bisimulation equivalence. *Theoretical Computer Science, 456,* 100–111.
33. Doukas, C., & Maglogiannis, I. (2012). Bringing IoT and cloud computing towards pervasive healthcare. In *2012 Sixth International Conference on Innovative Mobile and Internet Services in Ubiquitous Computing*. IEEE.
34. Alsebae, A., Leeson, M., & Green, R. (2013). The throughput benefits of network coding for SW ARQ communication. In *IEEE 2013 27th International Conference on Advanced Information Networking and Applications Workshops.*
35. Suraki, M. Y., & Jahanshahi, M. (2013). Internet of things and its benefits to improve service delivery in public health approach. In *2013 7th International Conference on Application of Information and Communication Technologies*. IEEE.
36. Deb, S., Chowdhury, N. F. A., & Claudio, D. (2014). Service quality improvement in an IT center: A simulation study. In *Proceedings of the 2014 Industrial and Systems Engineering Research Conference.*
37. Santos, A., et al. (2014). Internet of things and smart objects for M-health monitoring and control. *Procedia Technology, 16,* 1351–1360.
38. Helleno, A. L., et al. (2015). Integrating value stream mapping and discrete events simulation as decision making tools in operation management. *The International Journal of Advanced Manufacturing Technology, 80*(5–8), 1059–1066.
39. Hassanalieragh, M., et al. (2015). Health monitoring and management using Internet-of-Things (IoT) sensing with cloud-based processing: Opportunities and challenges. In *2015 IEEE International Conference on Services Computing*. IEEE.
40. Rangel, J. J. A., Costa, J. V. S., Laurindo, Q. M. G., Peixoto, T. A., & Matias, I. O. (2016, March). Análise do fluxo de operações em um servidor de e-mail através de simulação a eventos discretos com o software livre Ururau. *Produto & Produção, 17*(1), 1–12.
41. Almotiri, S. H., Khan, M. A., & Alghamdi, M. A. (2016). Mobile health (m-health) system in the context of IoT. In *2016 IEEE 4th International Conference on Future Internet of Things and Cloud Workshops (FiCloudW)*. IEEE.
42. Serror, M., Kirchhof, J. C., Stoffers, M., Wehrle, K., & Gross, J. (2017). Code-transparent discrete event simulation for time-accurate wireless prototyping. In *SIGSIM-PADS'17*, Singapore, May 24–26, 2017.

43. Muhammad, G., et al. (2017). Smart health solution integrating IoT and cloud: A case study of voice pathology monitoring. *IEEE Communications Magazine, 55*(1), 69–73.
44. Álvarez, D. C., Rodríguez, A. L., & Dono, J. A. M. (2018). Risk management and design of mitigation plans through discrete events simulation and genetic algorithms in offshore wind processes. *International Journal of Service and Computing Oriented Manufacturing, 3*(4), 274–292.
45. Elhoseny, M., et al. (2018). Secure medical data transmission model for IoT-based healthcare systems. *IEEE Access, 6*, 20596–20608.
46. Chakraborty, C. (2019). Performance analysis of compression techniques for chronic wound image transmission under smartphone-enabled tele-wound network. *International Journal of E-Health and Medical Communications (IJEHMC), 10*(2), 1–15.
47. Amit, B., Chinmay, C., Anand, K., & Debabrata, B. (2019). Emerging trends in IoT and big data analytics for biomedical and health care technologies. *Handbook of data science approaches for biomedical engineering* (Ch. 5, pp. 121–152). Elsevier. ISBN: 9780128183182.
48. Chakraborty, C., Gupta, B., & Ghosh, S. K. (2013). A review on telemedicine-based WBAN framework for patient monitoring. *International Journal of Telemedicine and e-Health, 19*(8), 619–626. ISSN: 1530-5627.

Chapter 4
Investigating Correlation of Tension-Type Headache and Diabetes: IoT Perspective in Health care

Rohit Rastogi, Parul Singhal, Devendra Kumar Chaturvedi, and Mayank Gupta

Abstract Digital technology has changed health care today. Much data refer to big data collected by digitizing everything. Information gathered from a variety of sources focuses on changing the way the health care has developed using technology. Health analysis is the ability to detect and suggest ways to reduce costs, improve patient outcomes, and prevent preventable diseases. Artificial intelligence, also called artificial intelligence, is information that is displayed by a machine in comparison to the natural information displayed by humans and other animals.AI technologies are now more common across the various industries in the world: finance, agriculture, car transportation, energy, and health care. Learning the machine is an evolved technological tool that uses artificial intelligence to capture insecure areas of business models. Diabetes is a major chronic disease. The disease is caused by blood sugar (glucose) caused by the inability to absorb energy from food, especially glucose. As time goes on, people with diabetes tend to have long-term problems in the hypertension, coronary artery disease, eye disease, etc. The purpose of this study was to investigate the diabetes analysis from coronary artery disease and other diseases using the latest technologies to analyze and the correlation between big data and stress on human health. Generally, people with tension-type headache generally have high blood pressure. Six out of eight subjects were reported to have hypertension with tension-type headache and 75% tension-type headache. These figures clearly show that hypertension is associated with tension-type headache. If a person develops diabetes or hypertension in one day, or develops diabetes, TTH is most likely to occur and is more likely to be a male.

Keywords Big data (BD) · Internet of things (IoT) · Artificial intelligence (AI) · Machine learning (ML) · Machine intelligence in health care · Diabetes types

---

R. Rastogi (✉) · P. Singhal
ABES Engineering College Ghaziabad and Dayalbagh Educational Institute, Agra, India
e-mail: rohit.rastogi@abes.ac.in

D. K. Chaturvedi
Dayalbagh Educational Institute, Agra, India

M. Gupta
Tata Consultancy Services, Noida, India

C. Chakraborty et al. (eds.), *Internet of Things for Healthcare Technologies*, Studies in Big Data 73, https://doi.org/10.1007/978-981-15-4112-4_4

(DT) · Stress · Tension-type headache (TTH) · Hypertension (HTN) · Coronary artery disease (CAD)

4.1 Introduction

4.1.1 Machine Vision

Machine vision is a method by which a computer can display and use one or more analog–digital video cameras (ADCs) and digital signal processors (DSPs). The obtained data are controlled by computer or robot. The complexity of the device is similar to the complexity of speech recognition. Each sensitivity and resolution system has two important characteristics. For example, electronic component analysis, signature identification, optical character recognition, and handwriting recognition. Although the term device is commonly referred to as industrial computer software, computer terms are often used to describe digital computers, data processing, and any kind of technology in which some of them are recorded.

4.1.1.1 General Application

Machine Vision can be broadly used in product inspection management, visual inventory management, barcode reading, counting, etc. The food and beverage industry uses automotive vision systems to monitor quality. In the medical field, machine vision systems are used in medical imaging and inspection methods.

4.1.2 Medical Imaging

Medical imaging uses techniques and processes used to process images of various parts of the human body for diagnostic and digital purposes. The term medical imaging includes various radiographic techniques.

For example, X-ray, fluorescence microscope, magnetic resonance imaging (MRI),medical ultrasound or ultrasound, medical and functional imaging techniques for positron emission tomography (PET), medical imaging involves techniques that not only generate images but also measure and record the data often displayed in charts and maps. These include electroencephalogram (EEG), magnetic electroencephalography (MEG), and electrocardiogram (EKG).

4.1.2.1 Medical Imaging Usage in Digital Health

Medical imaging is very important in all medical settings and levels. Medical imaging allows doctors to make more accurate diagnoses and make better treatment decisions. Without medical imaging, both digital health diagnosis and treatment are very accurate at every level.

4.1.2.2 Important Applications for Medical Imaging Techniques

Projector X-ray fractures detect pathological changes in the lungs and certain types of colorectal cancer. Fluoroscopy creates realistic images of internal and human structures. MRI scans to create 2D images of body and brain. Capturing a two-dimensional image of the radiation emitted by an intact radioisotope to detect biologically active areas of the scotography that may be related to the disease. Positron Emission Tomography (PET) is commonly used to serve this purpose.

For the identification and treatment of various diseases using radioactive isotopes and energetic particles, applications such as thermography, contact thermography, dynamic angiography can be used. Tomography technology—Imagine a thin film structure (CT, PET scan). Echocardiography—Examines the exact structure of the heart, such as room size, heart function, heart valves, and pericardium.

4.1.3 Biomedical Image and Analysis

Biomedical imaging measures the human body at various scales. These images are taken by a specialist (such as a radiologist) to perform a clinical task (such as a diagnosis) and have a significant impact on physician decisions [1] (Fig. 4.1).

4.1.4 Big Data & Internet of Things

Big data are a large amount of structured, semi-structured, and unstructured data that can extract information and be extracted by machine learning projects. BD also contains a variety of data including structured data from SQL databases and data warehouses, and structured or semi-structured SQL data such as Web server files and data streams.

BDs also contain multiple simultaneous data sources and cannot be integrated. For example, a large data analysis project can measure the success and sales of future products [2].

loT, an interconnected computing device, is a digital device, machine, animal, or personal device with a unique identifier (UID) that connects networks without interfering with people or people. Ability to send information via computer [3].

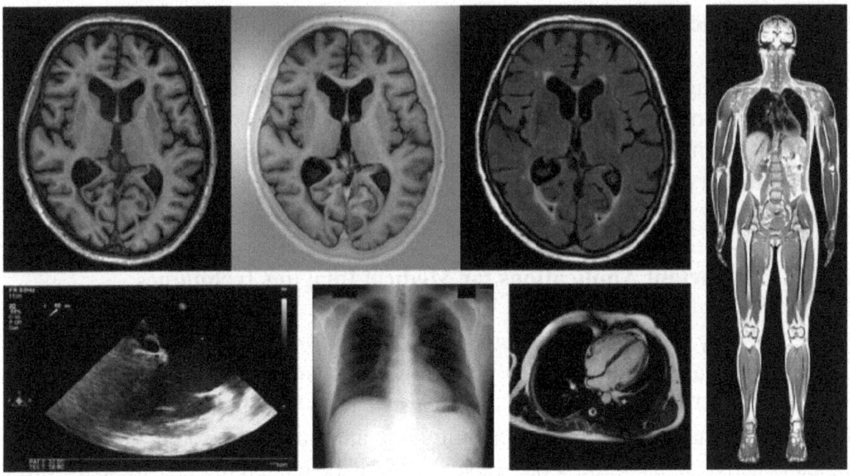

Fig. 4.1 Medical imaging example (upper left to lower right): MRI multiple brain distribution: T1 weight, reverse T1 recovery and FLAIR T2 channel; MRI total wrist; flat heart ultrasound; X-ray chest; MRI heart MRI [1]

4.1.5 Artificial Intelligence (AI) and Machine Learning (ML)

AI uses various devices; these free computer system features include notes (licenses for obtaining and using licenses) [4].

The goal of artificial intelligence is to mimic human cognitive functions. As the paradigm shifts to artificial medicine, it is changing rapidly and access to medical data analysis is changing. Review the current status of Al's plan in health care and talk about its future. Artificial intelligence can be applied to various types of medical data (structured and unstructured). Common artificial intelligence technologies include traditional machine learning techniques for structured data, such as support vector machines (SVM) and neural networks (N n/w), as well as advanced deep learning and natural language processing of raw data. Key areas of disease that use artificial intelligence tools include cancer, neurology, and natural language processing of raw data. Key areas of disease that use artificial intelligence tools include cancer, neurology, and heart disease. Next, the Al Stroke Program is tested in three major parts. Early diagnosis and diagnosis, treatment and outcome prediction, and prognosis. Finally, we describe pioneering Al systems, such as IBM Watson, and the real barriers to Al deployment. Medical machine learning recently introduced a new technology developed by Google machine [4].

4.1.5.1 Use of Machine Intelligence in Health care

Here are the top ten applications of machine learning in health care.

Learning cars in health care is one of the things that is seen in the gradual acceptance of the healthcare industry. Google has recently launched a machine learning algorithm to detect cancerous tumors in mammography, and Stanford researchers have used deep learning to identify skin cancer. The machine learning (ML) currently has various responsibilities in health management. ML helps healthcare analyze and analyze thousands of different data points, providing timely risk assessment, accurate resource allocation, and other applications. With the increasing use of automotive learning in health care, it will be possible to support millions of patients in the future without data, analysis, and innovation coming together.

Drug discovery and production: One of the clinical applications of machine learning is the early detection of drugs. It also includes R&D technologies such as next-generation sequencing and medical accuracy to help find alternatives to the treatment of multi factorial diseases. Currently, machine learning techniques include unmatched learning that can identify data patterns without prediction.

Intelligent health records: Keeping your health records up-to-date is a comprehensive process. Technology plays a role in reducing the data entry process, but most of the process still spends a lot of time completing. The main role of core learning in health care is to simplify the process of saving time, effort, and money. OCR detection technologies such as the Google Cloud Vision API and MATLAB's machine learning handwriting recognition technology are becoming increasingly popular.

Crowd-sourced data collection: Crowd sourcing is now upset by the medical community, allowing researchers and practitioners to access the wealth of information provided for individuals. These raw health data have a significant impact on how drugs are treated online. With the advancement of it, the healthcare industry continues to discover new ways to use this data, help with challenging diagnostics, and improve overall diagnostics and medications.

Better radiation therapy: One of the most used applications of ML in medicine is the radiology department. Medical image analysis has many individual variables that can occur at any given moment. There are many lesions, cancers, etc., that cannot be simplified using complex equations. ML-based algorithms are used in various instances in the hand, making it easy to find and find variables. The most common applications of ML in medical image analysis are to classify objects such as lesions into categories such as normal or abnormal, lesions or non-lesions [3–5].

4.1.5.2 Big Data and IoT Application in Health care

The main problem is that all patients, especially in remote areas, cannot receive medical treatment or treatment in critical situations. It has had unpleasant consequences for people with regard to hospital and doctor services. Today, these problems are mostly solved by using new technologies that use IoT devices to monitor health care.

Cost savings: Large amounts of data are the best way to save the cost of hospitals that are more or less of this book. Predictive analytics help to solve this problem by helping to predict admission rates and assigning employees. This reduces hospital investment and actually helps to maximize the investment potential. In the insurance industry, immunizing wearable health trackers can prevent patients from being hospitalized.

High-risk support: If all hospital records are digitized, this is the complete information that can be examined for many patient patterns. Take these patients to the hospital to identify chronic problems. Such an understanding helps to better manage such professionals and insights when modifying corrective actions to reduce frequent visits. This is a great way to maintain a list of at-risk patients and provide them with professional care.

Human error prevention: Experts are reported to believe that they mislead misleading drugs. In general, large amounts of data can be used to analyze user data and prescription drugs to reduce such errors. This can identify information and has great potential for prescribing alternatives to reduce errors and save lives. Such software is an excellent tool for doctors to be exposed to many patients [3, 5].

4.1.6 Diabetes and It's Types

Diabetes is a kind of problem which occurs due to increase of sugar level in our body. This problem increases with the age. That is why it is mainly seen in older people. The main cause of diabetes is taking high amounts of sugar on a regular basis. Then, if we neglect this problem, then it will cause serious damage to the body. So, for the prevention of this problem, we should have proper knowledge of diabetes and various preventive practices that we can do to cure this problem [6, 7].

Diabetes is also known as diabetes. In diabetes, there are basically two conditions: the body cannot make enough insulin, or the body cannot make insulin. There are different types of diabetes.

Type 1 diabetes: In type 1 diabetes, the immune system attacks and destroys pancreatic cells made with insulin.

Type 2 diabetes: In type 2 diabetes, the body becomes insulin resistance and blood sugar levels rise [8].

4.1.6.1 Diabetes and Headache

Not all diabetics experience a headache. People with recent diabetes tend to have headaches because they are still trying to control their blood sugar and eat their diet.

For diabetics, headaches are usually caused by changes in blood sugar levels.

A headache may indicate high blood sugar, which doctors call blood sugar. Instead, blood sugar levels could be too low, and one doctor called it hypoglycemia. Changes in blood sugar levels are likely to cause diabetes headache [6, 9, 10].

4.1.7 Tension-Type Headaches (TTH)

Today, headaches are the most common type of headache found in people. Various causes of tension headaches cause mild headaches on the back and head of the eyes. They can be observed once or twice a month [11–13].

4.1.7.1 Causes of TTH

A headache is a type of tension that can buy different types of foods, activities, and so on. The major causes of headache types are alcohol, eye strain, dry eye, fatigue, smoking, cold or flu, caffeine, and sinus infections.

4.1.7.2 Symptoms of TTH

Symptoms of tension headache include pressure around the forehead, dull headache, tenderness, and scalp. Tension headache pain is usually moderate, but sometimes it can be severe. Depending on the duration of the headache an individual can face anxiety, depression, sleeplessness, migraine and hypertension like symptoms [14].

4.1.7.3 Treatment

Massaging scalp, temples or bottom of your neck can help to relieve pain in a headache. Over the countries painkillers such as ibuprofen, aspirin, paracetamol and naproxen are mostly used by patients suffering from TTH. These painkillers are used when the condition of headache becomes uncontrollable and interferes with your physical activities. However, the treatment of TTH can vary according to the symptoms and triggers causing it.

4.1.7.4 Obesity

Obesity is defined as the disease which takes place when there is excessive body fat in our body. When the body burns more calories than it burns, excess fat is consumed and stored in the body, leading to obesity. Obesity is a long-term condition that can cause problems such as high blood pressure and diabetes.

Obesity can also be checked by evaluating the distribution of fat in our body. Therefore, determine the risk of obesity-related health problems. The first type is body fat distributed around the waist and the second type is fat distributed on the waist and thighs. The main causes of obesity are overeating and sedentary habits and not exercising regularly [15, 16].

4.1.7.5 Coronary Artery Disease (CAD)

If the coronary arteries are too narrow, cardiovascular disease (CHD) or coronary artery disease can occur. Coronary arteries are blood vessels that carry oxygen and blood to the heart and cause cholesterol in the walls of the arteries. These plaques can cause arterial occlusion and reduce blood flow to the heart. Thrombosis can disrupt blood flow and cause serious health problems. The coronary arteries form arteries on the surface of the heart where oxygen is supplied. If these arteries are narrow, the heart may not be supplied with oxygen-rich blood, especially during physical activity. Sometimes CHD causes a heart attack.

4.1.7.6 Symptoms

CHD can cause angina. A type of chest pain associated with heart disease. Angina can cause the following emotions in the chest: push pressure weight, etc. [17].

4.1.7.7 Treatment

There is no cure for CHD. However, there are ways in which one can manage the situation. Treatment includes changing your lifestyle including quitting smoking, eating a healthy diet, and regular exercise medicine. There are a variety of drugs available for treating cardiovascular disease [17].

4.1.7.8 Insulin

Insulin is a chemical messenger that allows cells to transfer glucose and glucose from one source. The pancreas is the abdomen, and the main cause of insulin in pancreatic cells is the hormonal component of the physical formation of blood sugar [9].

4.1.7.9 Novelty in Our Work

The Internet communicates, interacts, and identifies anytime, anywhere, making life more difficult and easier. This is one of the current trends and innovations in recent technology developments. Earth-based solutions are exploding in various fields such as cloud computing, connectivity, and data-driven medical systems. For example, in the healthcare sector, IoT monitors its performance for continuous heart rate monitoring (HR) and records HR data from pulse glasses created for Android smartphones. Stored seamlessly in the cloud. The goal of our research is to prevent and treat diabetes and improve the lives of all diabetics, by improving the classification method.

4.2 Literature Survey/Previous Findings

According to Alana Biggersa and her team members, Hypoglycemia is one of the most important complications of T2D and is associated with insulin and other hypoglycemic agents. The risk of hypoglycemia depends on diabetes, genes such as insulin and sulfonylurea's, loss of kidney function, aging and other complications.

They examined two groups of people with T2D to find out their relationship with depression, quality of sleep, and a history of low blood sugar [18]. They used to follow a methodology in which two adults in Chicago and Bangkok responded to a questionnaire to assess sleep quality, symptoms of depression, and the frequency of hypoglycemia with T2D. Effective barriers to regression models are established for each adjustment group for treatment duration, insulin and sulfonylurea management, and other factors.

They believe that people of both age groups with hypoglycemia respond more to long-term diabetes, lower insulin use, and less sleep quality. Chicago homosexual groups were less likely to use sulfonylurea's but had higher depression scores. In Thai groups, sulfonylureas are most commonly used. In Thailand's final regression model, depressive symptoms were independently associated with a higher incidence of hypoglycemia. In the final models of Chicago and Thailand, sleep quality was not associated with the prevalence of hypoglycemia. For more information on these complex relationships, Alana Biggersa and Lisa Carey Sharp use remote monitoring of blood glucose levels, sleep, and ecological momentum assessment. In the Thai group, symptoms of depression were associated with hypoglycemia [18].

Usama M. Alkholya and her colleagues have discussed the condition of Q10 and vitamin E in children with T1D was being studied [19].

They found that the levels of intracellular cell carcinoma of plasma Q10 and vitamin E in children with T1D and A1% C were significantly higher in children with diabetes. Children with low glycemic control showed platelet vitamin E, coenzyme Q 10.

They introduced the following method: It includes many children with T1D that have been selected and then compared to 48 healthy children. Each measurement was performed at an average of three consecutive measurements with a standard instrument and an international biological program.

The authors suggested that further research is needed on the therapeutic potential of both vitamin E and coenzyme Q10 in the prevention and prevention of vascular disease. They hypothesized that patients with mainly low-dose T1D had high levels of collagen vitamin E and Q10 and reduced platelet levels of the coenzyme Q10 vaccine.

Thus, patients with particularly weak T1D had elevated plasma levels of vitamin E and coenzyme Q10 and reduced redox status of platelet coenzyme Q10 [19].

Finn Diderichsena and Angelis Andersen told that there is not enough meaning to depression of diabetes and obesity. Low education and violence are also a major reason for obesity that can occur in an individual due to various reasons and of long term illnesses. Obesity is a major cause of diabetes. Low income is another issue. Violence against women also contributes to the economic crisis. They used the proposed method, a meticulous family study method using a three-step random sampling method [20].

According to Angelis Andersen the main unit head of the National Census Machine and vice chairman of Secondary unit-household, there are three levels of people in the Human development index. The Human Development Index was used in 27 states of Brazil to measure the content of socioeconomic development. Logistic regression is often used but here is a generalized binary linear model of IBM SPSS, V 25 for regression analysis. They recommended creating a better environment with less violence to educate the public about various issues decreased obesity.

Finally, they concluded that obesity also led to my wife and my depression. The diabetes and obesity cluster may be due to obesity. Both depression and diabetes, particularly in the case of adult women, are in connection with education and income [20].

The paper "Diabetes detection using deep learning algorithms" is written by the following authors Swapna G and her team members [21].

According to him, DM is a metabolic disease that affects many people around the world. The outbreak is great every year. Without treatment, many important pelvic visceral complications of diabetes can be devastating.

Early diagnosis of diabetes is important for timely treatment that can stop the disease before such effects. The RR parameter signal, known as the HRV (ECG) signal, can be used effectively to diagnose non-invasive diabetes. Extract planning and dynamic features of HRV input data using Swapna G and her team members by Long short-term memory (LSTM), convolution neural network (CNN), and combinations thereof. These features are supported by vectors.

They found that CNN and CNN-LSTM architectures show three and six% margins, respectively, compared to the recent work of non-SVM. The proposed classification scheme can help clinicians to use the ECG signal to diagnose diabetes with a very high accuracy of 96%. Thus, early diagnosis of diabetes is very important. Diabetic neuropathy affects neurological function.

In the proposed study, HRV BD was analyzed for the diagnosis of diabetes using deep learning techniques. CNN 5-LSTM achieved the highest accuracy value of 95.7% using the SVM network. This is the highest published value for the automated diagnosis of diabetes using HRV as input. A flexible, recyclable system without compromise can be a real tool for doctors to discover diabetes and improve accuracy with very large input data. If the input data are sufficient for research, the deep learning potential is truly terrible, and detection of anomalies in difficult and unpredictable areas in the future can be greatly improved. By extracting the dynamic nature of the input data, unexpected predictions of the input data that may not be unreasonable may be performed [21].

4.3 Our Implementation and Results

4.3.1 Experimental Setup

The selected subjects had diabetes suffered by a health insurance company without knowledge of personally identifiable information (PI) or confidential personally identifiable information (SPI). Sample samples, such as S1, S2, are assigned to individuals to identify individual cases.

We collected this BD and investigated people. We have studied their stress levels and have helped them cure it. In this chapter, we have done our best to analyze diabetes with coronary artery disease and other diseases. Samples of test data and medical reports are collected for the following specifications: gender, age, type of diabetes, insulin problems, obesity, coronary artery disease, and suffering from tension-type headache (headache)/migraine.

The area of interest is the tension-type headache/migraine parameter. This study focuses on the role of diabetes in the development of tension-type headache and the strange factors/patterns that lead to tension-type headache. I am interested in examining the data patterns and behaviors of people with coronary artery disease. First, we analyzed the collected sample data. Tableau software was used for the analysis.

4.3.1.1 About the Study and Analysis

The current analysis collected, estimated samples of 30 Indian random individuals and examined them under various medical parameters. Those people having diabetes and various other symptoms were recorded.

We investigated whether other diabetes could be similar. Patients with type I (T1D) and type II diabetes (T2D) were studied, and those who did not take insulin and those who did not take part in the study were also studied. This result suggests a correlation between tension-type headache and other diseases, such as obesity, hypertension, coronary artery disease, and direct prediction of their occurrence in the future.

4.3.2 Result and Discussion

Over all age groups are not categorized by tension-type headache and coronary artery disease subject numbers or stacked column charts. Very few cases of tension-type headache are seen in men younger than 60 but this number increases dramatically after the age of 60 (Fig. 4.2).

It also shows a direct relationship with tension-type headache and coronary artery disease with aging (as per Fig. 4.3).

Fig. 4.2 Tension-type headache and coronary artery disease distribution as per age groups in the sample

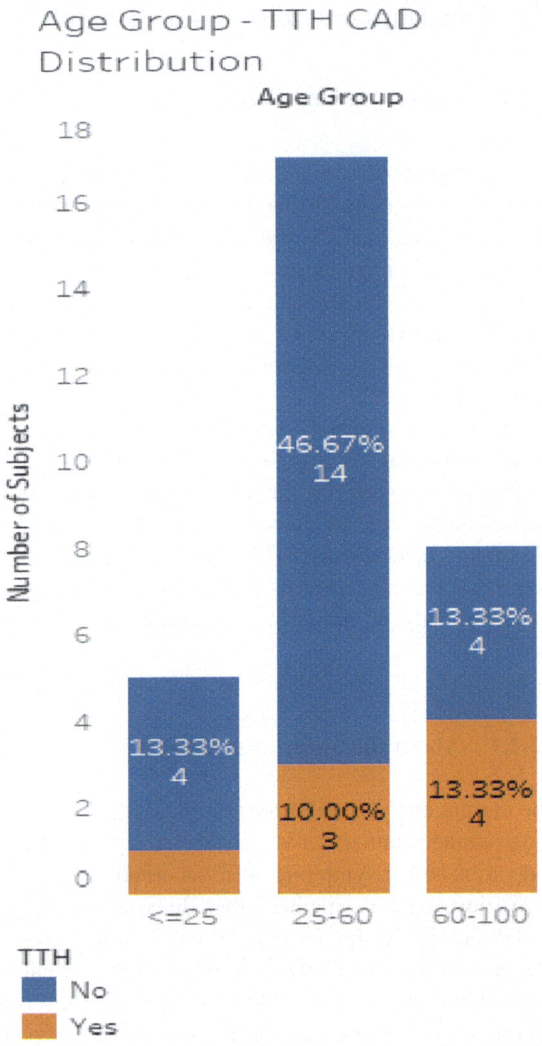

In the statistical samples collected, 31.58% of people with tension-type headache and coronary artery disease were reported. This number is important given that four patients with type 1 diabetes have a tension-type headache and coronary artery disease. Generally, diabetics are reported to have Tension-type headaches due to mental retardation caused by problems such as stress and diabetes. Analysis of the distribution of this ratio in gender shows that men are more susceptible to tension-type headache and, therefore, coronary artery disease than women. About 10.9% of men have a higher tension-type headache than women. After examining and discussing the data in detail, it was found that work stress could cause headaches because typical men work in the workplace and women do less work (as per Fig. 4.4).

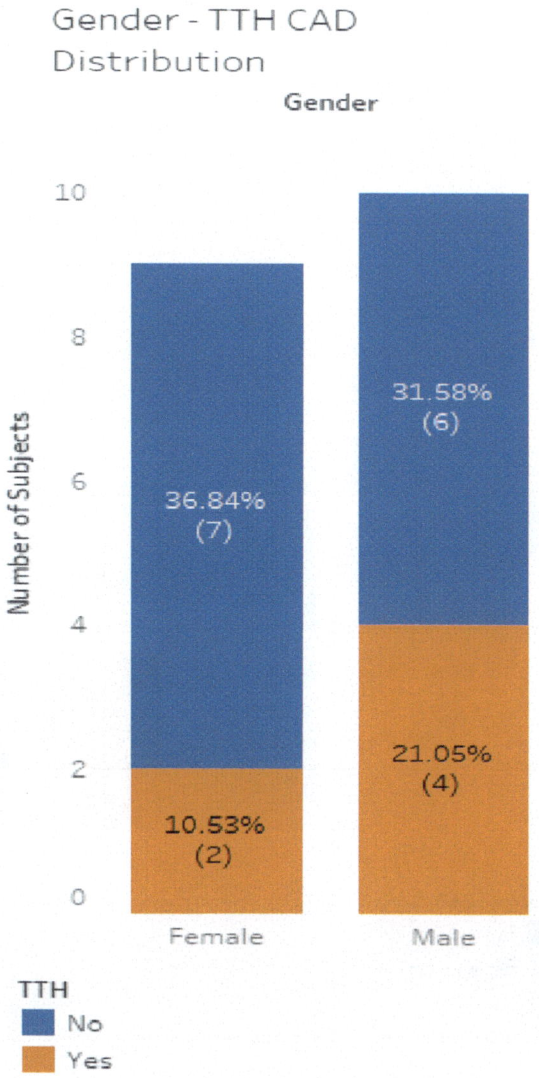

Fig. 4.3 Tension-type headache and coronary artery disease distribution as per gender groups in the sample

The overall age groups by gender and number of subjects with or without Tension-type headache and coronary artery disease have been described in the graphs through data analysis tools. It turns out that tension-type headache cases are very low in men younger than 60 but this number increases dramatically after the age of 60.

Also, for women, the increase in tension-type headache by age 60 is higher than tension-type headache with a decrease in coronary artery disease. This is consistent with the overall pattern of changing diabetes themes by age group. (As shown in Fig. 4.5). To fully illustrate this pattern, the chart above is for tension-type headache only for coronary artery disease people and is shown below.

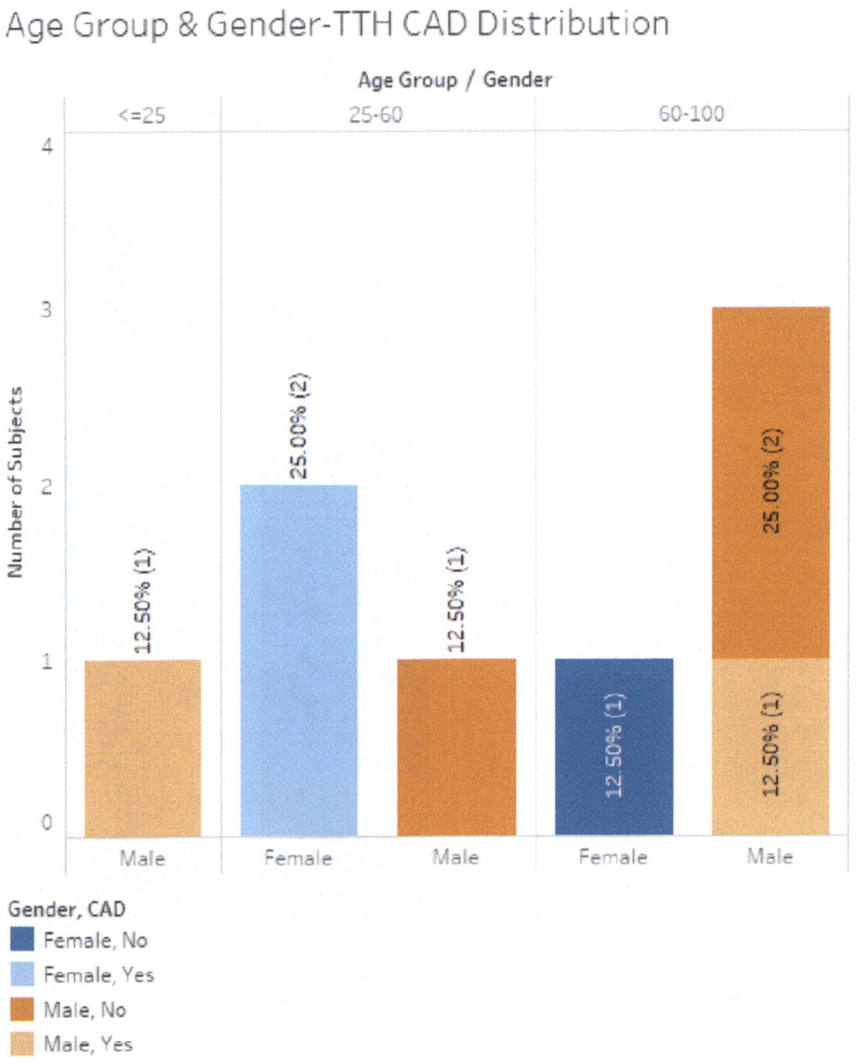

Fig. 4.4 Tension-type headache and coronary artery disease distribution as per age groups in terms of presence of coronary artery disease in different genders in the sample

As a result, tension-type headache and coronary artery disease cases increase with age in men and follow the pattern of change in diabetes with age, but if the tension-type headacheand coronary artery disease pattern in women is similar to diabetes, the trend increases to 60 years then decrease (as per Fig. 4.6) and (as per Fig. 4.7) Outline the relationship between type 2 diabetes and the tension-type headache stack bar to gain insight and additional information about the role of T2D diabetes in the development of tension-type headache—coronary artery disease.T1D diabetes has

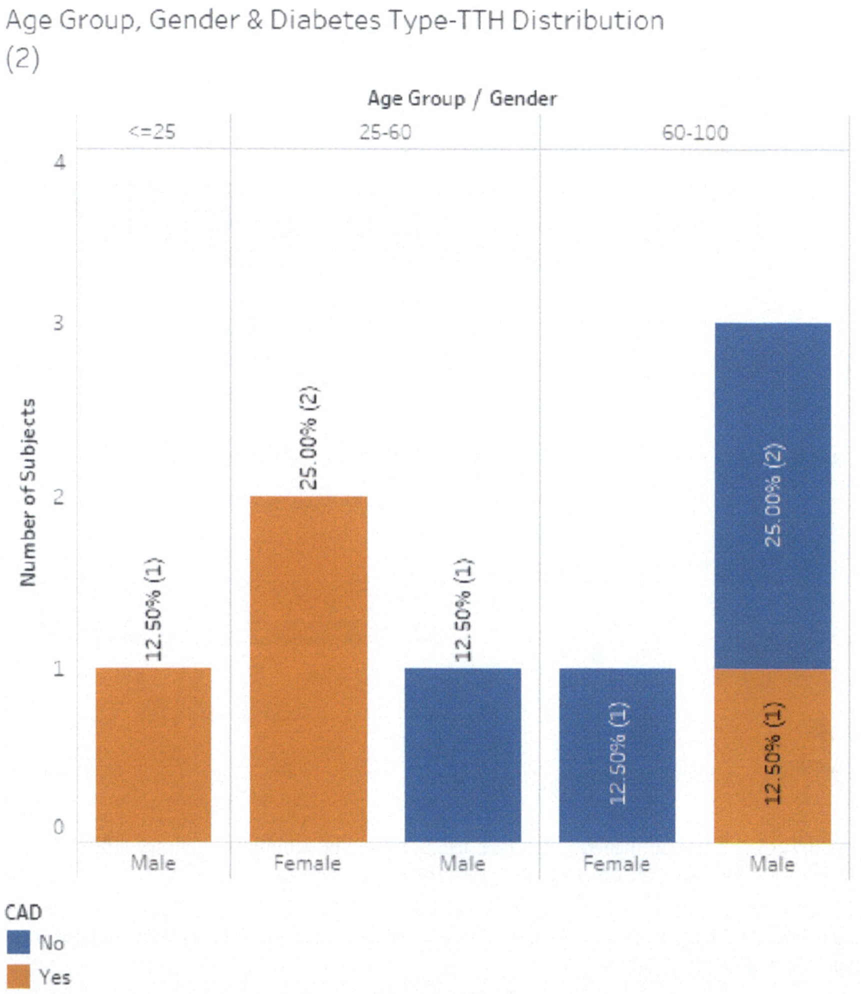

Fig. 4.5 Tension-type headache and coronary artery disease distribution as per age groups in terms of presence of coronary artery disease in the sample

been shown to have little involvement in tension-type headache and coronary artery disease. This means that T1D individuals report significantly less than a tension-type headache and coronary artery disease. Because T1D individuals are young, they may be able to cope with stressful situations or may not be as stressful for coronary artery disease that can cause tension-type headache and coronary artery disease (as per Table 4.1).

But the number increases significantly for type II diabetes patient. The summary data of various are as follows:

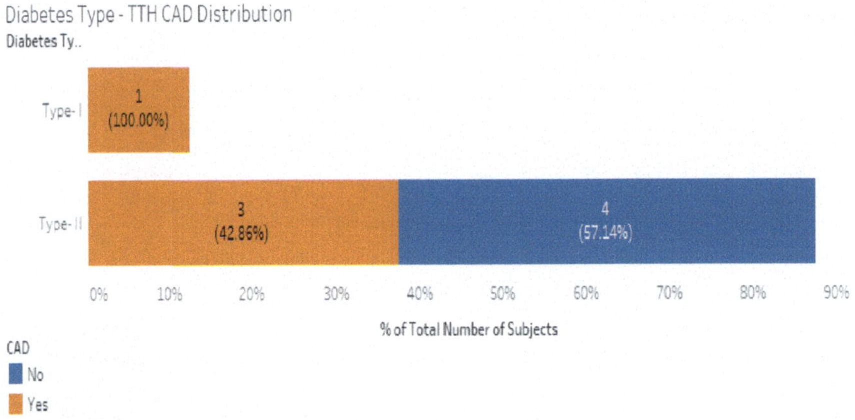

Fig. 4.6 Tension-type headache and coronary artery disease distribution w.r.t. presence of diabetes type

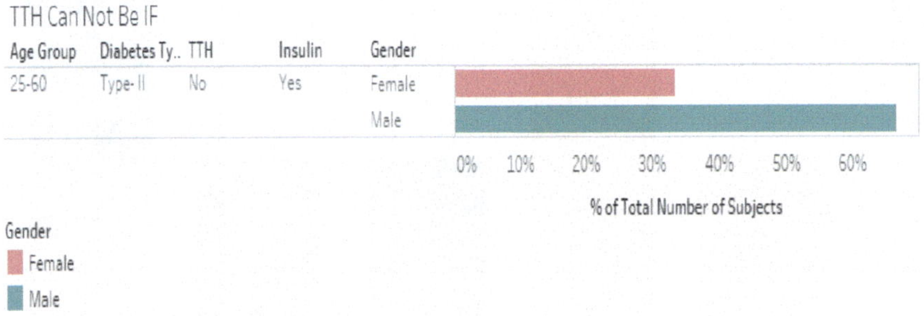

Fig. 4.7 Correlation of diabetes with type headache and possibility of coronary artery disease, hypertension, obesity, etc., diseases with insulin consumption

Table 4.1 Summary data for the diseases tension-type headache and coronary artery disease as per type I & II diabetes

Diabetes type	Tension-type headache	% of total number of subjects (%)	% of total number of subjects within each diabetic type (%)	Number of subjects
T1D	Yes	12.5	100	1
T1D	No	0	0	0
T2D	Yes	37.5	42.85	3
T2D	No	50	57.15	4

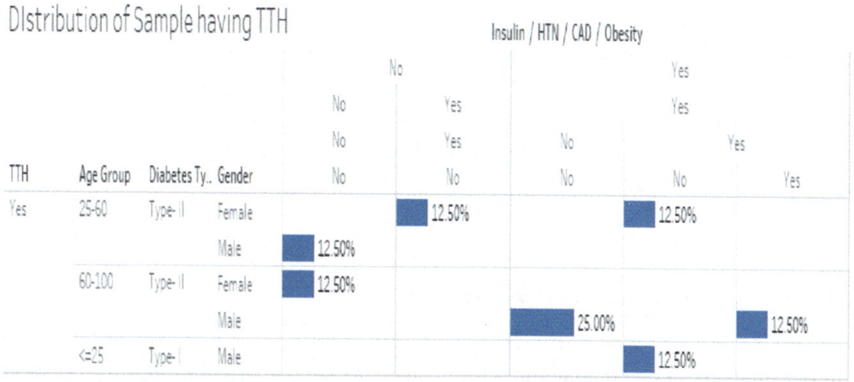

Fig. 4.8 Summary chart of analytical data for correlation of diabetes with tension-type headache and possibility of coronary artery disease, hypertension, obesity, etc., diseases with insulin consumption

4.3.3 TTH Cannot Be

The general presence of various diseases that cause or do not cause tension-type headache indicates that some people have insulin from tension-type headache and coronary artery disease but no blood pressure (hypertension). It is safe. Samples are found in men and women between the ages of 25 and 60 who meet these parameters. In such combinations, male advantage is easily seen. Two-thirds of the male population is in this combination (as per Fig. 4.8).

These people take insulin because they seem to have T2D diabetes. Subjects have no reported obesity problems and are not related to the digestive system. Thus, it can be concluded that a patient may not have a tension-type headache even if they have coronary artery disease, even if they have no problem with hypertension. This means that controlling blood pressure and blood pressure can remove tension-type headache even in heart disease. Analysis of the data showed that the percentage of women in these groups were low because depression problems were not reported in women. Male patients are evenly divided into depression and not depression. Therefore, these categories fall into three categories: women, men with depression, and men without depression. In the sample, women with mild depression have been observed to be one of the most important causes of tension-type headache decline in women compared to men.

Analyzing a sample that contains tension-type headache shows that the highest percentage of elderly people with tension-type headache is high and can easily be seen by examining the gender distribution of the age groups but this chart shows high blood pressure. Thus, if an elderly person is hypertensive and has T2D diabetes, he or she can clearly conclude that tension-type headache is needed. More specifically, the ratio of men with coronary artery disease to men without coronary artery disease is 1:3, and obesity is the same (as per Fig. 4.8).

In general, if the person is with a tension-type headache usually has hypertension. Six of the eight subjects reported to have a tension-type headache had hypertension and had 75% of tension-type headache subjects. These numbers clearly show that hypertension is associated with tension-type headache. If the subject has diabetes and hypertension, the risk of tension-type headache will increase sometime, and it is likely that they are male.

4.4 Future Scope and Limitations

Sample analysis showed that the sample had no sexual orientation; can be used to analyze large sample sizes in the future. Easily use tension-type headache by changing Tableau S/W in large collections by switching to other diseases that are in a different location than those listed, such as obesity, cancer and heart attack. (Table 4.2).

Because the sample size is smaller than the conclusion, a larger sample should be considered for patients T1D living in different areas. Using technology, you need to create and analyze large-scale diabetes data and create systems to predict potential risks.

Predictive analytics is the process of integrating various data mining techniques, machine learning, and statistical algorithms that integrate current and historical data sets to gain insight and predict future risks.

Symptoms may be due to low or high blood sugar, low blood sugar, or poor recognition of dehydration. When checking your blood glucose, if the symptoms do not match the reading system, or if you think the reading is incorrect, make sure that your blood glucose is set to glucose. This study does not include pregnant women, dialysis patients, or cancer patients.

Table 4.2 Tension-type headache variation with the variation of other disease

A	B	C	D	E	F	G	H	I	J
Subject	Age	Gender	Diabete	Insulin	Obesity	CAD	HTN	Headache/Migrar	
SI_04	36	F	Type- II	No	No	Yes	Yes	Yes	
SI_07	65	M	Type- II	Yes	No	No	Yes	Yes	
SI_10	62	F	Type- II	No	No	No	No	Yes	
SI_11	75	M	Type- II	Yes	Yes	Yes	Yes	Yes	
SI_17	18	M	Type- I	Yes	No	Yes	Yes	Yes	
SI_21	56	M	Type- II	No	No	No	No	Yes	
SI_23	65	M	Type- II	Yes	No	No	Yes	Yes	Migrane
SI_28	36	F	Type- II	Yes	No	Yes	Yes	Yes	

4.5 Recommendation and Considerations

The author sought to include an association with age, gender, insulin factor, and diabetes. Diabetics are being studied as health insurance without disclosing personal information. Finally, cases of tension-type headache and coronary artery disease varies by age in men and lack of diabetes patterns vary by age, but changes in tension-type headache and coronary artery disease patterns in women are similar to diabetes, increasing the incidence to 60 then it decreases [22].

The incidence of tension-type headache appears to be very low in men younger than 60, but reaches 60 and older. It is also directly related to age, tension-type headache, and coronary artery disease.

4.6 Conclusions

The current analysis collected, estimated samples of 30 Indian random individuals and examined them under various medical parameters. Those people having diabetes and various other symptoms were recorded. We investigated whether other diabetes could be similar. Analysis of the distribution of this sex ratio showed that men are more susceptible to tension-type headache and, therefore, coronary artery disease than women. About 10.9% of men have a higher tension-type headache than women. A close look at the data and discussions reveals that typical men work at work and women do not work very much, which can be a source of work stress that causes frequent headaches. Finally, the case of tension headache and coronary artery disease increases with age and following the pattern of diabetes changes with age, but the pattern of change in women with tension headache and coronary artery disease and diabetes tends to with age 60 then decrease [23].

This research will provide updates on new machine learning algorithms, optimization algorithms, and intelligent health applications. Discuss important topics such as privacy, previews, real projects, data analytics, and links between medical staff. These issues are essential for the development of health care. Otherwise, it is difficult to release machine learning algorithms to optimize real performance. As a result, people are expected to receive more and more healthcare programs in the coming decades. Medical care needs to be economically sustainable to protect patients' future health and access to future medical care.

Acknowledgements We would like to thank the seniors of ABES Engineering College, Ghaziabad, Dayalbagh Educational Institute, Agra, and experts from Tata Consultancy Services for their extraordinary support in this research process. The Infrastructure and research samples from different laboratories have been collected. We pay our sincere thanks to all direct and indirect supporters.

References

1. Martin, R., Ira Ktena, S., & Pawlowski, N. (2018, July 3). *An introduction to biomedical image analysis with tensorflow and DLT*. London: Imperial College London.
2. McAfee, A., Brynjolfsson, E., Davenport, T. H., Patil, D. J., & Barton, D. (2012). Big data: The management revolution. *Harvard Business Review, 90*(10), 60–68.
3. Amit, B., Chinmay, C., Anand, K., & Debabrata, B. (2019). *Emerging trends in IoT and big data analytics for biomedical and health care technologies* (Chap. 5, pp. 121–152). Elsevier: Handbook of Data Science Approaches for Biomedical Engineering. ISBN 9780128183182.
4. Panch, T., Szolovits, P., & Atun, R. (2018, December). Artificial intelligence, machine learning and health systems. *Journal of Global Health, 8*(2), 020303. Published online 2018 Oct 21. https://doi.org/10.7189/jogh.08.020303.
5. Murdoch, T. B., & Detsky, A. S. (2013). The inevitable application of big data to health care. *Journal of the American Medical Association*, (13), 1351–1352.
6. Nall, R. (2018, November 8). An overview of diabetes types and treatments, *Medical News Today*. https://www.medicalnewstoday.com/articles/323627.php.
7. Gabbe, S. G. (2018) Diabetes mellitus complicating normal pregnancy. In: *Obstetrics: Normal and problem pregnancy* (7th ed.). Philadelphia, Pa.: Saunders Elsevier. https://www.clinicalkey.com.
8. Cunningham, F. G. (2014). Diabetes mellitus. In: *Williams obstetrics* (24th ed.). New York, N.Y.: The McGraw-Hill Companies. http://accessmedicine.mhmedical.com.
9. Felman, A. (2018, November). An overview of insulin. *Medical News Today*. https://www.medicalnewstoday.com/articles/323760.php.
10. Rastogi, R., Chaturvedi, D. K., Satya, S., Arora, N., Yadav, V., Chauhan, S., Sharma, P. (2018, October 28). SF-36 Scores Analysis for EMG and GSR Therapy on Audio, Visual and Audio Visual Modes for Chronic TTH. In *Proceedings of the ICCIDA-2018 on 27 and 28th October 2018, CCIS Series*, Springer. Khordha, Bhubaneswar, Odisha, India: Gandhi Institute for Technology.
11. Sharma, A., Rastogi, R., Chaturvedi, D. K., Satya, S. A., Trivedi, P., Singh, A., & Singh, A. (2019) Intelligent analysis for personality detection on various indicators by clinical reliable psychological TTH and stress surveys. In *Proceedings of CIPR 2019 at Indian Institute of Engineering Science and Technology*, Shibpur on 19th–20th January 2019, Springer-AISC Series.
12. Sharma, P., Rastogi, R., Chaturvedi, D. K., Satya, S. A., Yadav, V., & Chauhan, S. (2018). Analytical comparison of efficacy for electromyography and galvanic skin resistance biofeedback on audio-visual mode for chronic TTH on various attributes. In *Proceedings of the ICCIDA-2018 on 27 and 28th October 2018, CCIS Series*, Springer. Khordha, Bhubaneswar, Odisha, India: Gandhi Institute for Technology.
13. Yadav, V., Rastogi, R., Chaturvedi, D. K., Satya, S. A., Gupta, M., Chauhan, S., Sharma, P. (2019). Chronic TTH analysis by EMG & GSR biofeedback on various modes and various medical symptoms using IoT. In: *Book-big data analytics for intelligent healthcare management: advances in ubiquitous sensing applications for healthcare*. ISBN 9780128181461.
14. Singhal, P., Rastogi, R., Chaturvedi, D. K., Satya, S., Arora, N., Gupta, M., Singhal, P., et al. (2019). Statistical analysis of exponential and polynomial models of EMG & GSR biofeedback for correlation between subjects medications movement & medication scores, ICSMSIC-2019, ABESEC, Ghaziabad, 8–9 March 2019, *International Journal of Innovative Technology and Exploring Engineering* (*IJITEE*), *8*(6S), 625–635. https://www.ijitee.org/download/volume-8-issue-6S/(2019b).
15. Marrie, R. A., Patel, R., Figley, C. R., Kornelsen, J., Bolton, J. M., Graff, L., Mazerolle, E. L., et al. (2019, January). Diabetes and anxiety adversely affect cognition in multiple sclerosis. *Multiple Sclerosis and Related Disorder satellites, 27*, 164–170.
16. Brazier, Y. (2018, November 2). What is obesity and what causes it? *Medical News Today*. https://www.medicalnewstoday.com/articles/323551.php.

17. Nordqvist, C. (2019, July 5). What to know about coronary heart disease. *Medical News Today.* https://www.medicalnewstoday.com/articles/184130.php.
18. Biggers, A., Sharp, L. K., Nimitphong, B., Saetung, S., Siwasaranond, N., Manodpitipong, A., Crowley, S. J., Hood, M. M., et al. (2019, January 2). Relationship between depression, sleep quality, and hypoglycemia among persons with type-2 diabetes. *Journal of Clinical & Translational Endocrinology, 15*, 62–64. https://doi.org/10.1016/j.jcte.2018.12.007.
19. Alkholy, U. M., et al. (2019, March–April). The antioxidant status of coenzyme Q10 and vitamin E in children with type 1 diabetes. *Jornal de Pediatria (Versão em Português), 95*(2), 224–230. https://doi.org/10.1016/j.jped.2017.12.005. Epub 2018 Feb 7.
20. Diderichsena, B. F., & Andersena, I. (2018, November). The syndemics of diabetes and depression in Brazil—An epidemiological analysis. *SSM Population Health*. https://doi.org/10.1016/j.ssmph.2018.11.002.
21. Swapna, G., Vinayakumar, R., & Soman, K. P. (2018). *Diabetes detection using deep learning algorithms*. ICT Express 4 September 2018; accepted 15 October 2018. Available online 8 November 2018, pp. 243–246. www.elsevier.com/locate/icte.
22. Saini, H., Rastogi, R., Chaturvedi, D. K., Satya, S. A., Verma, H., & Mehlyan, K. (2018). Comparative efficacy analysis of electromyography and galvanic skin resistance biofeedback on audio mode for chronic TTH on various indicators. In: *Proceedings of ICCIIoT-2018, 14–15 December 2018 at NIT Agartala, Tripura*, ELSEVIER-SSRN Digital Library. ISSN 1556-5068.
23. Gupta, M., Rastogi, R., Chaturvedi, D. K., Satya, S. A., Verma, H., Singhal, P., & Singh, A. (2019). Comparative study of trends observed during different medications by subjects under EMG & GSR biofeedback. *International Journal of Innovative Technology and Exploring Engineering* (*IJITEE*), *8*(6S), 748–756. https://www.ijitee.org/download/volume-8-issue-6S/. (ICSMSIC-2019, ABESEC, Ghaziabad. 8–9 March 2019).

Chapter 5
Machine Learning Applications for a Real-Time Monitoring of Arrhythmia Patients Using IoT

Rajendran Sree Ranjani

Abstract Real-time monitoring of life-threatening cardiovascular disease like arrhythmia using wearable sensors and Internet of things (IoT) devices paves ways to mobile health (m-health) systems. Smartphones with developed applications, wearable sensors and IoT devices are the major parts of the developed real-time arrhythmia monitoring system. In this work, an in-house round-the-clock cardiac monitoring is proposed with the use of machine learning techniques to predict the symptoms of arrhythmia by classifying the data obtained from UCI repository. The physiological signal electrocardiogram (ECG) is considered to characterize the anomalous behavior of the cardiac system. Our main novelty is to predict the symptoms of arrhythmia with the analysis and classification of data obtained from the patients using sensors or smartphones to the data classified at the repository. We establish the accuracy and efficiency of the proposed solution, by analyzing the large set of data with the field collected ECG signals.

Keywords Arrhythmia · Machine learning · Real-time monitoring · Anomaly detection · m-health · IoT

5.1 Introduction

Cardiac arrhythmia (a.k.a dysrhythmia) is a condition of irregular heartbeat, which causes a sudden life loss of the patient [1]. To overcome this sudden life loss, the cardiac behavior of the arrhythmia patients has to be monitored continuously to provide an appropriate medical procedure. Nowadays, Internet of things (IoT) plays a vital role in real-time monitoring of the modern healthcare domain. Supervision and access to medical care are the main pillars of any medical health (m-health) with a substantial reduction of the cost of monitoring with early detection and prevention

R. Sree Ranjani (✉)
RISE Lab, Department of Computer Science and Engineering, Indian Institute of Technology Madras, Chennai, India
e-mail: sreeranjanirajendran@gmail.com

C. Chakraborty et al. (eds.), *Internet of Things for Healthcare Technologies*, Studies in Big Data 73, https://doi.org/10.1007/978-981-15-4112-4_5

[2]. IoT devices like blood glucose monitor, blood pressure monitors, electrocardiogram (ECG) monitor, pulse oximeter, etc., promote remote healthcare management to monitor the wellness of patients. Nowadays, to promote an early prediction of any m-health conditions, machine learning techniques are introduced. Diagnosis and early prediction of disease, psychoanalysis, survival analysis and even hospital management are made much easier by the classification techniques of machine learning in healthcare domain. Automatic diagnosis system for earlier detection of disease is introduced in many leading countries. Data collected from various medical tests are analyzed by the machine learning techniques to provide an automatic diagnosis of disease [3]. Thus, machine learning becomes a supportive tool in the medical domain with trained algorithm which includes various features and class of a disease.

There are different causes of arrhythmia like sodium or potassium imbalance in blood, change in heart muscular, different coronary illness, healing process after surgery, etc. Since irregular heartbeat is a major cause of arrhythmia, irregularity in ECG plays a vital role in the prediction of arrhythmia. This sudden disorder may cause cardiac arrest if not diagnosed [4]. Ventricular tachycardia, atrial flutter, atrial fibrillation and supraventricular tachycardia are ECG-based classification of resuscitation cardiac rhythms for retrospective data analysis [5]. An automated categorization of arrhythmia can save life of many patients [6]. A random forest classifier is designed to diagnose arrhythmia among 16 types of it in [7]. Too many feature selection and excessive data set may degrade the performance of the classifier. The authors used correlation-based feature selection (CFS) and simple random sampling (SRS) classifying methods to overcome the above problem. The most appropriate feature selection is done by CFS [8] filtering approach, and the data set is resampled by SRS to get a uniformly distributed class data set. In this work, the machine learning technique to classify the arrhythmia data set proposed in [7] is used to develop a real-time arrhythmia monitoring system with the use of sensors and IoT devices.

The rest of the chapter is organized as follows: Sect. 5.2 describes related work in literature, and the proposed work is discussed in Sect. 5.3. The results are discussed in Sect. 5.4, and Sect. 5.5 concludes the work with future extension.

5.2 Related Work

ECG signal is represented in time-frequency space which is proposed by using a discrete cosine transform to get an efficient signal [4]. The feature set is reduced by the principal component analysis to classify the ECG signal and to improve the accuracy support vector machine (SVM) optimization was proposed. In [5], the artificial neural network classifier is used to annotate the rhythms of ECG signal and automatically classify the cardiac rhythms. The classifiers' accuracy is improved by the wrapper-based method. Heartbeat is classified using a reservoir computing machine learning approach [9]. EGC-based biometric recognition was proposed in [10], which uses multitask learning approach. In some studies, cardiac arrhythmia was classified based on neural networks. Block-based neural network classifier was proposed in [11], with the particle swarm optimization (PSO) algorithm for high efficiency. In [12], multilayer perception (MLP) algorithm is used for the arrhythmia classification, and the wavelet and Fourier features of ECG signals are given as input to the trained neural network with feedforward-based classifier. Multidimensional particle swarm optimization (MD-PSO) technique is used in neural network to optimize the process. Logistic regression and backpropagation algorithm are used in Bayesian neural network for arrhythmia detection in [13]. To improve the accuracy of arrhythmia detection, the deep learning-based arrhythmia classifier was proposed in [14].

Among the all, a joint feature extraction and classifier method were more effective than the conventional method of arrhythmia detection. To remove the noises in the extracted biomedical signal, the non-local means (NLM) approaches are proposed in [15]. Cardiovascular diseases are diagnosed by the forward search algorithm based on the parameters of ECG signals are proposed in [16]. The cardiodisorder is detected by the integrated circuit (IC) embedded in the mobile phones, along with the developed android application. To achieve 95% of accuracy in classifying heartbeat irregularity, a parallel general regression neural network (GRNN) method is proposed in [17]. The data processing time is greatly reduced due to the parallel GPU-based algorithm, and this saves the significant amount of time for the doctors also. An automatic detection framework is proposed in [18], which isolates the localization and classification of signals from the ECG noises. A long-term remote health monitoring system was proposed in [19], in which ECG signal is monitored in the residential environment using an IoT infrastructure. An IoT platform embedded with a wireless wearable ECG monitoring system [20] in which Bayesian filtering is used to separate the ECG signal from noises. ECG signal separation is efficiently done by the T/QRS ratio calculation. This extracts the ST, QT interval and PR interval of ECG signal. In [6], a survey of feature extraction and classification of detection algorithms of arrhythmia disease are discussed. The patient care and diagnosis can be improved by extending the patient monitoring in the casual environment of patient. This method enhances the quality of diagnosis as the condition of patient is monitored in normal house environment rather than a clinical setup. Physiological monitoring of patients has to be accurate, easy to use and available at nominal cost [21]. Ambulatory electrocardiography can be used for the remote patient monitoring as per the guidelines published by the American College of Cardiology (ACC) and the American Heart Association (AHA) [22]. Therefore, to monitor the patients in their usual environment, the wearable sensors can be used. The interest over the wearable sensors is rising in recent years. In order to achieve long-term recording of physiological information of patients and manage those data, the researchers have considered the application of wearable sensor technology [23–25]. A standardized Body Area Network (BAN) framework is being used for the incorporation of the wireless sensors, which is aimed at improving the free and casual mobility of the patients in a daily situation while being monitored by a wireless wearable system [26]. This concept is advantageous to the existing system as it does not need any technical skills to operate. The overall idea presented in this paper includes arrhythmia patient monitoring system, arrhythmia classification using machine learning and the data visualization. The existing frameworks either consist of the monitoring methods [27] or the classification algorithms as mentioned in [7]. Mostly, a complete system for arrhythmia that can be equipped in real time in hospitals is not proposed. Thus, in this paper, we propose a complete system for arrhythmia patient monitoring and categorization using IoT and machine learning algorithm.

5.3 Methodology

The ultimate aim of our concept is to provide a system for arrhythmia patient monitoring and arrhythmia classification to improve the diagnosis. This system can be used in the hospitals for extending health care to patients. In this method, patients having irregular heartbeats are assigned with unique number with which the mobile application can be accessed. The application has different views for doctors and patients with restricted access. Our proposed concept monitors the patients continuously using the wearable sensors and transmits the data to the android/iOS application which can be viewed by both doctors and patients. The patient who is suspected to have arrhythmia is continuously monitored for the physiological parameters like heart rate and temperature using the wearable sensors. In case of detection of irregular heartbeat, the android/iOS application notifies the patient to wear the wireless ECG sensor. The application classifies the state of patients into 16 groups of arrhythmias as in [28] automatically using machine learning algorithms. The application enables two different views for patients and doctor. The patients can only view their corresponding medical records while doctors can view records of all patients. The mobile application is designed with enhanced security and privacy. This architecture consists of five major components: data sensing, data transmission, cloud storage, classification and visualization as shown in Fig. 5.1.

- Data sensing method involves monitoring patients which is performed using the wearable sensors for monitoring ECG, pulse rate and temperature. The location of patients is also tracked using Global Positioning System (GPS), in order to provide medical services in case of emergencies. All the sensors are typically aggregated to a microcontroller which reads the data from sensors. The data sensing consists of wearable sensors and GPS.
- Data transmission component consists of a wifi module which acquires the data from the microcontroller and transmits it to the mobile application via the cloud. This transmission must be done in a secured way in order to achieve data privacy.
- Cloud storage includes the major component of the system storage. The system is designed in a way such that the biomedical information of patients is stored for a long time. This longtime storage also assists the health professionals in diagnosing arrhythmia.

5.3.1 Data Sensing

The data sensing that is being performed using the wearable sensors with the design qualities does not hinder the patient's mobility, lightweight and easy to operate. The wearable devices are aggregated to form a wireless personal area network (WPAN). The wearable devices acquire the physiological data—heart rate and temperature. The data from ECG are acquired when the application intimates irregular heartbeat detection. The location of patients is also tracked in order to provide services during medical emergencies. The heart rate, temperature and ECG of the patients are acquired continuously from the BAN, and the location is tracked using GPS. The values from the sensors are acquired by the microcontroller. This physical phenomenon of sensing data in the distributed fashion is stated as energy-efficient sensing mechanism [29]. In [30], the authors proposed a continuous status monitoring of wounds with 93.75% of accuracy. This is achieved by classifying wound tissues in the segmented regions. Whereas in [31], the tele-wound technology network (TWTL) is proposed to monitor the wound remotely using smartphones such that rural and urban people will be benefited by remote monitoring framework. Schemes, like energy-efficient sensing mechanism, are implemented using IoT-based sensing architecture. The decision-making process is made and intimated using the mobile application. In real time, the patient is assumed to be in normal condition. In this state, only heart rate and temperature are monitored by the microcontroller that can be programmed to compare heart rate value periodically. If the value varies from the threshold range, then the signal is sent to the application which intimates the patient to wear ECG monitor, and the microcontroller gets the data from the ECG sensor. Moreover, this method overcomes major issues like reliability, privacy issues and user interface as mentioned in wearable sensors [32]. This architecture is shown in Fig. 5.2.

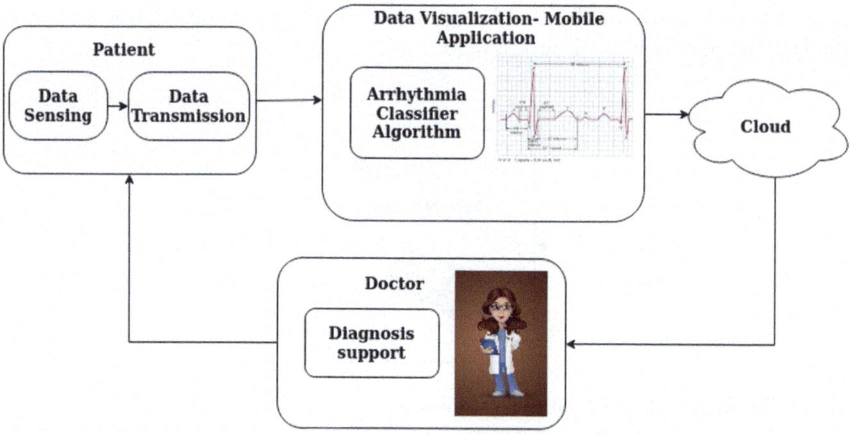

Fig. 5.1 Architecture of arrhythmia patient monitoring and classification

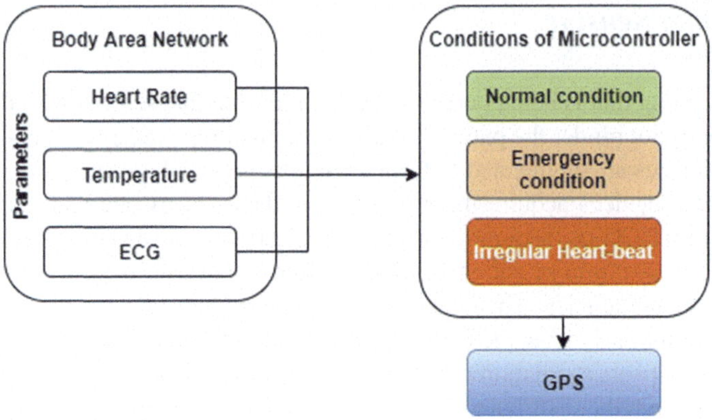

Fig. 5.2 Architecture for data sensing

5.3.2 Data Transmission and Cloud Storage

The components in this system are used for transmitting the data to the doctors and patients with the help of mobile application. The recordings of the physical parameters of the patient are transmitted via the cloud. The microcontroller transmits the data to cloud using the wifi module. The recordings of the patient are transmitted to the cloud for long-term storage as shown in Fig. 5.3. This method improves scalability and extends the benefits like data accessibility on demand both from patients and doctors. The cloud storage has to maintain data security and privacy. While storing electronic medical data of an individual, much importance should be given to data privacy. This is implemented by restricting the data access by users. That is, the patients can access their corresponding records only. And only authorized doctor can access the records via the mobile application. Our concept incorporates secured cloud storage methods as discussed in [33, 34].

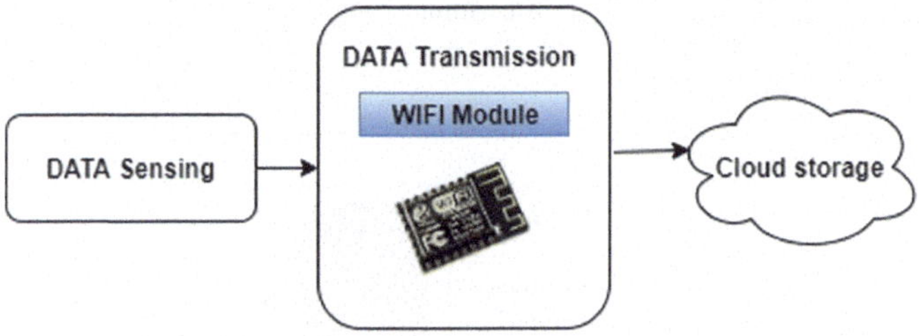

Fig. 5.3 Data transformation from sensor to cloud

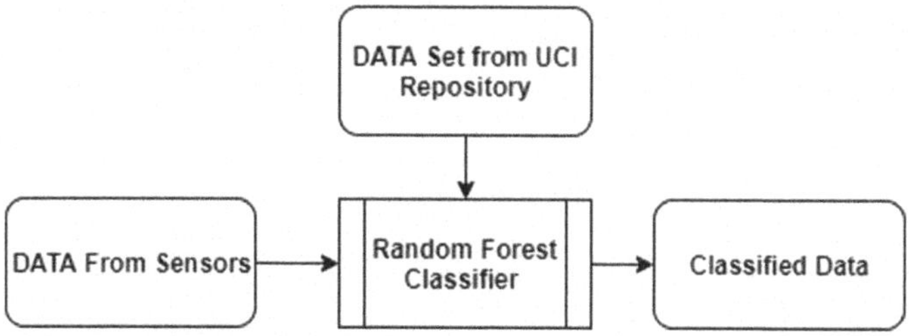

Fig. 5.4 Data classification using machine learning algorithm

5.3.3 Classification and Visualization

The data from the cloud are accessed by the mobile application which makes decisions on the sensors and classifies the arrhythmia as shown in Fig. 5.4. The mobile application processes the data from the sensors and makes the decision regarding the usage of sensors and intimates the patients about it. The classification of arrhythmia is done using the resampling method and random forest classifier with selected features [7]. The arrhythmia classification method involves training the classifier with the data set from clinical records and prior ECG sensor data. After the training process, the classifier is provided with the current sensor data which classifies arrhythmia into 16 categories and has 96% accuracy [7]. Visualization is necessary as it would be easy for both doctors and patients to access the voluminous data and analyses by the proposed system. The data visualization is considered as the independent and important research area [35]. The visualization of data is achieved using the interactive mobile application. The categorized data are presented using different colors. We are equipping this method as color distance and color categories enhance the identification and understanding of the differences in data [36].

5.4 Results and Discussion

This system is proposed for real-time implementation in the hospitals specifically for arrhythmia patients. Figure 5.5 shows the ECG sensor reading in a normal patient. The system is mainly controlled over the mobile application as shown in Fig. 5.6. Section verifies the accuracy and reliability of the proposed scheme through simulation and comparison of the performance with several well-known schemes.

This is how the home screen of the mobile application will look like where the patient has to enter the unique number and password in order to use the services. The classifier is trained using the original data set that is available in the UCI repository. The two images are samples depicting the visuals of the proposed system. The random ensemble classifier mentioned in [7] is incorporated in the mobile application as it is suitable for solving the particular problem. This is implemented using the open-

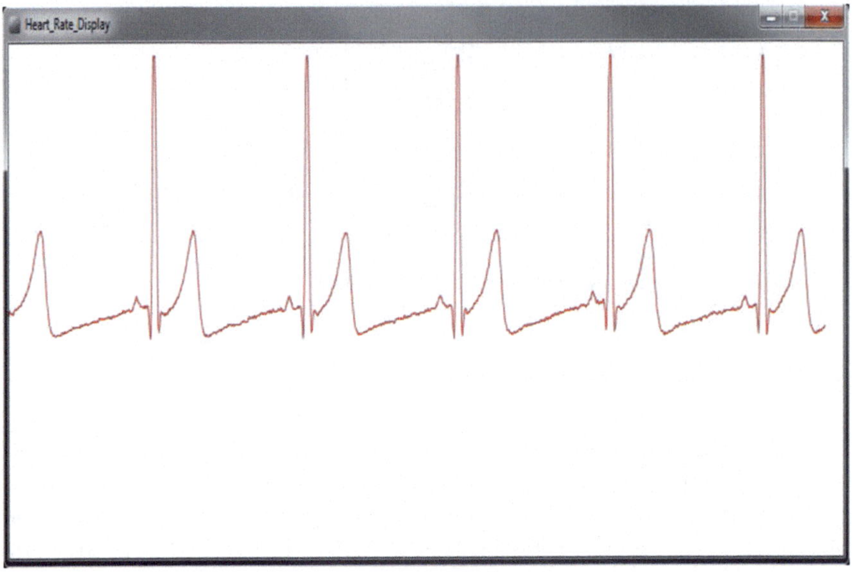

Fig. 5.5 ECG signal of normal patient

Fig. 5.6 Home screen of mobile application

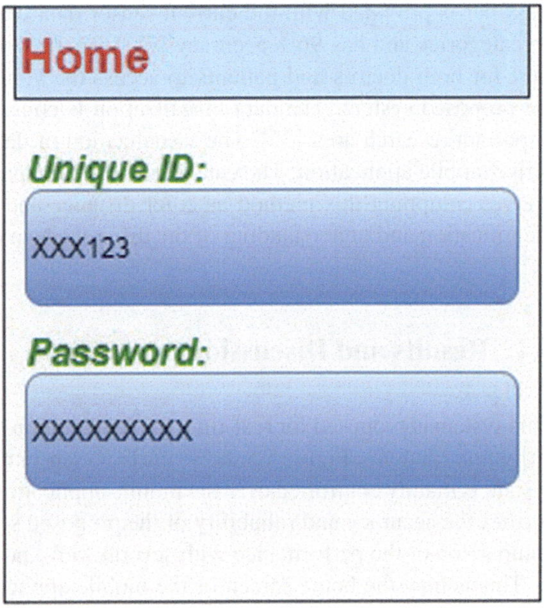

source software TensorFlow. The required libraries can be imported and develop the application which will be able to classify the arrhythmia. The sample data set is taken from the UCI repository [28], and Fig. 5.7 shows the different classes of arrhythmia before resampling of the data. This database consists of 452 samples and 274 features [28]. The sample data set is resampled using the methods mentioned in [7]. Data resampling is necessary to achieve accuracy over a small set of samples. The volume of patients varies, but the accuracy of application has to be maintained so the feature selection is done. There are several algorithms for the arrhythmia classification, but for the proposed system this algorithm is preferred to maintain the accuracy and reliability for varying volume of data. The heart rate of the patient is continuously monitored, and we can analyze the type of arrhythmia with respect to different heart rates. Figure 5.8 shows arrhythmia classes in the graph plotted with respect to heart rate. The sample data are processed to get the required details. Table 5.1 shows 16 classes of arrhythmia conditions used in this work.

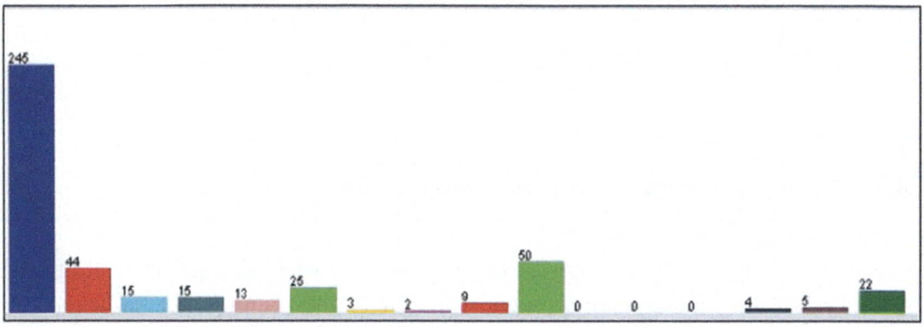

Fig. 5.7 Different classes of arrhythmia for the original data set of UCI repository

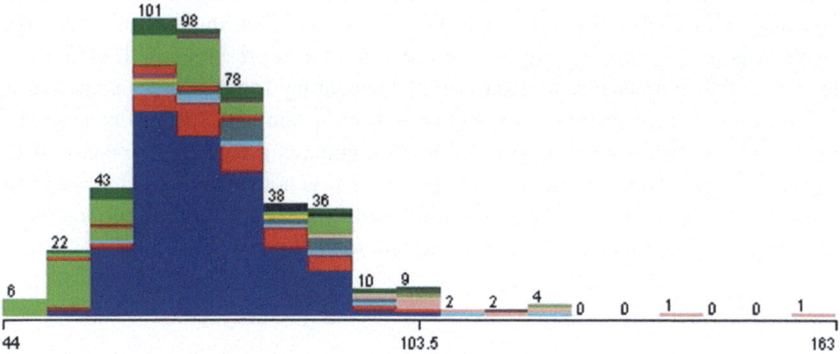

Fig. 5.8 Arrhythmia classes plotted with respect to heart rate

Table 5.1 Arrhythmia classes [28, 37]

Class code	Name of the class
1	Normal
2	Ischemic changes (coronary artery disease)
3	Old anterior myocardial infarction
4	Old inferior myocardial infarction
5	Sinus tachycardia
6	Sinus bradycardy
7	Ventricular premature contraction (PVC)
8	Supraventricular premature contraction
9	Left bundle branch block
10	Right bundle branch block
11	First degree atrio ventricular block
12	Second degree AV block
13	Third degree AV block
14	Left ventricular hypertrophy
15	Atrial fibrillation or flutter
16	Others

5.4.1 Scheme Evaluation and Comparison

The training data set and test data set are two subsets of the original data set of UCI repository, and they are chosen separately. Whereas, the training data set is used to train the classifier algorithm, and the test data set is validated for its performance by calculating the rate of the classifier. Confusion matrix measures the performance of the classifier. Tables 5.2 and 5.3 describe the confusion matrix of random forest classifier. Original data set contains 279 features, and by means of feature selection it is reduced to 23. Data resampling before and after is presented in Table 5.4, and the size of the sampler is also discussed. The accuracy for 16 classes is increasing from 0 to 94%, 96% and 98%, respectively. Data resampling method is applied to improve the accuracy of classifier. Table 5.5 compares the accuracy results of the proposed scheme with the existing schemes, and it is noted that the accuracy of the proposed scheme is 97.2%. Thus, the proposed method more accurately classifies the arrhythmia patients effectively from a remote distance.

5.5 Conclusion

m-health is an important healthcare application of IoT and prevention of cardiodisease like arrhythmia is a serious issue to be prevented. Our endeavor is to develop a proper system for arrhythmia patient monitoring remotely to enhance an early

Table 5.2 Random forest classifier confusion matrix before data resampling

Class code	1	2	3	4	5	6	7	8	9	10	11	12	13	14	15	16
1	225	8	0	0	1	4	0	1	0	0	2	0	5	0	0	0
2	11	26	1	4	0	0	1	0	1	0	1	0	0	0	0	1
3	2	2	13	1	1	0	0	0	1	0	2	0	1	1	1	0
4	3	0	0	8	1	0	1	0	0	1	0	1	1	0	0	0
5	7	1	3	1	3	0	0	1	0	1	0	0	0	1	0	0
6	3	0	1	2	2	19	0	0	1	1	0	1	1	0	0	0
7	2	5	0	0	0	1	0	0	1	0	0	0	1	1	1	2
8	0	2	0	0	1	0	0	0	0	1	0	1	0	1	1	0
9	10	0	2	0	0	1	0	0	7	0	0	1	0	1	1	0
10	0	3	0	0	0	0	0	0	0	34	0	1	1	0	0	0
11	0	6	1	5	4	0	0	1	0	0	0	0	1	0	0	0
12	0	0	0	9	0	0	2	1	4	1	0	0	0	0	0	1
13	2	0	0	4	0	1	1	0	1	3	0	1	0	1	1	0
14	3	0	0	0	3	0	0	0	0	0	0	0	0	0	0	0
15	11	1	0	0	1	0	0	0	0	0	0	0	1	0	0	1
16	2	2	1	1	2	0	0	0	1	1	0	1	0	1	2	0

Table 5.3 Random forest classifier confusion matrix after data resampling

Class code	1	2	3	4	5	6	7	8	9	10	11	12	13	14	15	16
1	201	4	0	0	1	0	0	1	0	0	2	0	0	0	0	0
1	52	1	0	0	0	0	1	0	0	0	0	1	0	0	1	0
3	2	2	17	1	1	0	1	0	1	1	1	0	1	1	0	1
4	3	0	0	11	1	0	0	0	0	0	0	0	0	0	0	0
5	0	0	0	0	3	0	0	1	0	0	0	0	0	0	0	0
6	2	0	0	0	0	5	0	0	1	1	0	1	1	0	0	0
7	1	0	0	0	0	1	3	0	0	0	0	0	1	0	1	0
8	0	2	0	0	1	0	0	6	0	0	0	1	0	0	0	0
9	1	0	1	0	0	0	0	0	7	0	0	1	0	0	0	0
10	0	3	0	0	0	0	0	0	0	3	0	1	1	0	0	0
11	0	6	1	5	4	0	0	1	0	0	47	0	1	0	0	0
12	0	0	0	9	0	0	0	1	4	1	0	0	0	0	0	0
13	2	0	0	4	0	1	1	0	1	3	0	1	0	1	1	0
14	3	0	0	0	0	0	0	0	0	0	0	0	0	7	0	0
15	1	1	0	0	1	0	0	0	0	0	0	0	1	0	6	1
16	2	2	1	1	2	0	0	0	1	1	0	1	0	1	2	11

Table 5.4 Evaluation of classifier before and after sampling

Class code	Name of the class	Before sampling		After sampling	
		Size of classifier	Accuracy (%)	Size of classifier	Accuracy (%)
1	Normal	245	92	210	94
2	Ischemic changes (coronary artery disease)	44	61	40	97
3	Old anterior myocardial infarction	15	93	16	100
4	Old inferior myocardial infarction	15	60	17	100
5	Sinus tachycardia	15	60	17	100
6	Sinus bradycardy	25	80	20	100
7	Ventricular premature contraction (PVC)	03	0	06	100
8	Supraventricular premature contraction	02	0	4	100
9	Left bundle branch block	9	88	6	98
10	Right bundle branch block	50	72	45	100
11	First degree Atrio ventricular block	0	0	0	98
12	Second degree AV block	0	0	0	90
13	Third degree AV block	0	0	0	97
14	Left ventricular hypertrophy	4	0	6	100
15	Atrial fibrillation or flutter	5	0	6	93
16	Others	22	0	25	94
	Average	28.25	0.962	25.75	0.972

Table 5.5 Performance comparison with existing method

Author	Accuracy (%)
Guvenir et al. [28]	68
Uyar and Gurgen [38]	76
Aliferis et al. [39]	65
Mohapatra and Mohanty [7]	96
Devadharshini et al. [37]	96.5
Proposed methodology	97.2

warning. IoT and machine learning equipped system offer observations and recordings for a longer period of time, and this continuous monitoring prevents the severity of arrhythmia. The classified data and visualizations improve the diagnosis process. Thus, the proposed real-time monitoring system for arrhythmia patients will reduce the risk of human life loss with wearable sensors and machine learning technique. In the future, some other parameters like blood pressure can be monitored in order to enhance the early detection and accurate diagnosis of arrhythmia patients.

References

1. Krasteva, V., & Jekova, I. (2007). QRS template matching for recognition of ventricular ectopic beats. *Annals of Biomedical Engineering, 35*(12), 2065–2076.
2. Niewolny, D. (2013). How the internet of things is revolutionizing healthcare, freescale semiconductors. In *Proceedings of International Conference on Healthcare* (pp. 211–219).
3. Hayashi, J., Kunieda, T., Cole, J., Soga, R., Hatanaka, Y., Lu, M., et al. (2004). A development of computer-aided diagnosis system using fundus images. In *Proceedings Seventh International Conference on Virtual Systems and Multimedia* (pp. 429–438). IEEE.
4. Raj, S., & Ray, K. C. (2017). ECG signal analysis using DCT-based DOST and PSO optimized SVM. *IEEE Transactions on Instrumentation and Measurement, 66*(3), 470–478.
5. Rad, A. B., Eftestøl, T., Engan, K., Irusta, U., Kvaløy, J. T., Kramer-Johansen, J., et al. (2017). ECG-based classification of resuscitation cardiac rhythms for retrospective data analysis. *IEEE Transactions on Biomedical Engineering, 64*(10), 2411–2418.
6. Luz, E. J. da S., Schwartz, W. R., Cámara-Chávez, G., & Menotti, D. (2016). ECG-based heartbeat classification for arrhythmia detection: A survey. *Computer Methods and Programs in Biomedicine, 127*, 144–164.
7. Mohapatra, S. K., & Mohanty, M. N. (2018, September). Analysis of resampling method for arrhythmia classification using random forest classifier with selected features. In *2018 2nd International Conference on Data Science and Business Analytics (ICDSBA)* (pp. 495–499). IEEE.
8. Ozcift, A., & Gulten, A. (2011). Classifier ensemble construction with rotation forest to improve medical diagnosis performance of machine learning algorithms. *Computer Methods and Programs in Biomedicine, 104*(3), 443–451.
9. Escalona-Morán, M. A., Soriano, M. C., Fischer, I., & Mirasso, C. R. (2014). Electrocardiogram classification using reservoir computing with logistic regression. *IEEE Journal of Biomedical and Health Informatics, 19*(3), 892–898.
10. Gutta, S., & Cheng, Q. (2015). Joint feature extraction and classifier design for ECG-based biometric recognition. *IEEE Journal of Biomedical and Health Informatics, 20*(2), 460–468.
11. Shadmand, S., & Mashoufi, B. (2016). A new personalized ECG signal classification algorithm using block-based neural network and particle swarm optimization. *Biomedical Signal Processing and Control, 25*, 12–23.
12. Ince, T., Kiranyaz, S., & Gabbouj, M. (2009). A generic and robust system for automated patient-specific classification of ECG signals. *IEEE Transactions on Biomedical Engineering, 56*(5), 1415–1426.
13. Gao, D., Madden, M., Chambers, D., & Lyons, G. (2005, July). Bayesian ANN classifier for ECG arrhythmia diagnostic system: A comparison study. In *Proceedings. 2005 IEEE International Joint Conference on Neural Networks, 2005* (Vol. 4, pp. 2383–2388). IEEE.
14. Xu, S., Mak, M. W., & Cheung, C. C. (2017, July). Deep neural networks versus support vector machines for ECG arrhythmia classification. In *2017 IEEE International Conference on Multimedia & Expo Workshops (ICMEW)* (pp. 127–132). IEEE.

15. Tracey, B. H., & Miller, E. L. (2012). Nonlocal means denoising of ECG signals. *IEEE Transactions on Biomedical Engineering*, *59*(9), 2383–2386.
16. Jain, S. K., & Bhaumik, B. (2016). An energy efficient ECG signal processor detecting cardiovascular diseases on smartphone. *IEEE Transactions on Biomedical Circuits and Systems*, *11*(2), 314–323.
17. Li, P., Wang, Y., He, J., Wang, L., Tian, Y., Zhou, T. S., et al. (2016). High-performance personalized heartbeat classification model for long-term ECG signal. *IEEE Transactions on Biomedical Engineering*, *64*(1), 78–86.
18. Satija, U., Ramkumar, B., & Manikandan, M. S. (2017). Automated ECG noise detection and classification system for unsupervised healthcare monitoring. *IEEE Journal of Biomedical and Health Informatics*, *22*(3), 722–732.
19. Spanó, E., Di Pascoli, S., & Iannaccone, G. (2016). Low-power wearable ECG monitoring system for multiple-patient remote monitoring. *IEEE Sensors Journal*, *16*(13), 5452–5462.
20. Roonizi, E. K., & Sassi, R. (2015). A signal decomposition model-based Bayesian framework for ECG components separation. *IEEE Transactions on Signal Processing*, *64*(3), 665–674.
21. American Heart Association. (2016). *Cardiac arrest statistics*. http://cpr.heart.org/AHAECC/CPRAndECC/General/UCM_477263_Cardiac-Arrest-Statistics.jsp. Accessed December 2, 2016.
22. Chen, X., Xu, D., Zhang, G., & Mukkamala, R. (2009, September). Forecasting acute hypotensive episodes in intensive care patients based on a peripheral arterial blood pressure waveform. In *2009 36th Annual Computers in Cardiology Conference (CinC)* (pp. 545–548). IEEE.
23. Deshmane, A. V. (2009). *False arrhythmia alarm suppression using ECG, ABP, and photoplethysmogram* (Doctoral dissertation, Massachusetts Institute of Technology).
24. Ganeshapillai, G., & Guttag, J. V. (2011). Weighted time warping for temporal segmentation of multi-parameter physiological signals. In *BIOSIGNALS 2011*.
25. Banerjee, R., Ghose, A., Choudhury, A. D., Sinha, A., & Pal, A. (2015, April). Noise cleaning and Gaussian modeling of smart phone photoplethysmogram to improve blood pressure estimation. In *2015 IEEE International Conference on Acoustics, Speech and Signal Processing (ICASSP)* (pp. 967–971). IEEE.
26. Sachpazidis, I., Stassinakis, A., Memos, D., Fragou, S., Nachamoulis, S., Vamvatsikos, A., et al. (2002). HOME ein neues Eu-projekt zum Tele Home Care. *Biomedizinische Technik/Biomedical Engineering*, *47*(s1b), 970–972.
27. Fensli, R., Gunnarson, E., & Gundersen, T. (2005, June). A wearable ECG-recording system for continuous arrhythmia monitoring in a wireless tele-home-care situation. In *18th IEEE Symposium on Computer-Based Medical Systems (CBMS'05)* (pp. 407–412). IEEE.
28. Guvenir, H. A., Acar, B., Demiroz, G., & Cekin, A. (1997, September). A supervised machine learning algorithm for arrhythmia analysis. In *Computers in Cardiology 1997* (pp. 433–436). IEEE.
29. Torfs, T., Leonov, V., Van Hoof, C., & Gyselinckx, B. (2006, October). Body-heat powered autonomous pulse oximeter. In *SENSORS, 2006 IEEE* (pp. 427–430). IEEE.
30. Chakraborty, C. (2019). Computational approach for chronic wound tissue characterization. *Informatics in Medicine Unlocked, 17*, 1–10.
31. Chakraborty, C. (2019). Mobile health (m-Health) for tele-wound monitoring. In *Mobile health applications for quality healthcare delivery* (Ch. 5, pp. 98–116). Hershey, PA: IGI. ISBN: 9781522580218. https://doi.org/10.4018/978-1-5225-8021-8.ch005.
32. Martin, T., Jovanov, E., & Raskovic, D. (2000, October). Issues in wearable computing for medical monitoring applications: A case study of a wearable ECG monitoring device. In *Digest of Papers. Fourth International Symposium on Wearable Computers* (pp. 43–49). IEEE.
33. Li, M., Yu, S., Zheng, Y., Ren, K., & Lou, W. (2012). Scalable and secure sharing of personal health records in cloud computing using attribute-based encryption. *IEEE Transactions on Parallel and Distributed Systems*, *24*(1), 131–143.
34. Ruj, S., Stojmenovic, M., & Nayak, A. (2012, May). Privacy preserving access control with authentication for securing data in clouds. In *2012 12th IEEE/ACM International Symposium on Cluster, Cloud and Grid Computing (CCGRID 2012)* (pp. 556–563). IEEE.

35. Tufte, E. R. (2001). *The visual display of quantitative information* (Vol. 2). Cheshire, CT: Graphics Press.
36. Healey, C. G. (1996, October). Choosing effective colours for data visualization. In *Proceedings of Seventh Annual IEEE Visualization'96* (pp. 263–270). IEEE.
37. Devadharshini, M. S., Heena Firdaus, A. S., Sree Ranjani, R., & Devarajan, N. (2019). Real time arrhythmia monitoring with machine learning classification and IoT. In *2019 Fifth International Conference on Data Science and Engineering (ICDSE).*
38. Uyar, A., & Gurgen, F. (2007, September). Arrhythmia classification using serial fusion of support vector machines and logistic regression. In *2007 4th IEEE Workshop on Intelligent Data Acquisition and Advanced Computing Systems: Technology and Applications* (pp. 560–565). IEEE.
39. Aliferis, C. F., Tsamardinos, I., & Statnikov, A. (2003). HITON: A novel Markov Blanket algorithm for optimal variable selection. In *AMIA Annual Symposium Proceedings* (Vol. 2003, p. 21). American Medical Informatics Association.

Chapter 6
Human Heart Arrhythmia Identification Using ECG Signals: An Approach Towards Biomedical Signal Processing

Ravina Dnyaneshwar Edake

Abstract ECG signals are widely used for detecting any abnormality related to the heart. ECG signal has a number of cardiac cycles, and each cardiac cycle has P–QRS–T waves. The aim behind implementing this project is to detect cardiac arrhythmia using KNN and SVM classifiers. In this work, a total data of 48 subjects ECG signals are used. Zero-phase filter is used to eliminate the baseline noise. Daubechies wavelet 4 is used for feature extraction. KNN and SVM classifiers are used to classify the signals into normal and abnormal groups. The performance evaluations (accuracy, sensitivity, specificity) are calculated for both the classifiers. Accuracy for KNN classifier is 76.92%, whereas accuracy for SVM classifier is 79.48%. Sensitivity of KNN is 82.35%, and for SVM, it is 71.42%. Specificity for KNN classifier is 72.72%, and for SVM classifier, it is 100%. The performance of both the classifiers is compared with the help of confusion matrix.

Keywords Electrocardiogram (ECG) · Cardiovascular disease (CVD)

6.1 Introduction

Literature Survey

The ECG is a non-invasive method and the record of variation of the bio-potential signal of the human heartbeats. Some of the feature extraction methods implemented are discrete wavelet transform, Karhunen–Loeve transform, Hermitian basis, etc. The parameters that must be considered while developing an algorithm for feature extraction of an ECG signal are simplicity of algorithm and the accuracy of the algorithm in providing the best results in feature extraction. Various techniques have been implemented for the analysis of ECG signals. Some of the methods explained are as follows:

R. D. Edake (✉)
MKSSS's Cummins College of Engineering for Women, Pune, Solapur, India
e-mail: ravinaedake@gmail.com

C. Chakraborty et al. (eds.), *Internet of Things for Healthcare Technologies*, Studies in Big Data 73, https://doi.org/10.1007/978-981-15-4112-4_6

(1) P.D Khandait, N.G Bawane and S.S Limaye proposed a method to extract the features for the detection of cardiac arrhythmia. The database of 48 records each of 30 min duration was used. To remove the baseline drift, median filters were used. Db4 wavelet was used to extract the features from the signals. The accuracy obtained was about 98.17%.
(2) Waqas Ahmed and Dr. Shehzad Khalid made a survey to recognise cardiovascular diseases. Methods such as adaptive filter, finite impulse response, wavelet decomposition, empirical mode decomposition, mean median filtering using DWT can be used to remove the baseline noise. Classifiers such as artificial neural network (ANN), K-nearest neighbour (KNN), fuzzy logic and support vector machine (SVM) can be used to classify the ECG signals.
(3) Shambhu D. and Umesh A.C. proposed a method to classify the ECG signals using SVM and extract the features using wavelet transform. 48 recordings (25 male and 25 female) of 30 min duration were used. Features were given to SVM for the classification purposes.
(4) Prof. Alka S. Barhatte, Dr. Rajesh Ghongade and Abhishek Thakare proposed a method for QRS complex detection and classifying arrhythmia by SVM. 48 records of 30 min duration with sampling frequency of 360 Hz were used. Db9 was used as mother wavelet. Classification was performed with the help of support vector machine and artificial neural network. Accuracy was about 99.78%.
(5) V. K. Srivastava and Dr. Devendra Prasad proposed a method to extract the features using DWT. ECG database was used from the Physio bank. Bandpass filter was used to eliminate baseline wander and motion artefact. DWT was used to extract the features from ECG signals. For classification of signals, neuro-fuzzy system was used.
(6) AswathyVelayudhan and Soniya Peter gave a survey to analyse noise and different denoising techniques for ECG signals. Different types of noise present in ECG signals are powerline interference, EMG, channel noise, baseline noise, etc. Filtering techniques used for the removal of powerline interference are IIR notch filters, FIR filtering, adaptive filtering, discrete wavelet transform, filtered residue method, empirical mode decomposition, etc.
(7) Prajakta S. Gokhale presented work on ECG signal denoising using DWT for the removal of powerline noise. The database was taken from MITBIH arrhythmia database and sampled at 360 Hz frequency range. Denoising of ECG signal is performed using Db4 wavelet. The effectiveness of the proposed algorithm was determined by MSE and output SNR values.
(8) Marco V. Gualsaqui Miranda, Ivan P. Vizcaino Espinosa, Marco J. Flores Calero presented a method to extract the features from ECG signals. Database of 24 signals was collected using CESL3 (time duration = 1 min, sampling frequency = 500 Hz, resolution = 16 bits, sample length = 30,000, file format = .scp). DWT was used for denoising of ECG signals. CWT Daubechies 5 was used for groups of ECG signals. The database of real ECG signals generated in this work allowed us to obtain the relevant features with sensitivity of 96%.

(9) Namita Thomas and Deepthy Mathew presented a method for KNN-based pattern analysis and classification. The data sets consist of 549 records of 290 subjects with 52 healthy controls and 148 MI patients. This work uses DWT-based decomposition and selective reconstruction for denoising and QRS detection. The ECG database is trained, classified using KNN method for accurate and positive results. It resulted in accuracy of 81.61%, sensitivity of 92.30% and specificity of 76.92%.

(10) TAN Yun-fu, Du Lei presented a method on wavelet transform in processing the ECG signals. This paper chooses 104 ECG signals (300 to 300.608 s) of MITBIH arrhythmia database to carry out the simulation. Coif4 is adopted to carry 9-scale wavelet decomposition. Use of threshold method to eliminate powerline and myoelectrical interference was performed. The conclusion said that all the noises were eliminated, and wavelet transform has a good filtering effect. ECG signals after filtering provide right basis for the wave detection and analysis of arrhythmia.

(11) Apurva Kulkarni, SnehalLale, PranaliIngole and SayaliGengaje have given a method to analyse the ECG signals. Database of 46 patients was taken from MITBIH arrhythmia database sampled at the rate of 360 Hz. To remove the interference, Pan–Tompkins algorithm was used with bandpass filter of pass-band of 5–12 Hz. K-nearest neighbour was used for classification. Accuracy of 86.95%, sensitivity of 87.09% and specificity of 86.66% were obtained for 60% training data set.

(12) A. Muthuchudar and Lt. Dr. S. Santosh Baboo proposed a method to analyse the ECG signals. This research involves denoising, data compression, feature extraction and classification of signals. To extract the features, the non-syntactic method is used. For classification purpose, the classifier named artificial neural network is used in this project. There are eight abnormalities detected in this project, and they are Dextrocardia, Tachycardia, Bradycardia, Hyperkalemia, Myocardial, Hypercalcaemia, sinoatrial block and sudden cardiac death.

Electrocardiogram is the representation of heart activity which can be easily recorded with the help of surface electrodes in contact with human chest used to detect and diagnose the cardiovascular diseases. CVDs are widely classified as rheumatic, congenital, hypertensive, peripheral artery diseases, heart failure, etc. One of the abnormalities related to heart is cardiac arrhythmia [1]. The ECG signal of the normal subject is shown in Fig. 6.1.

In cardiac arrhythmia, the heart rate is irregular. The rate of heart is higher than 120 beats per minute in cardiac arrhythmia. Symptoms such as fainting or collapse, chest pain, breathe shortness and dizziness can be observed if a person suffers from cardiac arrhythmia. It may result in heart failure or stroke development if it is not treated on time. ECG signal processing system comprises of three basic steps such as pre-processing, feature extraction and classification [1]. Table 6.1 shows time interval and amplitude range for the ECG signal containing P–QRS–T waves.

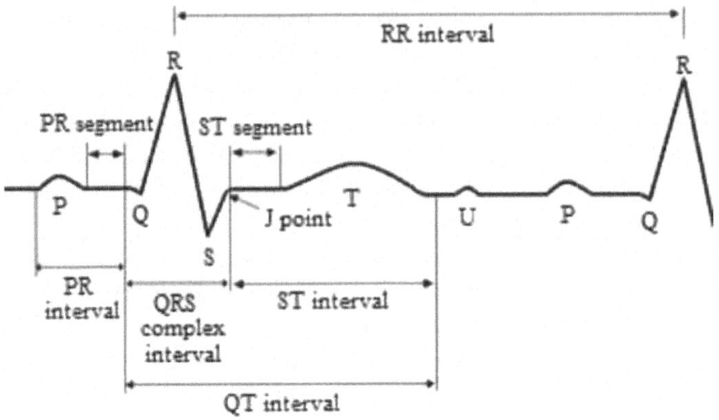

Fig. 6.1 ECG signal

Table 6.1 Time interval and amplitude range of P–QRS–T wave

Wave or interval	Function	Amplitude	Time interval
P wave	Corresponds to atrial depolarisation	0.25 mV	0.11 s
QRS complex	Corresponds to blood depolarisation	<6 mV	0.09 s
T wave	Corresponds to repolarisation of ventricles	0.1–0.5 mV	160 ms
RR interval	Calculated by finding difference of 2 RR peaks	–	0.6–1 s
PQ interval	Is the period of atrial contraction	–	0.12–0.20 s
ST interval	Calculated by finding difference of 2 ST peaks	–	0.05–0.15 s

mV millivolt, *s* seconds, *ms* milliseconds

6.1.1 ECG Signal Processing System

The basic block diagram of ECG classification system is shown in Fig. 6.2.

Fig. 6.2 ECG signal processing system

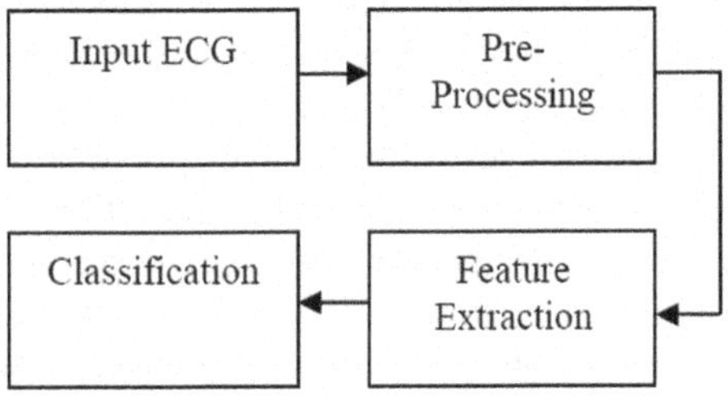

6.1.1.1 Input ECG

Any biomedical signals such as ECG, EEG and EMG can be applied as input to the system. These signals can be easily obtained from clinic, MITBIH site or direct recording from the humans. The most important task in signal processing is the removal of interference without affecting (increasing or decreasing) the signal amplitude. Defining of sampling frequency, time duration, file format of the signal is important for further processing in any application for biomedical signal processing domain [2].

6.1.1.2 Pre-processing

ECG signals have different types of noise such as baseline noise, powerline noise, high-frequency noise, electrode noise, instrumentation noise, burst noise, and electromyogram noise. These types of unwanted noise provide interruption in further processing and also reduce the overall quality of the signal. So it is very essential to remove the noise from the input signal. For the removal of these interference methods such as empirical mode decomposition, mean median filtering, discrete wavelet transform are used [2].

6.1.1.3 Feature Extraction

This step provides the relevant and desired information about the signal. Finding the right feature combinations is a hard task. Features of ECG signals are mean, variance, standard deviation, skewness, kurtosis, maximum amplitude, maximum frequency, etc. These features act an input to any particular classifier. More and more number of features can be given to the classifier as input. These features can be calculated by using mathematical equations (formulae) or by using direct commands (depends on which software tool is in use, for example, MATLAB, Python, etc.) [2].

6.1.1.4 Classification

The classifiers are used to categorise the signals into their appropriate group and then reach the final decision stage. Classifiers such as artificial neural network (ANN), K-nearest neighbour (KNN), support vector machine (SVM), fuzzy logic system and linear discriminant analysis (LDA) are used for ECG classification purposes. One classifier can be used to categorise various abnormalities respectively. More than one classifier can be implemented for one application which is further useful to compare which classifier works better for a particular application [2].

6.2 Methodology

The ECG signal processing consists of steps such as removal of artefacts/unwanted signals, extracting the features from the filtered output and finally the classification of signals into their appropriate group. To extract the useful information from the signals, the raw signal has been processed by removing the baseline noise from the input. For classification of signals, two classifiers are used which are K-nearest neighbour and support vector machine classifiers. To implement this experiment, flowchart shown in Fig. 6.3 is used.

6.2.1 ECG Signal

In this project, all the ECG signals are taken from MITBIH arrhythmia database. Total data set of 48 subjects ECG signals including normal and diseased subjects are considered for the implementation. Training set has 40 signals, and testing set has 8 signals. The time duration of all signals is 30 s, and sampling rate is 360 Hz. While recording the signals, all the signals were in .qrs format. In order to get it loaded into MATLAB, all the signals are converted to .mat format.

Fig. 6.3 Flowchart

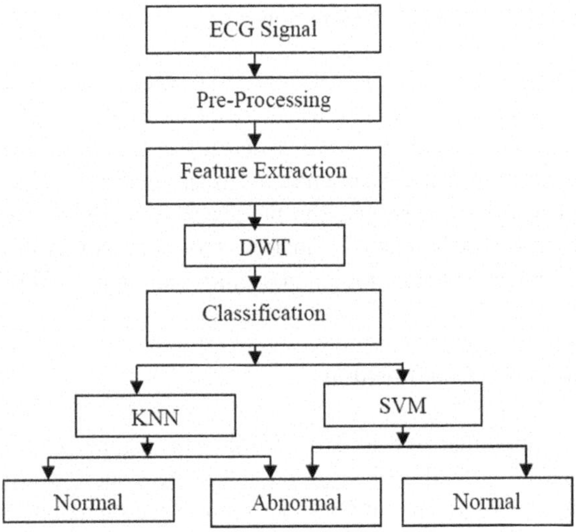

6.2.2 *Pre-processing*

ECG signal consists of different unwanted signals, and they are baseline noise, instrumentation noise, high-frequency noise, electrode noise, burst noise, muscle noise, etc. The presence of such noise in ECG signal degrades both the quality and the accuracy of the signal. So it becomes essential to remove this unwanted noise from the input signal. Different techniques such as IIR notch filtering, FIR filtering, adaptive filtering and filtered residue method are available for the removal of noise from the signals. With the help of zero-phase low pass-filter, the baseline noise is eliminated [3].
The following steps are followed:

(1) Zero-phase signal is passed to the input.
(2) The obtained signal is then subtracted from the input.
(3) After performing the above steps, the signal obtained is the filtered ECG signal.

6.2.2.1 Types of Noise in ECG Signal

(1) Powerline Interference: This noise causes problem in interpreting low amplitude waveform like ECG. In order to avoid wrong identification of the characteristic of ECG signals and its impact on analysis and diagnostic accuracy, it is necessary to remove the powerline interference effectively from the input signal [4].
(2) Electromyogram Noise: Contraction of muscles behind the heart contributes to this type of noise. When other muscles in the vicinity of the electrodes contract, generation of depolarisation and repolarisation waves takes place and these waves are picked up by the ECG signals. This noise is common in the subjects with uncontrollable tremor, disabled kids and persons [4].
(3) Baseline Wander: It is the low-frequency noise component present in ECG signals. It has a frequency greater than 1 kHz. It causes an interruption in detection and analysis of peaks. It is caused by changes in electrode to skin polarisation voltages, or by electrode movement or by respiration movement or by body movement. One possible cause is the movement of cables. This type of noise causes the base of signal to move up and down from its respective axis [4].
(4) Instrumentation Noise: Electrodes, probes, cables, signal amplifiers, analogue-to-digital converters are the major source for this type of noise. Unfortunately, instrumentation noise cannot be removed but it can be reduced with high-quality equipment and careful circuit design [4].
(5) Electrode Contact Noise: This type of noise is generated due to poor contact between the electrode and the skin. The larger the electrode-skin impedance, the smaller are relative impedance change which is required to cause a major shift in the baseline of ECG signals [4].
(6) Burst Noise: It is typically classified as white Gaussian noise (WGN) which appears on subset of leads for a very short duration. Examples of burst noise

are electrode pop noise, electrode motion artefact, electrode surgical noise, instrumentation noise, etc., and the frequency range of this noise is not well defined. Biomedical signals can be severely affected by this type of noise [4].

6.2.2.2 Methods for Removal of Noise from ECG Signal

(1) IIR Notch Filter: It is widely used for the removal of powerline interference at 50 Hz. Notch filters can be used to remove the stationary powerline noise. Stationary means which do not vary with amplitude, frequency and phase over time [4].
(2) FIR Filtering: Using the different windows such as rectangular, Hamming, Hanning, Blackman the low-pass and high-pass filters are designed with cut-off frequency of 3 and 100 Hz. The noisy ECG signals are passed through these filters for the removal of noise. FIR filters are stable and have linear phase characteristics [4].
(3) Adaptive Filter: It reduces the mean squared error between primary input and reference input. Here the filtering response is fast. It provides excellent performance with varying amplitude. This filter is used to remove the noise, extract the information from the signals and separate two or more combined signals. They are widely used to remove the powerline interference from ECG signals [4].
(4) Filtered Residue Method: Here the residue of noisy ECG signals is calculated. The residue is given as the difference between input ECG signal and corresponding signal average at every point. The main advantage of using this method is that it is easy to implement, stable, preserve high-frequency components, etc. [4].

6.2.3 Feature Extraction

Extracting the features from the signal is one of the important tasks in ECG signal processing system because it provides relevant information about the signal. To extract the features, different methods such as discrete wavelet transform, continuous wavelet transform and S transform can be used. Features of ECG signals can be classified as temporal, morphological, statistical features, etc. Calculating more and more number of features will enhance the performance evaluation of that particular application respectively. Features of ECG signal are calculated by using the direct mathematical equation in the software which is used for implementation purpose [5].

The following statistical features are calculated:

(1) Mean: Average value of total number of signals is termed as mean [6].

$$\text{Mean} = \frac{X_1 + X_2 + \cdots X_n}{N}$$

(2) Standard Deviation: It is the variation amount in ECG signal [6].

$$\text{Standard Deviation} = \frac{1}{N-1}\sum_{1-n}^{N}(X_n - \mu_x)$$

(3) Skewness: It is defined as the amount of deviation distribution (asymmetry) compared to normal distribution [6].

$$\text{Skewness} = \frac{3 * (\text{Measn - Median})}{\text{S.D}}$$

(4) Kurtosis: It is defined as the highest (peak) value of the ECG signal [6].

$$\text{Kurtosis} = \frac{\sum_{n=1}^{N}(Y_i - Y)}{N}$$

(5) Variance: It is calculated by subtracting the value of signal from its mean value, then subtracting it and finally dividing it by number of signals present in the data set [6].

$$\text{Variance} = \frac{\sum_{i=1}^{n} x_i - x_{\text{avg}}}{n-1}$$

(6) Maximum Amplitude: It is defined as the highest amplitude of the signal [6].
(7) Maximum Frequency: (1) It is defined as the highest frequency of the signal [6].

6.2.3.1 Types of ECG Features

(1) Temporal Features: This category of features mainly includes heart rate and interval features [5].
(2) Morphological Features: It gives characteristic morphology details that include coefficients from wavelet decomposition, their minima maxima, etc. [5].
(3) Statistical Features: This category of features includes mean, variance and other statistical moments [5].
(4) Time-Based Features: It has time interval in milliseconds representing RR interval, PR interval, PP interval, etc. The duration or amplitude of P wave, T wave

and QRS complex is used as time-based features in ECG signal analysis. These features do not provide high performance due to low sensitivity [5].

(5) Frequency-Based Features: They are mostly computed through Fourier transform. These features have increased sensitivity but time resolution is lost during the transformation process; therefore, it cannot specify in which portion of time the change has been occurred [5].

(6) Time-Frequency-Based Features: It provides frequency analysis with time resolution for analysed features. Here wavelet transform is used because of its computational simplicity and interpretability in a similar way as that of Fourier transform [5].

6.2.4 *Discrete Wavelet Transform*

To analyse the transients of aperiodic and non-stationary signals, DWT is widely used. It is an effective tool for extracting the features from the signals that act as the input to the classifier model. Discrete wavelet transform has various applications in biomedical signal processing, and some of them are cardiology research work (mostly for denoising as well as compression of different types of biomedical signals), ECG segmentation, to analyse the variability in heart rhythm, analysis of different types of abnormalities related to the heart (cardiac arrhythmias), etc. [7].

The wavelet technique provides a description of a signal in the timescale domain, analogous to a frequency-time domain allowing a representation of temporal features at multiple resolutions. The sampling frequency of ECG signal is 360 Hz, and this shows that maximum frequency present in the signal is 180 Hz, respectively. Wavelet transform is used for effective feature extraction which may be considered for the classifier model [8].

Daubechies wavelet 4 has properties such as asymmetric, orthogonal and biorthogonal. It belongs to a family of orthogonal wavelets which is characterised by maximal number of vanishing moment for the given support. Daubechies wavelet is chosen to have the highest number of vanishing moments. They are widely used to solve the problems such as signal discontinuities, self-similarity properties of a signal or fractal problems. They are not defined in terms of resulting scaling and wavelet functions, and they are not possible to write in closed form (Fig. 6.4).

6.2.4.1 Significance of Discrete Wavelet Transform

(1) ECG signals can be compressed into few features by spectral analysis of signals with wavelet transform [7].

(2) It provides good resolution at high-frequency and good frequency resolution at low frequency [7].

(3) It can be decomposed to wavelet filter banks [7].

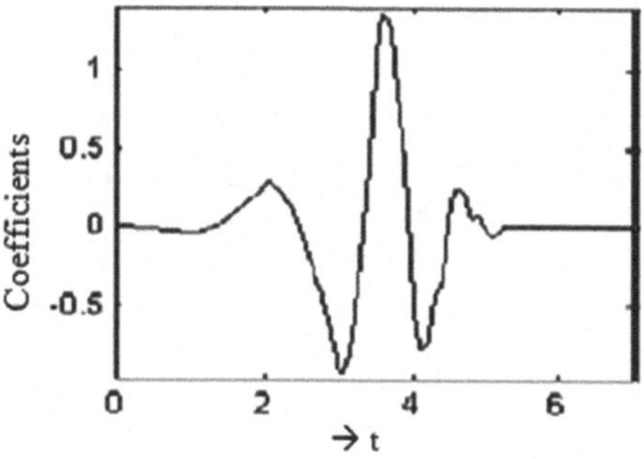

Fig. 6.4 Daubechies wavelet 4

6.2.5 *Classification*

In ECG signal processing, the classifiers play a very pivotal role to classify the signals into their appropriate group and reach the final decision stage. Different types of classifiers such as fuzzy logic system, linear discriminant analysis and ensemble-based classifiers are widely used for ECG signal classification purposes. In this application, two classifiers K-nearest neighbour and support vector machine is used [9].

6.2.5.1 K-nearest neighbour

K-nearest neighbour is one of the effective types of technique which is widely used for classification. K-nearest neighbour algorithm is flexible to all the types of features. In this algorithm, the value of "K" is called as "total number of nearest neighbour". The value of "K" should be as small as possible (small integer value). If we select a large value of "K", it may create misclassification for the signals. For the classification of signals, comparison between the training set and testing set is carried out. This classifier works effectively even if the training data set is large. This classifier is used because it is easy for implementation and calculation time is also small. K-nearest neighbour consists of two phases which are training phase and classification phase. In order for the classification to occur assume the availability of training data and size of the training data set (K) [10].

One of the disadvantages of using this classifier is that it needs all the available data which may sometimes create overhead. Figure 6.5 represents the K-nearest neighbour classifier model.

6.2.5.2 Applications of K-Nearest Neighbour

(1) K-nearest neighbour can be used for the motor imagery classification for EEG signals.
(2) In the classification of lymph node metastasis in gastric cancer.

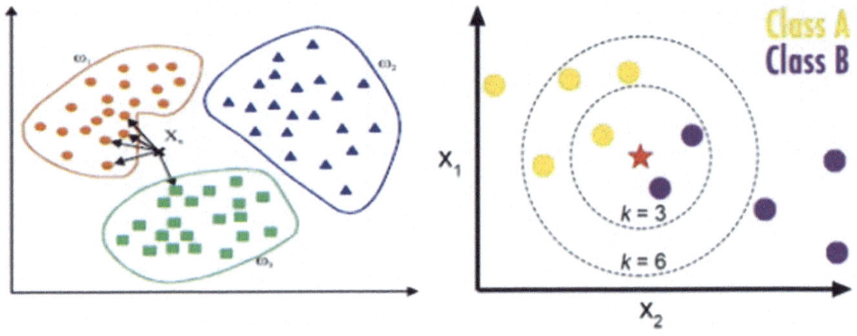

Fig. 6.5 K-nearest neighbour

(3) To retrieve images of brain.
(4) Detection and classification of lung cancer through MRI images.
(5) In brain balancing classification via spectrogram images.

6.2.5.3 Support Vector Machine

This method can solve both binary classification and multi-class problems. This technique constructs one or more than one hyper-planes in the infinite-dimensional space that is further used for classification purposes. The hyper-plane should be constructed in such a way that it should have the largest distance to the training data point. Thus, it can be said that for large margin it provides minimum error for the classification. These classifiers work well for the high-dimensional data. It also provides high performance if the data set is large such as in-text classification and tasks related to bioinformatics. The risk of overfitting is less in this classifier as compared to other classifiers. Figure 6.6 represents support vector machine classifier model.

6.2.5.4 Applications of Support Vector Machine

(1) In cancer classification with micro-array data [11].
(2) To analyse the biological data (protein and DNA sequence) [11].
(3) It is widely used for breast cancer diagnosis [11].

6.2.6 Types of Learners in Classifiers

Lazy learners and early learners are the two types of learners in classifiers.

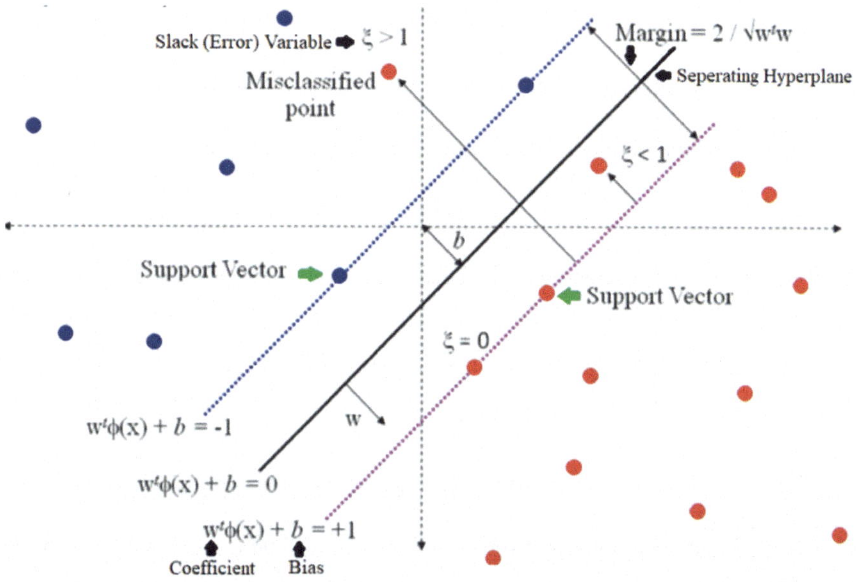

Fig. 6.6 Support vector machine

6.2.6.1 Lazy Learners

Here the training data is stored, and it waits for the presence of testing data. The training time required is less, whereas prediction time is more for this type of learners [12].

Example of lazy learners: K-nearest neighbour, case-based reasoning [12].

6.2.6.2 Early Learners

Here classification model is constructed based on training data. This type of learners requires long training time and less prediction time as it builds the classification model. Early learners acquire the entire instance space for classification purpose [12].

Example of early learners: Decision tree, Naive Bayes, artificial neural network [12].

6.3 Performance Evaluation

The statistical measures for the classification performance test are accuracy, sensitivity and specificity.

(1) Accuracy: The overall performance of any system is termed as "Accuracy" [10].

$$\text{Accuracy} = [(\text{TP} + \text{TN})/(\text{TP} + \text{TN} + \text{FP} + \text{FN})] * 100$$

(2) Sensitivity: It is defined as the actual positives which are detected correctly [10].

$$\text{Sensitivity} = [\text{TP}/(\text{TP} + \text{FN})] * 100$$

(3) Specificity: It is defined as the actual negatives which are detected correctly [10].

$$\text{Specificity} = [\text{TN}/(\text{TN} + \text{FP})] * 100$$

where

TP True Positive (if normal signal is classified as normal signal by both the classifiers)
TN True Negative (if abnormal signal is classified as abnormal signal by both the classifiers)
FP False Positive (if normal signal is classified as abnormal signal by both the classifiers)
FN False Negative (if abnormal signal is classified as normal signal by both the classifiers).

6.3.1 Confusion Matrix

Confusion matrix basically helps us to understand the performance of any classifier. It is also called as "Error Matrix". In confusion matrix, each row is predicted class, whereas each column is an actual class. Basically, it is a table with 2 rows and 2 columns which are named as True Positive, True Negative, False Positive and False Negative. Figure 6.7 represents the confusion matrix (along with the representation of predicted class and actual class). The confusion matrix explains the type of error that the classifier is making. This type of matrix is very easy to understand, and performing mathematical calculations also becomes easy [13].

After building a model, the work of checking the accuracy of that model is done by a confusion matrix. Confusion matrix is widely used in engineering field and also in all engineering domains such as biomedical signal processing, image processing and digital signal processing due to its easy behaviour for calculation purposes. This type of matrix provides accurate results for all the types of classifiers implemented for the particular application.

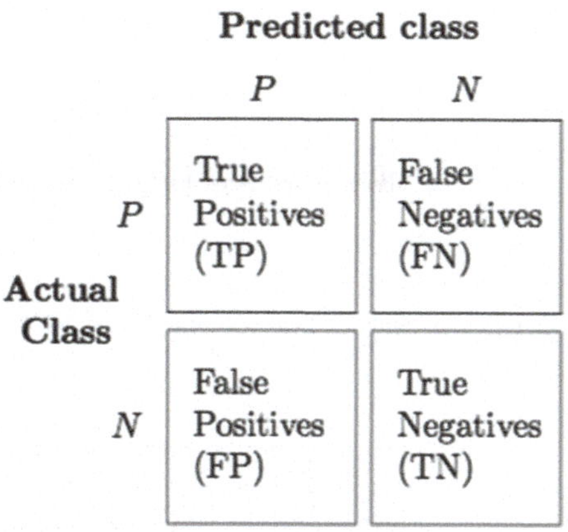

Fig. 6.7 Confusion matrix

6.4 Simulation and Experimental Results

Data set is downloaded from MITBIH database. Each of the ECG records has the following specifications: Sampling Frequency = 360 Hz, Time Duration = 30 s, File Format = .mat format. Below figure indicates the input ECG signal.

Figure 6.8 represents the input ECG signal.

In pre-processing stage, elimination of baseline noise is performed with the help of zero-phase filter. Below figures indicate zero-phase signal when passed to input ECG signal and filtered ECG signal.

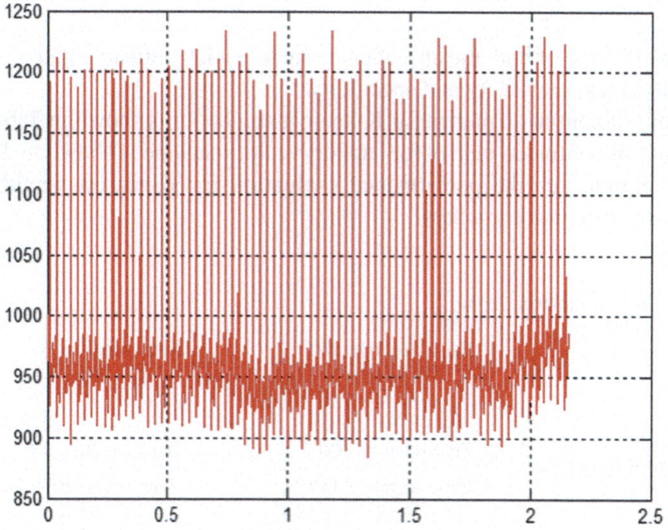

Fig. 6.8 Input ECG signal

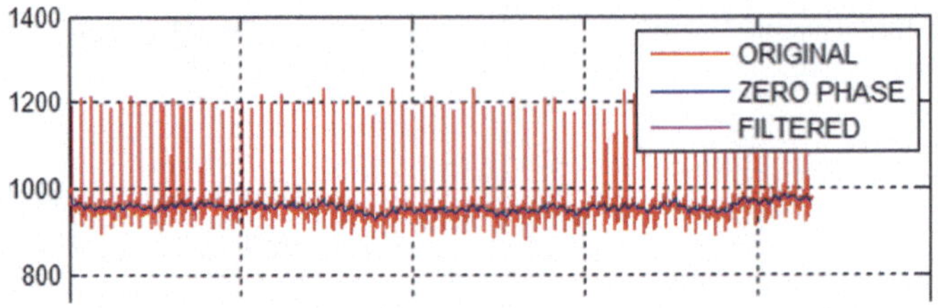

Fig. 6.9 Zero-phase signal with input ECG signal

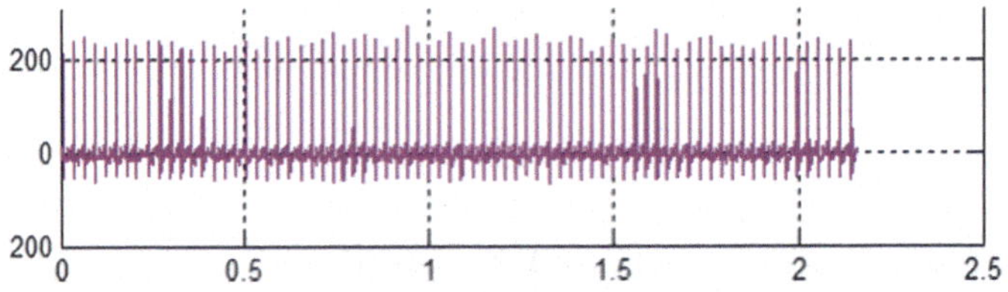

Fig. 6.10 Filtered ECG signal

Figure 6.9 represents the input ECG signal when a zero-phase signal is passed to it.

Figure 6.10 represents the filtered ECG Signal.

Extracting the features is one of the very important tasks for classification. Mean, variance, standard deviation, skewness, kurtosis, maximum amplitude and maximum frequency are the features' calculated.

All the features are then given to two types of classifiers that are K-nearest neighbour and support vector machine to classify the signals into normal and abnormal groups.

The performance of both the classifiers is calculated. Confusion matrix is used to calculate accuracy, sensitivity and specificity.

The result of confusion matrix for K-nearest neighbour is shown in Table 6.2.

The result of confusion matrix for support vector machine is shown in Table 6.3.

Table 6.4 indicates the performance evaluation for K-nearest neighbour and support vector machine classifiers.

Table 6.2 Confusion matrix for K-nearest neighbour

True positive 70%	False positive 30%
False negative 20%	True negative 80%

Table 6.3 Confusion matrix for support vector machine

True positive 100%	False positive 0%
False negative 45%	True negative 55%

Table 6.4 Performance evaluation (K-nearest neighbour and support vector machine)

Performance evaluation	KNN classifier (%)	SVM classifier (%)
Accuracy	79.92	79.48
Sensitivity	82.35	71.42
Specificity	72.72	100

6.5 Different Types of Classifiers

6.5.1 Artificial Neural Network

It works like a human brain. Here the term neural means "neuron" and network means "structure". These neurons are collected together in order to form layers. Different layers perform different transformations. The link between neurons is known as "Edges". This classifier effectively can handle unwanted information. This classifier can be used in biomedical signal processing domain for all types of biomedical signals (such as ECG, EMG and EEG). Applications of artificial neural network are pattern classification, clustering, optimisation, prediction, function approximation, speech recognition, computer vision, machine translation, social network filtering, medical diagnosis, etc. [14]. Figure 6.11 represents the basic diagram of artificial neural network.

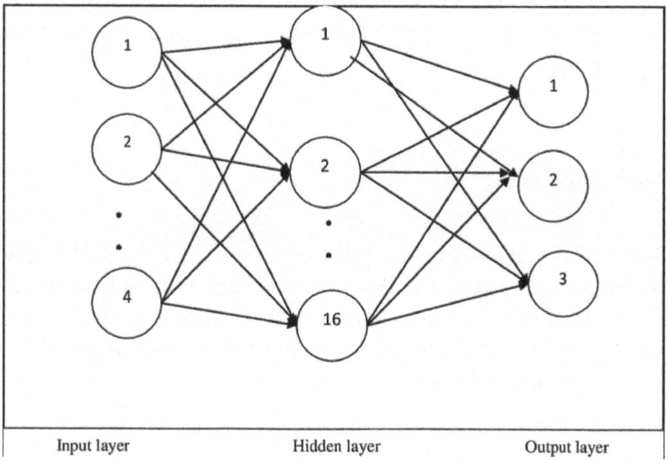

Fig. 6.11 Artificial neural network

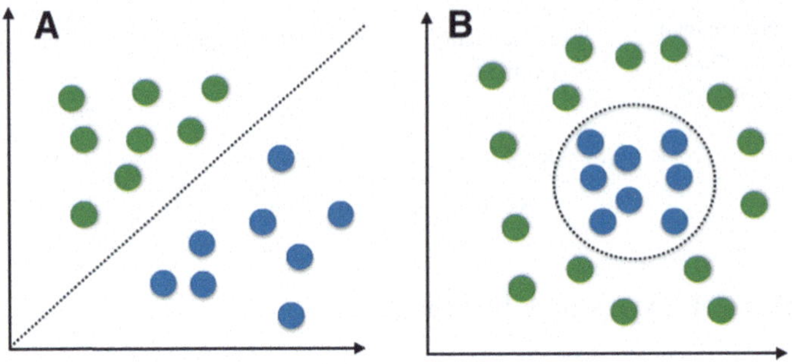

Fig. 6.12 Naïve Bayes classifier

6.5.2 *Naive Bayes Classifier*

Naive Bayes classifier is implemented by applying Bayes' theorem. This classifier can be trained for supervised learning. One of the advantages of using Naive Bayes classifier is that it requires less number of training data. Types of Naive Bayes classifier are multinomial Naive Bayes, Bernoulli Naive Bayes, Gaussian Naive Bayes. Multinomial Naive Bayes classifier is used for the classification of document problems. Bernoulli Naive Bayes uses Boolean variables as their predictors. Gaussian Naive Bayes uses continuous predictor values. This classifier is typically used for sentiment analysis, spam filtering, recommendation systems, etc. This classifier works fast, and it is easy for implementation. One of the disadvantages in using this classifier is that it requires independent predictors [15]. Figure 6.12 represents Naive Bayes classifier model.

6.5.3 *Decision Tree*

It uses the structure (similar to tree) to make decisions (reach the final decision stage). This classifier has three types of nodes which are decision node, chance node and end node. This classifier is simple to interpret. If we change small amount of data, it corresponds to change large amount of data of the decision tree. Figure 6.13 indicates the decision tree classifier model.

6.5.4 *Ensemble-Based Classifiers*

It is a type of supervised learning algorithm (firstly trained and then predictions are performed). Types of ensemble-based classifiers are stacking, blending, bagging and boasting. Supervised learning algorithms are described as performing the task of

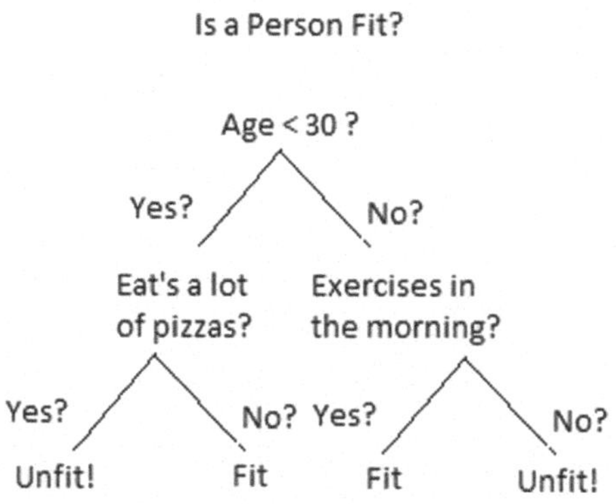

Fig. 6.13 Decision tree

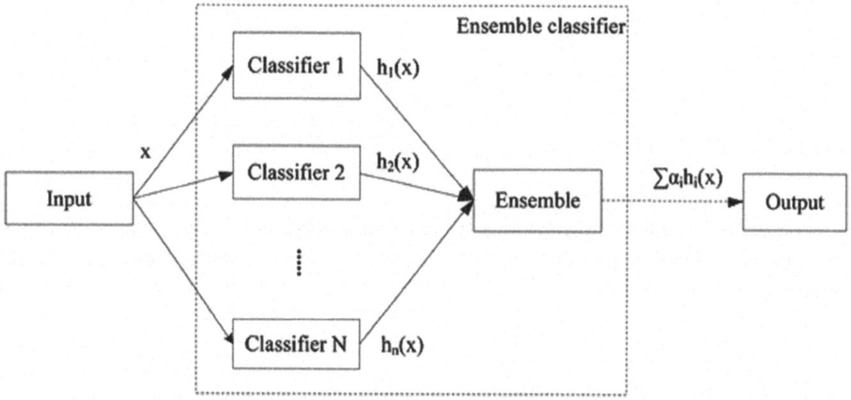

Fig. 6.14 Ensemble-based classifier

searching through a hypothesis space that will make good predictions with a particular problem. Ensembles combine multiple hypotheses to form a better hypothesis. Figure 6.14 represents a basic diagram of ensemble-based classifier. Ensemble classifiers have successfully applied in neuroscience, proteomics, medical diagnosis and facial emotion recognition [16].

6.6 Wavelet Selection

Haar, Daubechies, biorthogonal, Coiflets, Symlets, Morlet, Mexican hat, Meyer, etc., are the different types of wavelets which can be used for the analysis of the ECG signals. The wavelet selection is completely depended on the type of signal to be analysed for the particular application. The Daubechies wavelet shows similarity

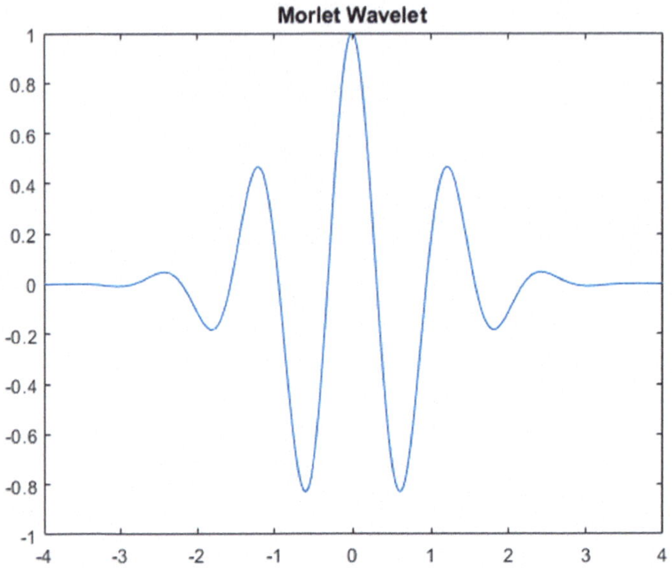

Fig. 6.15 Morlet wavelet

with the QRS complex and provides more details accurately as compared to other wavelets. Here Daubechies wavelet 4 was used to decompose the signals into four frequency scales [17].

6.6.1 Morlet Wavelet

Complex version is called as "Gabor wavelet" whereas the real-valued version is called as "Morlet wavelet". The application of the Morlet wavelet analysis is used to discriminate abnormal heartbeat behaviour in the electrocardiogram (ECG). Since the variation of abnormal heartbeat is the non-stationary signal, this signal is suitable for wavelet-based analysis [18]. Figure 6.15 indicates the Morlet wavelet.

6.6.2 Haar Wavelet

This wavelet was proposed by Alfred Haar in the year 1909. Haar wavelet is a square-shaped wavelet which shows similarity with Fourier analysis. This wavelet is also called as "Db1", and it is one of the easiest forms of wavelet. This type of wavelet is widely used in the domain like image processing, pattern recognition, digital signal processing and image compression. Haar wavelet was discovered by Alfred Haar in the year 1909. Discontinuity is one of the disadvantages of the Haar wavelet. Haar

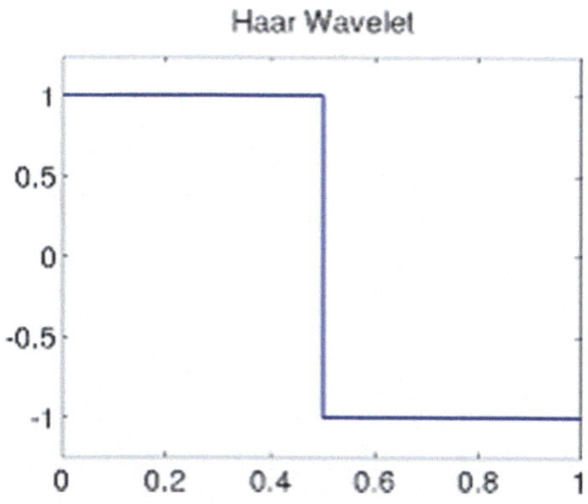

Fig. 6.16 Haar wavelet

wavelet supports the scaling function. One of the most important properties of Haar wavelet is its orthogonality in nature. Some other applications of Haar wavelet are image coding, edge extraction and binary logic design. VLSI designers also take interest in using this wavelet to implement their own application [19]. Figure 6.16 indicates the Haar wavelet.

6.6.3 Meyer Wavelet

Meyer wavelet was discovered by Yves Meyer. It is one of the types of continuous wavelets which can be differentiated infinitely. This wavelet can be applied to the adaptive filters, fractional random fields, multi-fault classification, etc. This type of wavelet is smooth; it supports fast attenuation, and it has a finite spectrum. Numerical calculations become easy with the help of Meyer wavelet so it is used in engineering fields more frequently [20]. Figure 6.17 represents Meyer wavelet.

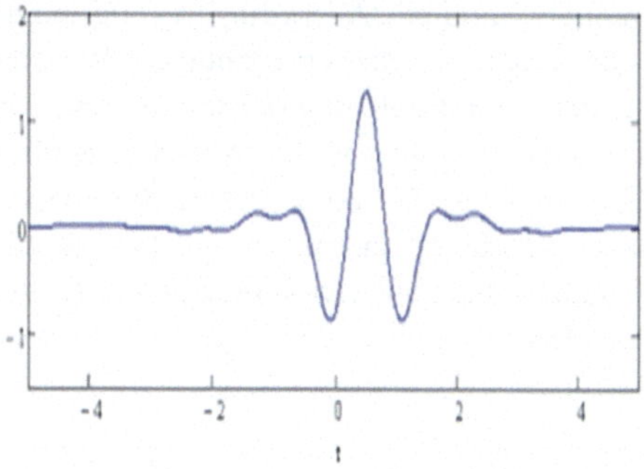

Fig. 6.17 Meyer wavelet

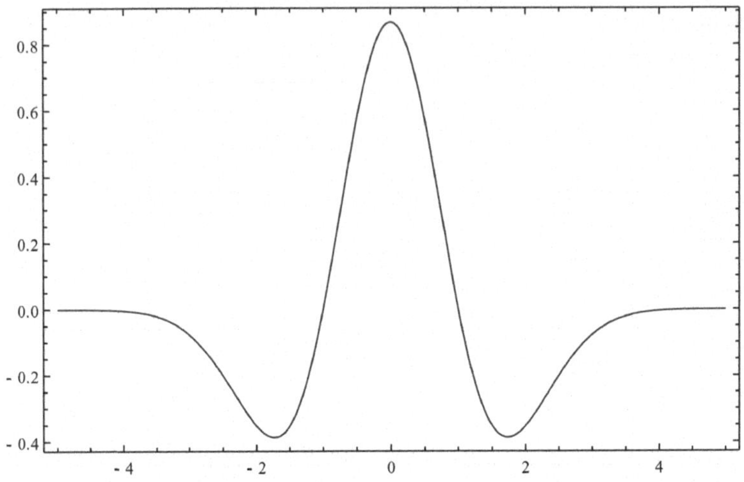

Fig. 6.18 Mexican hat wavelet

6.6.4 Mexican Hat Wavelet

Mexican hat wavelet is also called as "Ricker wavelet" which is the second derivative of the Gaussian function. Sometimes it is also referred to as "Marr wavelet". To get a new type of wavelet, we can apply the Laplacian to the Mexican hat wavelet. This wavelet can also be used to extract the relevant features from images and signals [21]. Figure 6.18 represents the Mexican hat wavelet.

6.6.5 Advantages of Wavelet Transform

Any signal in wavelet transform can be represented in both time domain and in frequency domain. According to scale and resolution, the data can be analysed which is used for timescale representation. Wavelet transform provides compact support. It means that it is able to represent the functions or signals that have localised features. This type of support is widely used in applications like compression, signal detection and denoising. For compressing the image, the property of wavelet transform such as de-correlation, energy compaction, multi-resolution decomposition is very useful to analyse the non-stationary signals and to identify the periods, and phase of signal wavelets is widely used.

6.7 Issues in ECG Classification

(1) Lack of ECG features:
Feature extraction method temporary selects ECG features so accuracy of this method depends on the detected features. A small variation in the values of these features may cause misclassification over large data sets [22].

(2) Variability of ECG features:
Stress, excitement, exercise and other physical activities may vary the heart rate. The changes in heart rate accordingly vary the features such as RR interval, PR interval and QT interval. These features need to be carefully transformed, and the impact of varying heart rate needs to be eliminated [22].

(3) Finding out most appropriate classifier:
Finding out the classifier which is capable of classifying the arrhythmia on real-time is an issue because classification accuracy depends on many parameters such as type of arrhythmia, diversity in arrhythmia, selected arrhythmia database [22].

(4) Removal of noise:
The presence of noise in ECG signal degrades the quality of signal and also affects the accuracy of overall experiment. It provides interruption in further processing. So it becomes essential for the removal of noise. Various methods are available for removing this type of interference. The accuracy of any application is also depended on the amount of noise removed from the input signals [22].

(5) Selection of database:
Database selection for implementing a particular application is a very important task. Different signals have different time duration and frequency, different amplitude and file format. Selection of database is completely depended on the type of application to be implemented. The classification accuracy is depended on the database set. It can be highly affected if the wrong database set is selected [22].

(6) ECG recording analysis:
While recording any biomedical signals, they are in .qrs or in .mat format. The most important task for biomedical signal processing is reading the biomedical signals in the software used (e.g. MATLAB and Python). Defining the sampling frequency, time duration of the signal is also important in further processing [22].

(7) ECG computer simulations:
The ECG recordings that we download are in finite number which directly means that there are limited number of types of heartbeats as well as cardiac conditions. Simulations of electrical activity of heart can also be proposed with the help of graph-based theory (which is one of the fast algorithm techniques) [22].

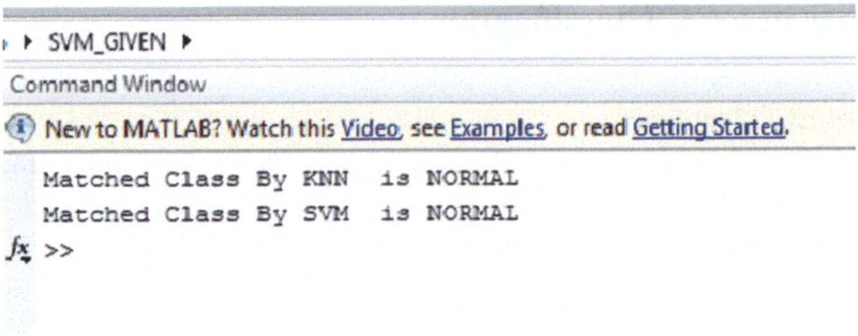

Fig. 6.19 Classification results (MATLAB image)

(8) Comparison of classifiers:
More than one classifier can be implemented for a single application. After overall designing of two or more than two classifiers, we can easily conclude which classifier works well and good for a particular type of application [22].

This algorithm has been tested on 48 ECG signals obtained from MITBIH website. Standard database is available on site called "Physio net". Physio net provides free access to large collections of recorded physiologic signals (Physio bank) and related open-source software (Physio toolkit). ECG features that extracted play a very pivotal role in the diagnosis of cardiac diseases. Daubechies wavelet proves to be the best in analysis of ECG signals due to its similarity with QRS complex. K-nearest neighbour and support vector machine classifier are applied for the classification of ECG arrhythmias. Confusion matrix proved to be a very easy method to calculate the performance measures for both K-nearest neighbour and support vector machine classifiers. The obtained results of the pre-processing, feature extraction and classification are used to conclude the proposed technique. The experimental results of support vector machine-based classifier provided the maximum accuracy of 79.48% for classifying normal and abnormal signals.

Figure 6.19 represents the classification results by using both the classifiers in MATLAB software.

6.8 Discussion Under IoT in Healthcare Domain

Nowadays, many people (young as well as old age people) across the globe are suffering through different types of cardiac problems. This condition mainly arises due to many reasons such as lack of physical exercise, consumption of unhealthy food, stress and consumption of alcohol. Due to the above reasons, the cholesterol (or fats) from our body gets collected within the arteries or veins of heart which leads to the generation of heart blockages. To get over this serious condition, various techniques such as open-heart surgery, bypass surgery, angioplasty are widely used in the medical field. These operational methods are depended on the percentage of blockages created in the heart. If this condition is not treated on time, it may lead to loss of life as well. In order to avoid this abnormality, early precautions should be taken (e.g. consuming healthy food, avoid alcohol, regular physical exercise, performing stress test, avoidance of stress, etc.). This algorithm is mainly implemented to classify all the types of ECG signals whether they are normal ECG signals or abnormal ECG signals. Here the same algorithm can be used for large number of ECG signals. As the number of signals will increase the percentage of performance evaluation (accuracy, sensitivity and specificity) will also increase.

The only problem which can arise during implementation of this algorithm is downloading of ECG signals. As in MITBIH arrhythmia database, all the ECG signals are present in .qrs format. So hence if you are implementing this algorithm in MATLAB software, you first need to convert the signals into .mat format. This step can be done by using online source.

In order to examine which classifier works well for ECG signal processing, various classifiers can be implemented for a single application. The same algorithm can be used for other biomedical signals (such as EEG, EMG). For PhD researchers, this concept can be expanded by detecting various different types of cardiac problems and implementing large number of classifiers. The ECG signals of animals can also be considered if needed. This algorithm is completely implemented in software. But the hardware interface is also possible for this application. We can design a Graphical User Interface (GUI) in order to show the real-time recorded ECG signals and also the classification result (whether the signal is a normal signal or abnormal signal) can also be displayed on the display screen. This algorithm can also be implemented in OpenCV Python software. If Python software is used, the length of code increases because direct commands (such as display ECG signal, mathematical equation for feature extraction and designing of different types of classifiers) are not available in Python as it is available in MATLAB software. If this algorithm is used in real-time basis, more number of lives can be saved without undergoing a type of surgery. The only thing needed to be kept in mind is early precautions should be taken to avoid any kind of cardiovascular diseases. The only good thought which I would like to share with my dear readers is: "Self Care Is The Best Care and Necessity For All The Individuals".

6.9 Conclusion and Future Scope

Support vector machine along with K-nearest neighbour classifier also provided promising classification results in case of arrhythmia and myocardial infarction detection. In addition to this, recognition system can be developed for fast and reliable diagnosis of cardiovascular diseases, which can extend number of heart diseases that can be recognised with better classification accuracy. Wavelet transform can be implemented with multi-resolution analysis using a suitable wavelet family to obtain highly detailed features from signals. This research work can be further extended to test large amount of data to reduce processing time and increase the classification accuracy. Exploration of application of ECG signal is processing for other medical signals. The database can be improved by taking signals of different time duration and selecting different sampling frequency. The variations in the database can increase the performance measures such as accuracy, sensitivity and specificity. More powerful classification algorithms can be used to achieve good results. We can ensure good training by increasing the size of database. Adaptive multiwavelet transform technique can be implemented to perform signal decomposition and to extract the features. To classify more varieties of arrhythmias, advanced soft computing techniques can be included for more clarification. To detect the QRS complex of ECG signals, Adaptive multiwavelet transform can be used. As we have collected the ECG data from MITBIH arrhythmia data sets, the electrodes can be used to collect the signals directly from humans and further identify the cardiac illness by using the same data sets. For the security of stored data, the method known as cancellable biometrics or cryptosystems can be adapted for ECG signals. The P–R and R–R variability analysis can also be used to identify some of the physiological abnormalities. Wearable equipment can regulate information as well as collect the information. It will detect various physiological and psychological parameters along with the resolution of the human body.

References

1. Kulkarni, A., Lale, S., Ingole, P., Gengaje, S. (2016, April). Analysis of ECG signals. *SSRG International Journal of Electronics & Communication Engineering (SSRG-IJECE), 3*(4).
2. Ahmed, W., & Khalid, S. (2016). ECG signal processing for recognition of cardiovascular diseases: A survey. In *The Sixth International Conference on Innovative Computing Technology (INTECH 2016).*
3. Gokhale, P. S. (2012, May). ECG signal de-noising using discrete wavelet transform for removal of 50 Hz PLI noise. *International Journal of Emerging Technology and Advanced Engineering,* 2(5). ISSN 2250-2459.
4. Velayudhan, A., & Peter, S. (2016). Noise analysis and different denoising techniques of ECG signal—a survey. *IOSR Journal of Electronics and Communication Engineering (IOSR-JECE),* 40–44. e-ISSN 2278-2834, p-ISSN 2278-8735.
5. Khandait, P. D., Bawane, N. G., & Limaye, S. S. (2012). Features extraction of ECG signal for detection of cardiac arrhythmias. In *National Conference on Innovative Paradigms in Engineering and Technology (NCIPET-2012) Proceedings published by International Journal of Computer Applications (IJCA).*
6. Miranda, M. V. G., Espinosa, I. P. V., & Calero, M. J. F. (2016). ECG signal features extraction. In *Proc. 2016 IEEE Ecuador technical Chapters Meeting*, 1–6. ISBN: 978-1-5090-1629-7/16.
7. Srivastava, V.K., & Prasad, D. (2013). Dwt based feature extraction from ECG signal. *American Journal of Engineering Research (AJER), 2*(3), 44–50. e-ISSN 2320-0847, p-ISSN 2320-0936.
8. Sambhu, D., & Umesh, A. C. (2013, December). Automatic classification of ECG signals with features extracted using wavelet transform and support vector machines. *International Journal of Advanced Research in Electrical, Electronics and Instrumentation Engineering,* 2(Special Issue 1). (An ISO – 3297:2007 Certified Organisation).
9. Barhatte, A. S., Ghongade, R., & Thakare, A. S. (2015). QRS complex detection and arrhythmia classification using SVM 2015. In *International Conference on Communication, Control and Intelligent Systems (CCIS).*

10. Thomas, N., & Mathew, D. (2016, May). KNN based pattern analysis and classification. *International Journal of Science, Engineering and Technology Research (IJSETR), 5*(5), 1–5. ISSN: 2278–7798.
11. https://monkeylearn.com/blog/introduction-to-support-vector-machines-svm/.
12. https://towardsdatascience.com/machine-learning-classifiers-a5cc4e1b0623.
13. Chakraborty, C. (2017). Chronic wound image analysis by particle swarm optimization technique for tele-wound network. *Springer: International Journal of Wireless Personal Communications, 96*(3), 3655–3671. ISSN: 0929–6212.
14. https://en.wikipedia.org/wiki/Artificial_neural_network.
15. Chakraborty, C. (2019). Computational approach for chronic wound tissue characterization. *Elsevier: Informatics in Medicine Unlocked, 17,* 1–10. https://doi.org/10.1016/j.imu.2019.100162
16. https://link.springer.com/article/10.1007/s10462-009-9124-7.
17. Tan, Y., & Du, L. (2009). Study of wavelet transform in the processing for ECG signals. In *World Congress on Software Engineering.*
18. https://en.wikipedia.org/wiki/Morlet_wavelet.
19. https://en.wikipedia.org/wiki/Haar_wavelet.
20. https://www.mathworks.com/help/wavelet/ref/meyer.html.
21. https://en.wikipedia.org/wiki/Mexican_hat_wavelet.
22. Rangayyan, R. M. (2015). *Biomedical signal analysis—a case study approach.*

Chapter 7
Deep Learning and Its Applications in Medical Imaging

Farzaneh Mansouri Musolu, Saeid Sadeghi Darvazeh, and Iman Raeesi Vanani

Abstract Big data are information assets characterized by high volume, velocity, variety, and veracity. Large, multilevel, and integrated datasets offer the promise of unlocking novel insights and accelerating breakthroughs. According to an increasing interest in artificial intelligence around the world, deep learning has attracted a great deal of public attention. Deep learning techniques increase learning capacity and provide a decision support system at scales that are transforming the future of health care. Every day, deep learning algorithms are used broadly across different industries. The latest advances in deep learning technologies provide new effective paradigms to obtain end-to-end learning models from intricate data. This chapter explains what deep learning is and why it is so important. We provide several examples where deep learning techniques find applications and what kind of problems can be solved using deep learning in medical imaging. This chapter also introduces a particular type of deep learning algorithm, including autoencoders, restricted Boltzmann machines, deep belief network, recurrent neural networks, and convolutional neural networks with practical variant case studies, which are at the basis of deep learning.

Keywords Artificial intelligence · Deep learning techniques · Decision support system · Medical imaging

7.1 Introduction

The healthcare industry historically has generated large volumes of high velocity, complex, and variable data, driven by record keeping, compliance and regulatory requirements, and patient care. These big data require advanced techniques and technologies that provide the possibility of the capture, storage, distribution, management, and analysis of the information. Big data are overwhelming not only because

F. Mansouri Musolu (✉) · S. Sadeghi Darvazeh · I. Raeesi Vanani
Faculty of Management and Accounting, Department of Industrial Management, Allameh Tabataba'i University, West End Hemmat Highway, Dehkadeh-ye-Olympic, 1489684511 Tehran, Iran
e-mail: Farzane_mansouri@atu.ac.ir

C. Chakraborty et al. (eds.), *Internet of Things for Healthcare Technologies*, Studies in Big Data 73, https://doi.org/10.1007/978-981-15-4112-4_7

of its volume but also because of the diversity of data types and the speed at which it must be managed [1].

Machine learning, a popular sub-discipline of artificial intelligence, utilizes large datasets and identifies interaction patterns among variables. These techniques can discover previously unknown associations, generate novel hypotheses, and drive researchers and resources toward most fruitful directions. Machine learning can be applied in various fields, including financial, automatic driving, smart home, etc. In medicine, machine learning is widely used to build automated clinical decision systems. Most machine learning approaches fall into two main categories: supervised and unsupervised methods. Supervised methods are great for classification and regression. Unsupervised learning does not require labeled data. It aims to identify hidden patterns present in the data and is often used in data exploration and novel hypotheses generation. There are other algorithms, such as reinforcement learning, which can be viewed as a combination of supervised and unsupervised learning to maximize the accuracy using trial and error [2].

One of the applications designed in neural networks in medicine was developed by [3], and the idea behind it was to store a large number of medical records containing information about symptoms, diagnose a disease based on the symptoms, and treatment for each case. This uses the auto-associative memory neural network, and network is trained to make predictions on the best diagnosis and treatment based on the different symptoms. Various types of huge datasets are created in modern biomedical, including imaging, electronic health records, sensor data, and text, which are high-dimensional, poorly annotated, complex, heterogeneous, and generally unstructured. Therefore, it is a key challenge in transforming health care to extract knowledge and actionable insights from this complex, heterogeneous and high-dimensional biomedical data. Traditional data mining and statistical learning approaches typically focus on the final mapping and need to first perform feature engineering to create smart representations of the data and then make prediction or clustering [4]. Some challenges exist on both steps of feature engineering and prediction or clustering in a scenario of poorly annotated, complex, heterogeneous, and generally unstructured data. The latest advances in deep learning technologies provide new effective paradigms to obtain end-to-end learning models from intricate data. Deep learning is a class of machine learning techniques where information is processed in hierarchical layers, to understand representations and features from the data in increasing levels of complexity. In deep learning (DL) technologies, the networks do not simply learn to predict outputs given input examples, but they also learn basic aspects of the data structure. One of the reasons why deep neural networks can succeed than other traditional machine learning techniques is the neural network capable of making abstractions features that comprise the input examples, learning the basic characteristics of the examples, and making predictions based on those characteristics without needing (much) human and domain knowledge. In addition, deep models learn diffused basic features of the input examples, which empower generalization to new combinations of the values of learned features beyond those seen during the training process. The other reason for the popularity of deep learning today is the drastically increased processing capacity of graphical processing units

(GPUs). In a deep neural network with many layers and a large number of neurons, bandwidth becomes the bottleneck, and this is the reason why GPUs perform are used to optimize the bandwidth. Recent advances in DL show that computers can extract more information from images, more reliably, and more accurately than ever before [4].

Recently, deep learning techniques have been applied to a wide range of medical image analysis tasks (classification, segmentation, registration, detection, enhancement, image reconstruction, etc.) across a wide range of anatomical sites (brain, heart, lung, abdomen, breast, prostate, musculature, etc.) [5]. IBM by using deep learning techniques is Intend to make prediction on possible heart failures, reading doctor's notes, and prescription, similarly to an experienced cardiologist.

This chapter purposes to present some of the most fundamental and recent applications of the deep learning techniques in the medical imaging and their experimental analysis with advantages and disadvantages. Regarding this purpose, first, the key concepts and general principles of deep learning and its application in medical imaging are presented. Second, a review on the application of deep learning in medical imaging such as image classification, image detection, image segmentation, image registration is presented. Third, we pay to various deep learning algorithms and their advantages and disadvantages in medical imaging. Fourth, some of the challenges of deep learning in healthcare data and developed techniques for tackling them are noticed. Fifth, in this chapter some insight about the future application of deep learning in medical imaging are presented, and lastly, the chapter ends with the conclusion, some managerial implications, and recommendations for the future research.

In the healthcare industry, an extremely large amount of data has been created that increases the training time. On account of large, multilevel, and integrated imaging datasets, deep learning joined with computerized reasoning could enhance the reliability of clinical choice decision supportive networks. Although more data are available than ever, only a fraction is being curated, integrated, understood, and analyzed; therefore, techniques and technologies are required to enable the capture, storage, distribution, management, and analysis of the information. In terms of big data aspects, the volume of medical data which is needed to train a robust and effective deep learning model could be more than other media [6]. Healthcare data are very redundant, noisy, incomplete, heterogeneous, and vague. Training a fine DL model is correlated such as massive and variety datasets are challenging, and many issues like data redundancy, missing value, and sparsity are required to considered [7]. Data need to be extracted, transform, and loaded into a data warehouse and combines data from multiple sources into a coherent store. The integration of medical image analysis methods and other patient data such as demographics, patient history, and age could further improve the performance of clinical decision-making aids. Moreover, preprocessing techniques seem to contribute substantially to good performance and robustness of analysis techniques [8].

Although artificial intelligence increases learning capacity and provides a decision support system at scales that are transforming the future of healthcare, we should never lose sight and experience of experts. The aim of the application of deep

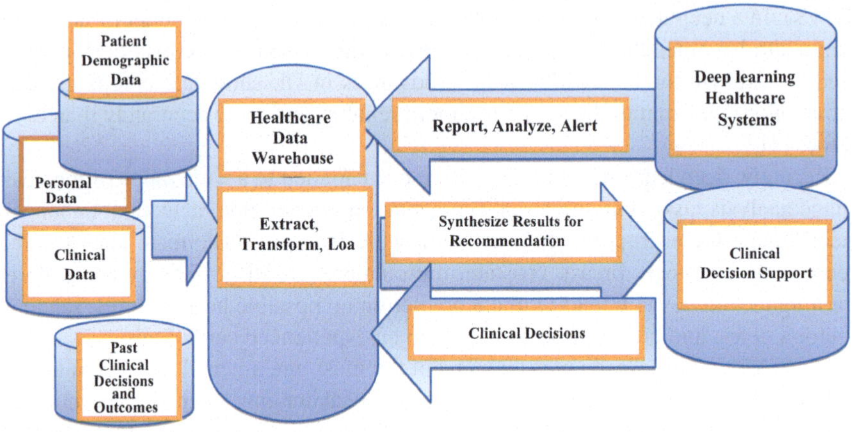

Fig. 7.1 Process of data analysis

learning techniques or other artificial intelligence techniques is to provide a decision support system. "Conventional" image analysis methods were never intended to replace radiologists but rather to serve as a second opinion [8]. Expert knowledge about the clinical task can provide advantages that go beyond adding more layers to a CNN, and incorporating expert medical knowledge with artificial intelligence techniques to optimize methods, for example, through novel data preprocessing or augmentation techniques and for a specific clinical task is often crucial in obtaining good performance. It is possible to combine the outputs of deep learning methods with the knowledge of the field of medical imaging analysis which has accumulated with computer-extracted and handcrafted features [8]. Analysis of medical data is a process that begins with extracting, transforming, and loading data into a healthcare data warehouse, and data from multiple sources into a coherent store are combined. Analysis should be performed on this large, multilevel, and integrated datasets if necessary. Figure 7.1 shows the process of data analysis in the healthcare industry.

The analysis of medical data is a process that begins with extracting, transforming, and loading data into a healthcare data warehouse, and data from multiple sources into a coherent store are combined. Analysis should be performed on this large, multilevel, and integrated datasets if necessary. Then expert medical knowledge with outputs of deep learning methods combines to optimize methods. Finally, the results and outputs load into the healthcare data warehouse.

7.2 Deep Learning

Deep learning algorithms have become a successful approach for automated extraction of complex data representation for end-to-end training [9]. Deep learning algorithms consist of layered and hierarchical architectures of neurons, which automatically extract features and abstractions from the underlying data [10]. The key difference between deep learning and traditional machine learning techniques is that the former can automatically learn effective and more robust features of the data, thereby eliminating the need for handcrafted features. In deep learning, the neural network can learn representations, deep learning algorithms are less sensitive to noise, and deep learning can be a generative algorithm. What is more interesting is that deep learning has the transfer learning property and this means that the effective and abstraction features learned from one dataset can be useful even when they are applied to a different set of data. Because deep learning requires large training data, the transfer learning property is particularly useful in cases where relevant data for a particular task are scarce. Deep learning is a multilayer neural network that has at least two hidden layers between the input and output layers. The hidden layers work similarly for a deeper understanding of the complex features of the data. Deep learning refers not only to the depth of the network (number of hidden layers of the neural net), but also to the level and depth of learning [4].

Deep learning techniques have yielded prominent results in analyzing health-related data, such as speech recognition, ICU mortality prediction, phenotype discovery, and disease prediction. Recently, deep learning techniques have been applied to train a wide range of medical natural images to learn proper feature representations that allow it to see. The trained technique can subsequently use these representations to produce an encoding of a medical image that is used for classification.

This chapter highlights the till date progress of the thirteen deep learning techniques, namely autoencoders, stacked autoencoders, recurrent neural networks (RNNs), LSTMs, gated recurrent unit (GRU), variants of RNN, Boltzmann machines (BM), restricted Boltzmann machines (RBM), deep belief networks (DBN), convolutional neural networks (CNN), and variant of CNNs. This chapter tries to reflect some of the most fundamental and recent applications of deep learning techniques in medical imaging and also to identify some of the challenges and opportunities of these techniques.

7.3 The List of Basics of Various Deep Learning Algorithms

In the previous paragraph, we have given an intuitive introduction to deep learning. In this section, we will give a more precise definition and introduction of key concepts of deep learning algorithms. Deep learning is a class of machine learning techniques where information is automatically processed in hierarchical layers, to extract features and representations from the data in increasing levels of complexity [4]. In this class of algorithms, we can generally include.

7.3.1 Autoencoders

Autoencoders are a class of powerful unsupervised learning algorithms, which are getting popularity in fields such as feature engineering or anomaly detection, using the output of intermediate layers as features to train a supervised model instead of the raw input data. Denoising, contractive, and autoencoders are great techniques for building an autoencoder network to achieve robustness in order to avoid wrong representations; but at the same time, not limit the capacity of the network by compressing the information through smaller sequential layers [4].

Contractive autoencoders make the model to be more stable to small deviations from the training distribution and also reduce false alarms. Contractive autoencoders are very good at compression the data. For example given an image of 128×128 pixels, a representation of a 14×14 pixel may be learned, which is easier to handle. Denoising autoencoder is also used to reproduce corrupted data, which is often in image form data. On the other hand, the stacked denoising autoencoder is used to pre-train deep networks. Stack autoencoder (SAE) is a deep learning model that is used to optimize deep learning solutions and avoid being stuck in local minima. Sparse autoencoders provide a good tradeoff between low reconstruction error and stability, and they are used in case of second-order optimizers [4].

7.3.2 Restricted Boltzmann Machines

Boltzmann machine (BM) is a symmetric network with a well-defined energy function. BM can be applied in fields such as recommendation and optimization systems. They are very computationally expensive. Correlation must be measured between every single node, and then a range of Monte Carlo samples must be generated from the model for every training step. Also, the kinds of patterns it can learn are limited. Restricted Boltzmann machines (RBM) are used as a pre-training process as a feature extractor for classification problems in the unsupervised learning approach. Restricted Boltzmann machines (RBM) are widely used in collaborative filtering, topic modeling, feature learning, dimensionality reduction, and classifications [7]. However, the RBM is not suitable in the supervised learning approach and also because of the complications of choosing variables. In addition, because of RBM model is not suitable for multiclass classification tasks, CRBM can be applied as nonlinear generative models for high-dimensional time series data. It also can be applied to get rich distributed representation in order to certain efficiency of precise inference. However, the RBM model is not robust to noise present in the data when they are used for image processing and speech recognition.

7.3.3 Deep Belief Network

Deep belief networks (DBNs) are a combination of unsupervised networks (RBMs) and sigmoid belief networks. DBN is widely used to design a strong generative model applying training data, learn features, and classify. DBNs are stochastic generative models where the top layers have symmetric connections between them (undirected, unlike feed-forward networks), while the bottom layers receive the processed information from directed connections from the layers above them. DBN is a combination of each two adjoining layer structure an RBM. The visible layer of every RBM is joined to the hidden layer of the antecedent RBM, and the top two layers are undirected symmetric connections between them. In DBN the distinct layer of RBM is trained sequentially. Firstly, the input layer of RBMs is trained subsequently followed by higher layers. After extracting the feature from top RBM layer, they can be propagated back to the top-down layers using the conditional probabilities. The stacked RBM will enhance the top limit of the log-likelihood compared to the single RBM, which intimates powerful learning capabilities.

7.3.4 Recurrent Neural Networks

Recurrent neural network (RNN) is an ANNs which consist of many hidden neurons capable of examining streams of information [4]. RNN is used in many fields such as text data and speech data. This generally uses the training data that have strong meaningful representation and interdependencies to preserve data about what occurred in the previous time steps. Another variation of RNN is gated recurrent unit (GRU) which was presented to resolve the vanishing gradient problems of RNNs. LSTM and GRU are designed similarly to resolve the vanishing gradient problems, and they have two gates named as reset and update gate. LSTM and GRU are designed similarly to resolve the vanishing gradient problems, and they have two gates named as reset and update gate, which take the decision of what information should be given to the output. The important advantage of GRU is that it can be trained to keep data from a long time without washing it through time or remove data which is irrelevant to the prediction [9]. Bidirectional LSTM is a new deep LSTM model based on wavelet sequences that it was proposed by Yildirim (2018) to classifying ECG signal database [10].

7.3.5 Convolutional Neural Networks

Convolutional neural networks (CNN) are DL techniques which they are inspired by the natural visual perception techniques. CNNs apply filters to the input image (or sound) by sliding this filter all across the incoming signal to produce a bi-dimensional activation map. These networks are able to extract all the features hidden from the inputs. CNNs are capable of providing powerful and accurate representation of the real images which construct visual patterns precisely from the raw images with no preprocessing and make the identification of real images possible from the visual patterns. Since 2006 numerous techniques have evolved to overcome problems encountered in training of deep CNNs, recursive convolution networks are novel techniques that they can be observed like CNNs with a similar quantity of feature maps in whole layers and bind filter weight across layers. ZFNet is a visualization method that takes the insight into a function in between feature layers and the operation of classifiers [11].

Each of these deep learning algorithms has its own advantages and disadvantages, and they can be easier or harder to train depending on the number of layers and neurons in each layer. Numerous techniques have evolved to overcome problems encountered in deep learning algorithms. Different variants of these algorithms will be shown in Table 7.1.

Table 7.1 Brief description of deep learning techniques in the medical healthcare system

Deep learning techniques	Variant of techniques
Autoencoder (AE) and stack autoencoder Advantage 1. No need for labeled data for training of AE 2. Presenting to make a robust representation like denoising autoencoders, contractive autoencoders, K-sparse autoencoder, separable deep autoencoder Disadvantage 1. Not widely used in real-world applications 2. A need of pre-training of model 3. The trained model also suffers from the vanishing gradient problem	DAE/ CAE/ SDAE/ SAEs Used for 1. Unsupervised learning techniques to efficient data coding 2. Output values to be equal to the input values 3. Goal to reproduce the input vector 4. Most intuitive use of AE is data compression
Restricted Boltzmann Machine (RBM) Advantage 1. RBM generally transform high-dimensional raw 2. Healthcare data into a uniform representation 3. Fast algorithms can be applied because of restrictions put on connections between hidden-hidden and visible-visible units Disadvantage 1. RBM is trained in an unsupervised manner, so there is no guarantee that the feature derived from the hidden layer of RMB will eventually be useful for supervised work 2. RBM accept unstructured input data but ignores explicit structures inherent in the healthcare record	convRBMs/DRBM/(CRBM) Used for 1. Initially proposed by Ackley et al. [12] is a kind of stochastic neural network 2. Information flows bilaterally during the training 3. To train RBM, the most algorithm performs Gibbs sampling and to speed up the sampling used contrastive divergence process

(continued)

Table 7.1 (continued)

Deep learning techniques	Variant of techniques
Deep Belief Network Advantage 1. The main advantage of DBN is its capability of learning features which is achieved by a layer-by-layer learning strategies 2. DBN processes unlabeled data effectively and the problem of overfitting and underfitting may also be avoided Disadvantage 1. When the DBN is pre-trained by using CD algorithms, the performance is not satisfactory because of input information is clamped 2. Increasing run-time complexity	DBN-softmax/ARIMA & DBN/DBN & RBM/DBN & Gaussian kernel Used for 1. DBN can be viewed as a combination of RBM + sigmoid belief networks 2. It learns to extract a deep hierarchical representation of the training data 3. The learning process of a DBN has been split into two steps: pre-training step and discriminative fine-tuning step
Recurrent Neural Networks (RNNs) Advantage 1. RNN stores information over time in the form of activations 2. It can handle sequential information of random the length and has shown great success in many NLP applications	LSTMs/GRU/deep LSTM model/RNN-LSTM/two-layer LSTM/LSTM Used for 1. The aim of RNN is to use sequential data 2. Network output also depends on previous computations
Convolutional Neural Networks (CNNs) Advantage 1. Sparse representation (CNN extracts only relevant features from input dataset) Parameter sharing (CNN reuses the same parameter across different functions) 1. Parameter sharing (CNN reuse the same Disadvantage 1. Hyper-parameter tuning is non-trivial 2. Need a large database	Recursive convolution networks/ZFNe/ILSVRC/GoogLeNet and winner of ILSVRC 2014/deep CNNs Used for 1. The idea of CNN is motivated by time-delay neural network where the weight sharing is limited 2. CNN is an NN which used convolution operation in place of simple matrix multiplication in at least one of their layers 3. CNN is used basically to classify image dataset

Denoising autoencoders (DAE) for denoising the normal; autoencoders; contractive autoencoders (CAE); separable deep autoencoder (SDAE); stack autoencoder (SAEs); convolutional RBMs (convRBMs); discriminative restricted; Boltzmann machine (DRBM); conditional RBM (CRBM); DBN with Gaussian kernel (DBN & Gaussian kernel); DBN with multiple layers of RBM (DBN & RBM); DBN and a Softmax classifier (DBN-softmax); combination of autoregressive integrated moving average (ARIMA) model and DBN (ARIMA & DBN); long short-term memory (LSTM); gated recurrent unit (GRU); deep LSTM model; ImageNet large-scale visual recognition challenge (ILSVRC)

7.4 Application of Deep Learning in Medical Healthcare System Medical Imaging

Deep learning techniques are used in the medical imaging field in various ways. The most prolific but crucial task in modern time is to survey medical imaging in modern medicine [7]. Medical imaging is the main reason for the development of the classification, segmentation, regeneration, detection, diagnosis, and characterization. Deep learning has contributed a lot to the image analysis in the medical imaging field. Since utilizing tremendous information applications, it is exceptionally hard to acquire named informational collection; the regulated learning calculations can barely give attractive execution in such cases. In light of these deep learning compositions, unsupervised learning calculations are now used to process the unlabeled information. The most recent use of deep learning techniques in segmentation and lesion detection has shown to be the best performance. So far, two types of strategies have been applied to these tasks in the research literature. First is to use deep learning networks for estimating a similarity measure between two images for driving an iterative optimization strategy and the second one is by directly predicting transformation parameters using deep regression parameters [7].

7.4.1 Image Registration

Medical image registration (via spatial alignment) is a common image analysis task which involves transforming a coordinate by calculating from one medical to another [7]. Cheng [13] applied two types of SAE for estimating the local similarity between CT and MRI. To assess a similarity cost between two matches from differing modalities, CNNs are used by Simonovsky [14]. Deep learning techniques such as CNN facilitate and improve classification by providing the ability to automatically extract features. The authors identify the uses of discriminative local appearance for training are much accurate than the training based on global image context. Hybrid methods where CNNs combine with other deep learning compositions are also introduced [15]. Deep learning composition is combined with deformable models to evolve and estimate a whole automatic segmentation for the left ventricle (LV) from short-axis cardiac MRI [16]. CNNs are enrolled to automatically recognize the LV chamber in MRI database, and stacked AEs are employed to deduce its shape. More detailed interpretation of many CNN compositions introduced in medical image analysis is shown in the survey [17].

7.4.2 Image Classification

Deep learning technology was first used in the medical image to image classification [7]. Deep learning techniques that are generally used in multiclass classification include SAEs, RBM, and DBN. SAEs and DBN are used to classify Alzheimer's disease patients data based on MRI [12, 18, 19]. Tacked autoencoder (SAE) is utilized to enhance the classification accuracy in brain disease diagnosis and prognosis [18]. Sergey [12] applies deep learning methods that include deep belief networks and their building block that restricted Boltzmann machine to structural and functional brain imaging data. Their results show that deep learning methods are able to learn physiologically important representations and detect latent relations in neuroimaging data. Recently, CNN technique is widely applied for classification. From 2015 to 2017 based on multiclass classification, 36 papers that used CNN for classification have been published. The application of these models is very different ranging from brain MRI to retinal imaging and digital pathology to lung CT imaging. Recently, CNN technique is widely used for imaging classification. Synergic deep learning (SDL) model (by applying multiple deep convolutional neural networks (DCNNs) has allowed for significant gains in the ability to classify images and detect objects in a picture [2].

7.4.3 Image Segmentation

Segmentation in medical imaging is one of the common subjects of researches that have seen a great influx of methods related to deep learning. Segmentation of organs and their substructures may be used to calculate clinical parameters such as volume as well as to define the search region for computer-aided detection tasks to improve their performance [8]. Recently, RNNs have been used to segmentation task. For example, Xie [20] applied a spatial RNN clockwork for segmenting the perimysium in images of H&E histopathology. The results obtaining from deep convolutional neural networks (DCNN) for the segmentation task compared to results obtains with CNNs were promising [21]. The deep learning platform for medical imaging (NiftyNet) provides a modular deep learning pipeline for a range of medical imaging applications including segmentation, regression, image generation, and representation learning applications [22]. Components of the NiftyNet pipeline including data loading, data augmentation, network architectures, loss functions, and evaluation metrics are tailored to and take advantage of the idiosyncrasies of medical image analysis and computer-assisted intervention. NiftyNet is built on the TensorFlow framework and supports features such as TensorBoard visualization of 2D and 3D images and computational graphs by default [22]. Wang and co-worker propose a novel deep learning-based interactive segmentation framework by incorporating CNNs into a bounding box and scribble-based segmentation pipeline [23]. In the recent research, patch-based CNNs, end-to-end 3D CNNs, and fully convolutional network (FCN) architectures have been applied to semantic segmentation tasks in medical imaging. Another new deep learning structure that is being used for the segmentation of organs is holistically nested networks (HNN). HNN has been successfully implemented in the segmentation of the prostate and brain tumors [22].

7.4.4 *Image Detection*

Detecting and localizing the location of the anatomical object (in space or time) such as landmarks, organs, and various other images are a fundamental step of preprocessing in the clinical workflow of therapy planning or in segmentation tasks as this helps in simplifying the process of segmentation. Medical image processing requires parsing of 3D volumes of data. Various deep learning techniques have been proposed to solve the problem of 3D information parsing problem. Landmark of the 3D position can be described as three 2D slices intersection with the greatest classification results [8]. Despite the importance of the problem of direct detection and localization of objects and landmarks in 3D pictures, a limited method has been proposed to solve it. A sparse adoptive DNN powered by marginal space learning has been employed to detect and localize the aortic valve in 3D transesophageal echocardiogram [24]. CNNs are famous for being used in the recognition of scan planes or keyframes in temporal information available. To detect and recognize the temporal information in medical videos of high dimension information, various deep learning models are used such as CNNs and RNNs, specifically LSTM-RNNs. For example, Chen [25] has used an LSTM algorithm for the detection of fetal standard plane. Dong [26] proposes a CNN and graph cut optimization in order to segment femur and locate the anatomical landmarks from the 3D MR images. Chen [25] proposes a novel knowledge transferred recurrent neural network (T-RNN) to explore spatiotemporal feature learning. T-RNN incorporates a deep hierarchical visual feature extractor and a temporal sequence learning model. It is possible to combine the outputs of deep learning methods with the knowledge of the field of medical imaging analysis which has accumulated with computer-extracted, handcrafted features [8]. Some studies suggest that combining deep learning with traditional information already known to be useful can improve the performance of these deep learning models [27].

7.4.4.1 Organ Detection

Detecting and localizing the anatomical structure is an important step of preprocessing in medical image analysis as this helps in simplifying the process of organ segmentation, radiotherapy planning, and lesion detection. Anatomical structure detection involves computing the location information of organs and landmarks in 2D or 3D image data [8]. Deep learning techniques and modern techniques (e.g., reinforcement learning) are two approaches adopted to tackle the organ/landmark detection problem [24]. Deep learning techniques for organ/landmark detection similar to traditional machine learning can be divided into two categories: regression-based ones and classification-based methods. Classification-based methods for organ/landmark detection focus on discriminating body parts/organs on the image or patch level but regression-based methods target at recovering more detailed location information, for example, coordinates of landmarks [8]. Baumgartner [28] presented a CNN framework to classify 12 standard scan planes and also localize fetal anatomy using a series of ultrasound fetal mid-pregnancy scans. Adapting and applying the CNN network with other advanced architecture and components significantly improve performance. Ghesu [24] tackles the 3D heart detection task problems with regression analysis techniques. This approach is integrated marginal space learning into the DL framework and learned sparse sampling to reduce computational cost in the volumetric dataset.

7.4.4.2 Lesion Detection

Detection of abnormalities (including tumors and other suspicious growths) is a difficult task because their locations are often initially unclear; therefore, the physician should look for across the 2D image or 3D volume to find deviations compared to surrounding tissue. Then physician should determine whether that deviation is an abnormality that requires follow-up and investigation procedures or something that can be dismissed from further investigation. Due to errors that may occur at this difficult task, therefore, automated computer detection algorithms have been of great interest for shortening reading times, reducing reading costs, and thereby simplifying the clinical workflow, and providing more quality and precise care for those living in deprived areas and have limited access to specialists [8]. Deep learning approaches are used to tackle the time-consuming pipeline design approach. Many of the papers apply transfer learning with architectures from computer vision in order to detect tasks [8]. For example, this approach is used for the detection of the third lumbar vertebra slice in a CT scan, for the detection of bowel obstructions in radiography, and for lesion detection in breast ultrasound.

7.4.5 Diagnosis

Computer-aided diagnosis (CADx) is a characterization/classification task that first characterizes the suspicious region or lesion and/or then estimates the likelihood of being diseased or non-diseased. Recently, characterization of diseases has been attempted with deep learning methods to disease diagnosis. Features that used to the interpretation of a medical image include shape, tumor size, texture, and/or kinetics (for dynamic contrast-enhanced imaging). DL characterization methods may take as input a region of the image around the potential disease site, such as a region of interest (ROI) around a suspect lesion. How that ROI is determined will likely affect the training and performance of the DL. Some of the techniques used to characterization of diseases include CNN architecture, conventional texture analysis, and deep learning, conventional CAD/radionics computer algorithms, radiomic texture analysis, DCNNs. More deep learning techniques have been used to diagnose breast cancer [8]. Given the variations in tumor presentations and initial limited datasets, training CNNs from scratch on this data is often not possible, so the methods of CNNs trained on nonmedical tasks (transfer learning) are used to extract tumor characteristics and in addition augment CNN performance by exploiting the four-dimensional nature of DCE-MRI (3D and temporal). Incorporation of temporal information into the DL efforts has resulted in the use of RNN, such as LSTM recurrent networks. Combining CNN-based CADx and conventional radiomics CADx methodology gave a statistically significant level of performance in distinguishing between malignant and benign breast lesions [8]. Investigators have used transfer learning for fine-tuning by either (a) freezing the earlier layers of a pre-trained CNN and training the later layers, that is, fine-tuning or (b) training on one modality, such as digitized screen/film mammography (dSFM), for use on a related modality, such as full-field digital mammography (FFDM) [8]. Recently, Samala [29] has been shown that multitask transfer learning may be an effective approach for training DCNN in lesion diagnosis on FFDMs. An artificial intelligence (AI) using a deep learning approach can classify retinal images from optical coherence tomography for early diagnosis of retinal diseases and has the potential to be used in other image-based medical diagnoses [30]. Kermany [31] develops an AI framework for detecting CNV, DME, and drusen from OCT images. Their AI framework used the transfer learning approach Inception V3 on a training set and was repeated for 100 iterations using three different approaches.

Figure 7.2 shows the four-section graph of analysis of the medical image. This process involves understanding the task, preprocessing operations, selecting appropriate deep learning models, as well as evaluation, concluding and interpreting it.

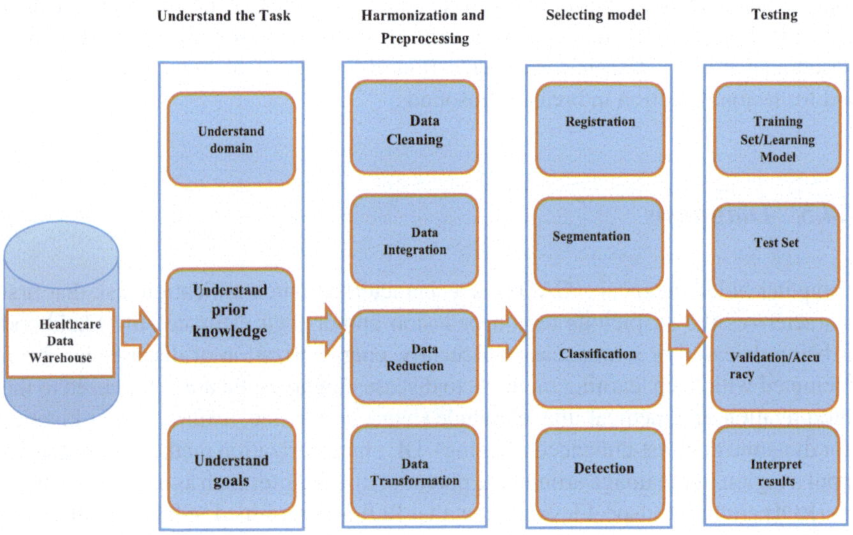

Fig. 7.2 Four-section graph of analysis

7.5 Conclusion and Managerial Implications

Deep learning techniques increase learning capacity and provide a decision support system at scales that are transforming the future of healthcare. In this chapter, unequivocally recent variants of the five models of deep learning techniques named the autoencoders, restricted Boltzmann machines, deep belief network, recurrent neural networks, and convolutional neural networks are illuminated in medical imaging. A review of the literature revealed that models of hybrid deep learning often work well than single models because they have the combined feature of techniques or learning methods. Combining the outputs of deep learning methods with the information of the field of medical imaging analysis already known to be useful may improve the performance of these deep learning models.

Since utilizing tremendous information applications, it is exceptionally hard to acquire named informational collection; the regulated learning calculations can barely give attractive execution in such cases. In light of these deep learning compositions, unsupervised learning calculations are now used to process the unlabeled information. Massive and variety datasets are challenging and advanced techniques, and technologies are required to enable the capture, storage, distribution, management, and analysis of the information. Moreover, we need to investigate and improve, develop standards for reporting as well as experiments, and have better access to annotated image data such as publicly available datasets to serve as independent benchmarks. On account of the availability of big data, advances in deep learning algorithms, and processing power, deep learning revolution could enhance the reliability of clinical choice decision supportive networks. In any case, few specialized difficulties remain to be settled. First, understanding and acquiring clinical information are expensive. Second, deep learning technique calculations have for the most part been applied in applications where the datasets were integrated, adjusted, and large, or, as a work-around, in which manufactured information was added to attain value. Another difficulty is that deep adapting dominatingly depends upon a lot of information processing. Thus, these difficulties lead to the improvement of consistent and quick gear for well-being observing and analyses will assume a noticeable part in the future research. Incorporating expert medical knowledge with deep learning techniques to optimize methods, for example, through novel data preprocessing or augmentation techniques, for a specific clinical task is often crucial in obtaining good performance. A wide variety of techniques have been developed for tackling the data shortage problem for both the general computer vision and medical image analysis domain. We need to investigate and present abundant new methods aimed at alleviating the limited dataset size problem. Data augmentation is the most straightforward way to increase the size of a dataset for training purposes.

References

1. Sadeghi Darvazeh, S., Raeesi Vanani, I., & Mansouri Mosolu, F. (2020). Application of big data analytics in supply chain management. *New Trends in the Use of Artificial Intelligence for the Industry 4.0.*
2. Noorbakhsh-Sabet, N., Zand, R., Zhang, Y., & Abedi, V. (2019). Artificial intelligence transforms the future of healthcare. *The American Journal of Medicine, 132,* 795–801.
3. Anderson, D. Z. (1986, August). Optical resonators and neural networks. In *AIP Conference Proceedings* (Vol. 151, No. 1, pp. 12–16). American Institute of Physics.
4. Zocca, V., Spacagna, G., Slater, D., & Roelants, P. (2017). *Python deep learning*. Packt Publishing Ltd.
5. Litjens, G., Kooi, T., Bejnordi, B. E., Setio, A. A. A., Ciompi, F., Ghafoorian, M. … Sánchez, C. I. (2017). A survey on deep learning in medical image analysis. *Medical Image Analysis, 42,* 60–88.
6. Najafabadi, M. M., Villanustre, F., Khoshgoftaar, T. M., Seliya, N., Wald, R., & Muharemagic, E. (2015). Deep learning applications and challenges in big data analytics. *Journal of Big Data, 2*(1), 1.
7. Pandey, S. K., & Janghel, R. R. (2019). Recent deep learning techniques, challenges and its applications for medical healthcare system: A review. *Neural Processing Letters, 50*(2), 1907–1935.
8. Sahiner, B., Pezeshk, A., Hadjiiski, L. M., Wang, X., Drukker, K., Cha, K. H., et al. (2019). Deep learning in medical imaging and radiation therapy. *Medical Physics, 46*(1), e1–e36.
9. Shie, C. K., Chuang, C. H., Chou, C. N., Wu, M. H., & Chang, E. Y. (2015, August). Transfer representation learning for medical image analysis. In *2015 37th Annual International Conference of the IEEE Engineering in Medicine and Biology Society (EMBC)* (pp. 711–714). IEEE.
10. Yildirim, Ö. (2018). A novel wavelet sequence based on deep bidirectional LSTM network model for ECG signal classification. *Computers in Biology and Medicine, 96,* 189–202.
11. Zeiler, M. D., & Fergus, R. (2014, September). Visualizing and understanding convolutional networks. In *European Conference on Computer Vision* (pp. 818–833). Cham: Springer.
12. Plis, S. M., Hjelm, D. R., Salakhutdinov, R., Allen, E. A., Bockholt, H. J., Long, J. D. … Calhoun, V. D. (2014). Deep learning for neuroimaging: A validation study. *Frontiers in Neuroscience, 8,* 229.
13. Cheng, X., Zhang, L., & Zheng, Y. (2018). Deep similarity learning for multimodal medical images. *Computer Methods in Biomechanics and Biomedical Engineering: Imaging & Visualization, 6*(3), 248–252.
14. Simonovsky, M., Gutiérrez-Becker, B., Mateus, D., Navab, N., & Komodakis, N. (2016, October). A deep metric for multimodal registration. In *International Conference on Medical Image Computing and Computer-Assisted Intervention* (pp. 10–18). Cham: Springer.
15. Majumdar, A., & Singhal, V. (2017, May). Noisy deep dictionary learning: Application to Alzheimer's Disease classification. In *2017 International Joint Conference on Neural Networks (IJCNN)* (pp. 2679–2683). IEEE.
16. Avendi, M. R., Kheradvar, A., & Jafarkhani, H. (2016). A combined deep-learning and deformable-model approach to fully automatic segmentation of the left ventricle in cardiac MRI. *Medical Image Analysis, 30,* 108–119.
17. Havaei, M., Dutil, F., Pal, C., Larochelle, H., & Jodoin, P. M. (2015, October). A convolutional neural network approach to brain tumor segmentation. In *BrainLes 2015* (pp. 195–208). Cham: Springer.
18. Brosch, T., Tam, R., & Alzheimer's Disease Neuroimaging Initiative. (2013, September). Manifold learning of brain MRIs by deep learning. In *International Conference on Medical Image Computing and Computer-Assisted Intervention* (pp. 633–640). Berlin, Heidelberg: Springer.
19. Suk, H. I., & Shen, D. (2013, September). Deep learning-based feature representation for AD/MCI classification. In *International Conference on Medical Image Computing and Computer-Assisted Intervention* (pp. 583–590). Berlin, Heidelberg: Springer.

20. Xie, Y., Zhang, Z., Sapkota, M., & Yang, L. (2016, October). Spatial clockwork recurrent neural network for muscle perimysium segmentation. In *International Conference on Medical Image Computing and Computer-Assisted Intervention* (pp. 185–193). Cham:Springer.
21. Soltaninejad, M., Zhang, L., Lambrou, T., Yang, G., Allinson, N., & Ye, X. (2017, September). MRI brain tumor segmentation and patient survival prediction using random forests and fully convolutional networks. In *International MICCAI Brainlesion Workshop* (pp. 204–215). Cham: Springer.
22. Gibson, E., Li, W., Sudre, C., Fidon, L., Shakir, D. I., Wang, G. … Whyntie, T. (2018). NiftyNet: A deep-learning platform for medical imaging. *Computer Methods and Programs in Biomedicine, 158*, 113–122.
23. Wu, G., Kim, M., Wang, Q., Gao, Y., Liao, S., & Shen, D. (2013, September). Unsupervised deep feature learning for deformable registration of MR brain images. In *International Conference on Medical Image Computing and Computer-Assisted Intervention* (pp. 649–656). Berlin, Heidelberg: Springer.
24. Ghesu, F. C., Krubasik, E., Georgescu, B., et al. (2016). Marginal space deep learning: Efficient architecture for volumetric image parsing. *IEEE Transactions on Medical Imaging, 35*, 1217–1228.
25. Chen, H., Dou, Q., Ni, D., Cheng, J. Z., Qin, J., Li, S., & Heng, P. A. (2015, October). Automatic fetal ultrasound standard plane detection using knowledge transferred recurrent neural networks. In *International Conference on Medical Image Computing and Computer-Assisted Intervention* (pp. 507–514). Cham: Springer.
26. Dong, C., Loy, C. C., He, K., & Tang, X. (2015). Image super-resolution using deep convolutional networks. *IEEE Transactions on Pattern Analysis and Machine Intelligence, 38*(2), 295–307.
27. Li, N., Huynh, B. Q., & Giger, M. L. (2017). A deep feature fusion methodology for breast cancer diagnosis demonstrated on three imaging modality datasets. *Medical Physics, 44*(10), 5162–5171.
28. Baumgartner, C. F., Kamnitsas, K., Matthew, J., Smith, S., Kainz, B., & Rueckert, D. (2016, October). Real-time standard scan plane detection and localisation in fetal ultrasound using fully convolutional neural networks. In *International Conference on Medical Image Computing and Computer-Assisted Intervention* (pp. 203–211). Cham: Springer.
29. Samala, R. K., Chan, H. P., Hadjiiski, L. M., Helvie, M. A., Cha, K. H., & Richter, C. D. (2017). Multi-task transfer learning deep convolutional neural network: Application to computer-aided diagnosis of breast cancer on mammograms. *Physics in Medicine & Biology, 62*(23), 8894.
30. Ting, D. S., Liu, Y., Burlina, P., Xu, X., Bressler, N. M., & Wong, T. Y. (2018). AI for medical imaging goes deep. *Nature Medicine, 24*(5), 539–540.
31. Kermany, D. S., Goldbaum, M., Cai, W., Valentim, C. C., Liang, H., Baxter, S. L., et al. (2018). Identifying medical diagnoses and treatable diseases by image-based deep learning. *Cell, 172*(5), 1122–1131.

Chapter 8
Brain Tumor Classification Using Deep Learning

Vishal K. Waghmare and Maheshkumar H. Kolekar

Abstract The computer-assisted study for improved deciphering imageries has been long-lasting topics in the field of medical imaging. Normally, various imaging techniques like ultrasound images, Magnetic Resonance Imaging (MRI) and Computed Tomography (CT) can be used for assessment of the tumor for prostate, lung, brain, breast, liver, etc. For this research, we have used brain MRI images for identification of tumor. The vast volume of data which is generated by MRI scan foils physical tumor classification versus non-tumor for specific period. Brain tumor is almost common and violent sickness, which leads to a very shorter life. Hence instinctive and reliable classification scheme is important to prevent this rate of deaths of human being. Deep learning is speedily evidencing to be the state-of-the-art foundation, achieving enhanced performances by extracting features through a convolutional neural network (CNN) and then classifying via fully connected networks. In this research work, automatic classification of brain tumor is anticipated with the help of CNN because they are companionable to do the task of image classification, including image recognition, localization, segmentation, registration and detection. As segmentation gulfs the image into different regions on some similarity bases because of which we can abstract different features from the images. This research has increased the accurateness of classifying brain tumors. Experimentation results show that the designed model can detect tumor up to the accuracy of 95.71% on an online dataset. We have implemented the CNN architectures for detection and classification of tumors by the use of various models such as basic CNN architecture, VGG-16 architecture.

Keywords Brain tumor · Convolutional neural network · MRI · Data augmentation · VGG16

V. K. Waghmare (✉) · M. H. Kolekar
Department of Electrical Engineering, Indian Institute of Technology Patna, Patna, India
e-mail: vishalkwaghmare@gmail.com

C. Chakraborty et al. (eds.), *Internet of Things for Healthcare Technologies*, Studies in Big Data 73, https://doi.org/10.1007/978-981-15-4112-4_8

8.1 Introduction

A brain tumour may be a mass or accumulation of biological cells within the brain. These cells are classified as abnormal cells that differ from the cure brain cells. These cells grow and increase in size inside the rigid skull that encloses the brain. This growth of the cells mass inside the hard structure of the skull forces the brain cells and causes serious pains and problems. Generally, tumors of the brain or any tumor are often classified into two sorts of tumor. The primary is named a benign tumour or non-cancerous tumor; whereas the second is extremely dangerous and cancerous that's said to be a malignant neoplasm. The expansion of those two sorts of tumor inside the skull forces the brain and may be very harmful to the lifetime of the patient. Human brain tumour is vivacious organs present within the physical body, which has billions of cells. It forms an irregular cluster of cells from the unrestrained cell segmentation, which we commonly call as a tumor.

Brain tumour is one among the foremost deadly sorts of cancer infections. It's its high effects because it's very caused to the most neuronal motor of the human being where every small defect can cost tons. For this reason, it's important to seek out methods of early detecting or alarming the likelihood of the existence of a brain tumour. This importance comes from the very fact that early detection increases significantly the likelihood of curing the disease and saving the lifetime of patients. Recently, the treatments of cancer have greatly developed, especially within the early stages of infection. Survival possibilities are very high for those patients receiving early treatments compared to those people that don't have this opportunity within the early stages of sickness (Fig. 8.1).

The persuasion for the study within the era of bio-medical image researches on brain tumors is the foremost ones among all. Nowadays, brain tumour occurs approximately to 2.5 lakhs people yearly globally which covers up but 2% of cancers. Dropping the burden on human verdicts we are aiming at building an interface which

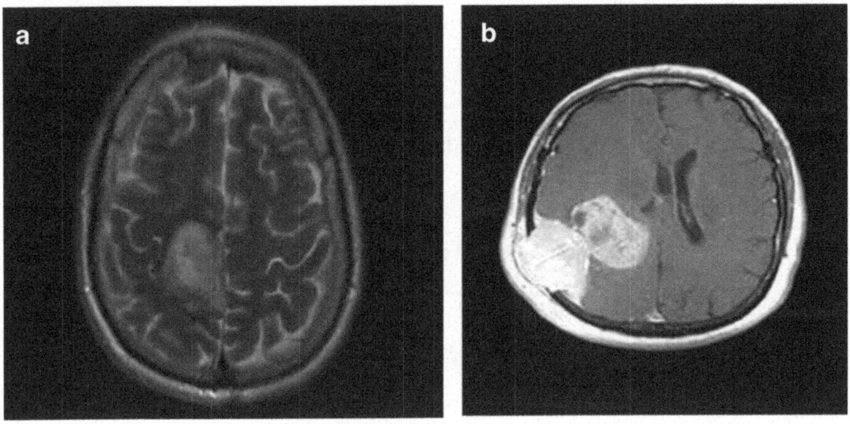

Fig. 8.1 Tumor types: **a** benign, **b** malignant [1]

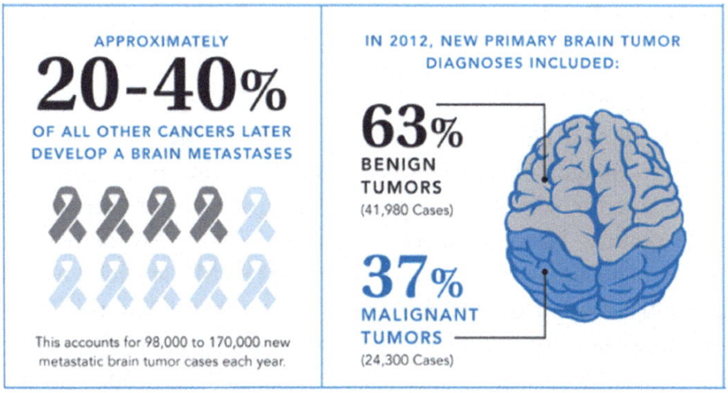

Fig. 8.2 Worldwide statistics for brain tumor [2]

may recognize the cancerous cells and thereby, restricting the mortality rate at its early stage. Brain tumors don't discriminate, it can affect the humankind irrespective of their genders, all ages and races. Last year eighty thousand individuals were being marked as a primary tumour. With medical imaging, we find moderately 120 diverse types of brain and Central nervous system (CNS) tumors [2] (Fig. 8.2).

Though there are numerous methods of brain tumour classification, but these need firm restrictions which necessitates to be measured while working for brain tumour classification and segmentation. Primary limitation of these systems for classification of tumor in their binary class, which is leading to several worries for the radiologist. This causes it to classification into benign and malignant tumor i.e., binary classification isn't enough for the radiologist to make a preventions decision and treatment for the person who is suffering. For a clear and better analysis for radiotherapist, this classification essentially should be multi-class, for categorizing tumour to its related scores and kinds. Additionally, absenteeism of knowledge is the key challenge to scholars for achieving specific results. For addressing these important restrictions, we have anticipated a convolutional neural network (CNN) based framework with the help of various techniques of data augmentation to accomplish current consequences for multi-grade classification brain tumour.

This chapter is premeditated in following manner: Sect. 8.2 the literature study for classification of brain tumour is expounded. Section 8.3 describes the background and Sect. 8.4 gives the thought about pre-processing and CNN layers. Section 8.5 contains all the specification of dataset, which is comparing experimental results with other methods. Also, the former section concludes and gives the idea of future work.

8.2 Literature Study

The main challenging and forthcoming field of MRI brain tumour images are Assessment and processing. MRI technique is called as intricate medical imaging technique which produces a images of high-quality confined within physical body which is really vital process for deciding the proper treatment at the correct period for a tumor infested person. Various techniques are anticipated for the classification of tumors in MR images like support vector machine (SVM), artificial neural network (ANN), fuzzy clustering means (FCM), expectation-maximization (EM), algorithm technique and knowledge-based techniques which are number of the favored methods used for region-based segmentation then to extract the important information from the medical imaging modalities.

In this section, our focus is going to be on earlier studies of brain tumour classification. Once we have checked out previous research on this medical imaging field, we are coming to understand that the majority of those pre-existing work is for the automatic segmentation for brain tumour region of MRI images. Lately, several researchers are presenting diverse methods to get and classify the brain tumour in MRI images.

In [3], the Fuzzy C-Means segmentation is amalgamated to differentiate the tumor and non-tumor region of the brain. However, the wavelet feature is extracted by employing a multilevel Discrete Wavelet Transform (DWT). Eventually, Deep Neural Network (DNN) is applied to the brain tumour classification with a high degree of correctness. The aforementioned practice is compared with Sequential Minimal Optimization (SMO) classification, Linear Discriminant Analysis (LDA) and KNN. Accuracy rate of 96.97% was obtained through DNN based brain tumour classification. However, the complexity was high and therefore the execution was very poor.

In [4], a special bio-physio-mechanical tumor advancement modelling is introduced for analyzing step by step advancement of the person who is having tumor. This had been being applied for gliomas and solid tumors with separate margins to capture the remarkable tumor mass effect. Discrete and continuous methods are used simultaneously for model tumor growth. This projected scheme provided the possibility to segment tumor possessing brain images supported atlas-based registration tacitly. The technique was just for the segmentation of brain tissue and therefore the problem with this method is its computational time is extremely high.

In [5], new brain tumour segmentation is introduced, which we will call as a multimodal brain tumour segmentation structure. They need combined diverse segmentation algorithms so as to accomplish good performance than the prevailing method the sole drawback is its complexity is high. In [5], the survey of brain tumour segmentation is presented discussing different segmentation methods like Margo Random Field (MRF), Region-based segmentation, Atlas-based segmentation, threshold-based segmentation, deformable model, geometric deformable model. In it, the correctness, precision and determination are analyzed for all the methods.

In [6], they need proposed an innovative CNN centered multi-grade brain tumour arrangement with segmenting the regions of tumor from an MRI image using deep learning models. They need performed widespread data augmentation to meritoriously train the proposed model. Data augmentation may be a tactic that permits practitioners to expressively upturn the variability of knowledge accessible for training models, bereft of indeed gathering new data. This is often due to the unavailability of datasets handling MRI images for the multi-grade brain tumour classification and eventually a pre-trained CNN model (VGG-16) is fine-tuned using augmented data for the classification of brain tumour.

We've proposed a deep learning-based algorithm with the help of data augmentation technique to achieve good results for the classification of brain tumour. We are using the Convolutional neural networks since we can not achive this accuracy with models like Hidden Markov Model, Support Vector Machine, Bayesian Networks, etc. [7–9].

8.3 Background

In past few years, Artificial Intelligence (AI) is becoming a topic for strong media excitement. AI, Machine learning (ML) and deep learning (DL) came up in immeasurable publications, frequently outside the journals of technology minded. What is mean by AI, ML and DL (understand Fig. 8.3). How these fields can narrate to each other?

Artificial intelligence

The inventors from the embryonic field of computing began to ask whether computers might be made to imagine that point AI came into the picture. AI may be a widespread field which incorporates ML and DL, also it embraces many methods which don't encompass any learning. To solve more complex fuzzy problems like

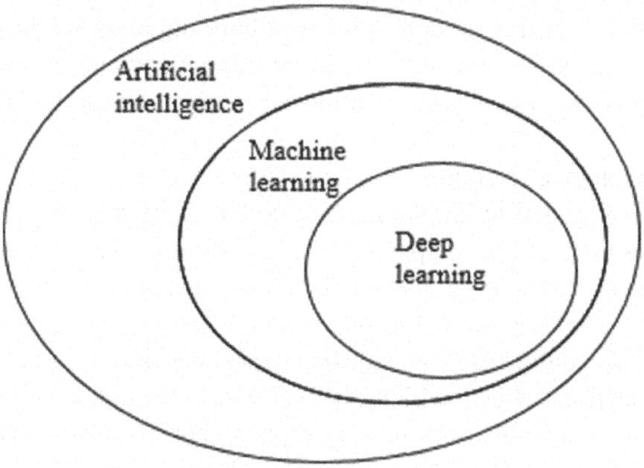

Fig. 8.3 An introduction to AI-ML-DL

language translation, speech recognition, and image classification method appear to need emblematic AI's place that is ML [10].

Machine learning

Machine learning has evolved with this query: can computer surpass "what we all know the way to order it to perform" also understand solitary the way it performs a particular task? Can computer wonder us? instead of computer programmer making rules for data-processing, will computer on its own learn some of these rules with the help of data? The ML system is trained instead of unequivocally programmed. As an example, if we have a wish of automating task for tagging pictures of trip, you will define a ML system with various models of pictures which are already tagged by humans, therefore the system is learning various arithmetical instructions for combining and tagging specific pictures to specific.

Deep learning

In simple words the DL may be a particular subfield of ML: It is a replacement combat learning representation from the data which puts a stress on learning of consecutive layers of progressively evocative depictions. The word deep in case of deep learning is not a regard to any relatively deeper understanding accomplished by the method; instead, it is standing for the concept of succeeding layers of representations. What percentage layers provide to a model of the info is named the strength of the model. However proper names for the region could be hierarchical and layered representations learning.

Now a days, deep learning repeatedly involves tens or maybe many consecutive layers of illustrations which they've all cultured inevitably from coverage to training data. It Means, other methods to machine learning tend to focus on learning just one or two layers of representations of the data; hence, they're sometimes called shallow learning. Models called neural networks, organized in literal layers weighted on top of every other. The term neural network may be a regard to neurobiology, but although a number of the central concepts in deep learning were created partially by gaining encouragement from our perception of the brain. There is no proof that the brain executes whatsoever just like the learning mechanisms exploited in contemporary deep-learning models. The most building block of those operations may be a neural network which is defined as an info science model that's encouraged by the brain nervous system which employs brain neuron model [1].

Biological Neuron

The human brain, signals are collected by neurons from others with the help of a number of fine shapes that we call as dendrites. These neurons send out spears for electrical activity with the help of an extended, slim stand that is called as an axon, it is divided into numerous branches. At the top of every branch, there is a structure that is called as synapse which translates the movement from the axon converting to electrical effects which obstruct within the connected neurons.

Neural networks are very rapid and precise thanks to the very fact that the completion of coaching the processing, optimization and time-consuming calculations are not any more needed. The generation of outputs of the network is straight for-ward from the provided inputs. The network is made by teaching the network how the precise system behaves with all of the inputs. There exist different network types implemented for various applications. Neural networks are utilized in engineering, forecasting of weather and financial markets, oil prices forecasting, business, and medical fields. Generally, artificial neural applications are often divided into the categories of knowledge clustering, and data arrangement. Data clustering is that the process of finding relationships be-tween different data inputs and arranging them into categories supported com-mon features between them. Within the classification applications, different inputs are assigned to defined classes to which they belong. Within the regression, a curve is made such it is often considered because the best fit between training sets. the foremost common regression neural networks are feed-forward networks and recurrent neural networks. The neural specification and main sorts of ANN are going to be discussed during this chapter of the work. Different variables which will affect the function of ANN and used as parameters are going to be dis-cussed also. The human mind is that the main decision motor within the human being. It consists of billions of nerves that are interconnected during a very complex structure. The brain as we will imagine its structure is quicker and more powerful than any computer that was manufactured. It can easily handle complicated problems with minimum effort and during a parallel manner that can't be handled by any computer. The biological analysis of the brain shows that it's multiple sets of layers of neurons connected between one another to perform multiprocessing tasks. The multiprocessing is extremely important for fast and accurate processing of knowledge of data 8 like images. The human brain is extremely fantastic in recognizing and memorizing images of things and humans with the minimum effort and time interval. All the neurons within the brain is connected to many other neurons to interchange the info within the best manner. Each neuron receives and sends information to all or any surrounding neurons. The biological neuron is shown in Fig. 8.4 consists of various parts that help it to finish its function. Main parts of the biological neuron are cell body (Soma), Dendrites, Synapses weights, and axon. All the billions of biological cells are connected with all surrounding neurons. The axon is that the output of the neuron through which it can transmit the knowledge to subsequent neurons.

We can define an artificial neuron as a device which has multiple inputs with single output, same as typical neuron. It works in two modes for operation mainly training mode and testing mode. Within training mode, we are training a neuron often to fireside (or not), for specific input forms. However, for the testing mode, when a trained input pattern is detected at the input, its related output becomes the present output. In case of in neural networks, the firing rule is a crucial concept and accounts for his or her high flexibility. It helps in determining or calculates whether a neuron should fire for any input pattern (Fig. 8.5).

As we said earlier, the neural network consists of multiple simple neurons. Different inputs of the neuron are being collected and fed to the body of the neuron. These inputs are summed together then fed to an activation function to get an appropriate output. The dynamics of the signal are often modelled as discrete or continuous. The

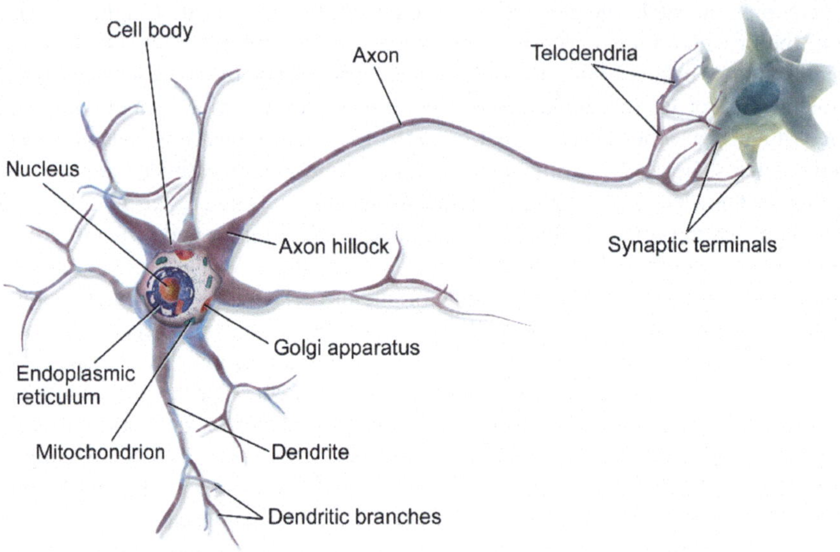

Fig. 8.4 Biological neuron

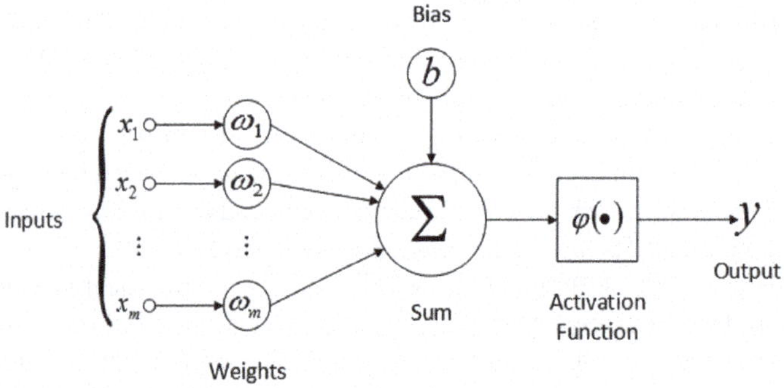

Fig. 8.5 Structure of the artificial neuron [1, 11]

transfer or activation function decides whether to get an output or deactivate it. Some transfer functions generate proportional signals with their inputs.

These neural networks explicitly uses convolution operation instead of general matrix operation in a minimum of one among their layers therefore they're called as Convolutional networks. They are used for the processing of data.

Imaging Modality

Bio-medical imaging systems helps medical experts and scholars to have insight to a physical body and examine internal activities without incisions. Diagnosis of cancer, class assessment, action response calculation, patient prediction and planning of surgery are the most crucial steps and challenges for cancer cure. We have different kinds of medical imaging techniques which are being employed by hospitals worldwide for various treatments. The brain imaging techniques are every so often considered into 2 categories: i.e., functional and structural imaging. Structural imaging entails of several measures allied with the brain structure, tumor position, damages and other brain ailments. The practical imaging techniques distinguishes the metabolic fluctuations, lesions on a finer scale and envision brain activities. This activity conception is feasible because of the metabolic changes in a certain portion of the brain which are gets imitated during the scans.

Computed tomography imaging (CT) and MRI are used for brain tumour analysis also they are equipped to capture distinct cross-sections of the body without doing surgical treatment. Different imaging techniques are designed to get the images of brain in order that tumor is often prognosed and diagnosed with its location and size of tumor like X-rays, CT scan and MRI.

Computed Tomography Imaging

CT is a significant imaging system within the boundaries of medical image analysis which provides information within seconds. It helps in giving more clearer perception tumours than X-rays, but the danger of radiation revelation is extremely high. During an X-ray, a CT scan beam mingles about a selected a part of the body and a sequence of images are depicted from several angles. The computer uses this data to produce a series of two-dimensional (2D) cross-sectional image of the body parts and blends them to make a three-dimensional (3D) image via mathematical modeling tools and applications, which is providing a far improved picture of the organs. Positron emission tomography (PET) may be a modified version of CT where a disparity agent is inserted into the body so as to focus irregular provinces. This scan is suggested by doctors in various conditions like hemorrhages i.e., internal blood clotting or cancer. Since, CT scans make the use of X-rays which is nothing but ionizing radiation thus potentially to distress existing tissues, by this means growing the risk of cancer. Study says that the threat of radiation in CT is hundred times above in normal X-ray analysis [12, 13].

Magnetic Resonance Imaging

Magnetic Resonance Imaging (MRI) is alternate technique which employs the frequency signals to extract the brain image. We are focusing on this image extraction technique. This technique is widely used and facilitates the prognosis and diagnosis of brain tumors in numerous neurological ailments. Standard MRI sequences usually do not discriminate among different kinds of brain tumors supported with different visual behavior and contrast grain analysis of the soft tissue. It creates unique pictures supported pixel by pixel. MRI is especially useful in neurological, musculoskeletal, and oncological imaging as it offers far more noteworthy intricacy amid the various delicate body tissues. Brain MRI image exclusively utilized for tumor recognition and treatment progressions.

MRI image gives more info about given medical image than the CT or ultrasound image. MRI isn't quite an equivalent as CT, and it doesn't utilize radiation of X-Rays

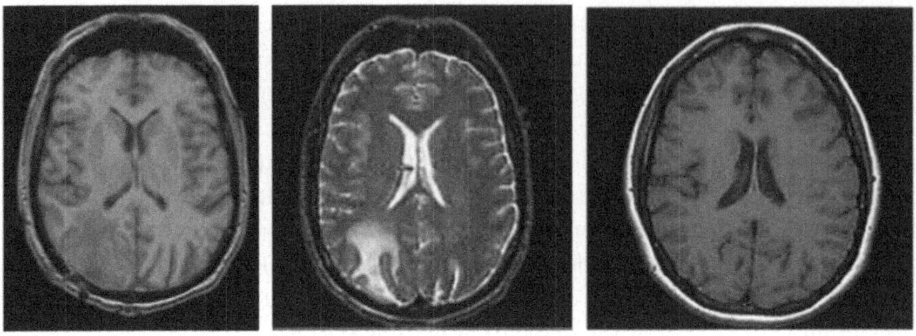

Fig. 8.6 Tumor images for T1 weighted, T2 weighted, FLAIR respectively

but uses a thriving attractive field to rearrange the atomic charge of hydrogen iota within the fluid present within the body [2].

MRI may be a radiation free and thus a harmless or even less threatening imaging procedure than CT. It gives clearer details of the brain, medulla spinalis and vascular anatomy because of its good quality of contrast. Axial, coronal and sagittal are the vital planes of MR images for visualization of the brain anatomy as shown in Fig. 8.6. The top frequently used MRI sequences for brain analysis are FLAIR, Tl weighted and T2 weighted. Tl weighted scans provides contrast in grey and substantia alba whereas T2-weighted is responsive to water content and is thus attuned to disorders where water gets accumulated into brain tissues. Both the images do not to discriminate spinal fluid [14, 15].

PET stands for Positron Emission Tomography in which a material is injected into the blood stream and the scanner detects the materials characteristics to produce an image. This system provides us with a thought of how the brain works and what are its activity and performance. X-rays are used in imaging technique which does not provide us with the detailed information about the organ. X-rays may root to carcinoma if used several periods of time on an same body portion. Apart from all these the technique is a cheaper option and uncomplicated to employ.

World Health Organization

World Health Organization has given some rules for Tumor Grading Cancer detection and proper grade guesstimate which are vital for the identification procedure. This is helping a doctor in choosing a bespoke action proposal which can rise the subsistence belief of the patients. The WHO classifies brain tumors using 4 basic features like nuclear atypia, microvascular proliferation, necrosis and mitoses [2].

In our chapter, we've proposed a singular deep learning algorithm which classifies brain tumour types, categorized by the quality of the planet Health Organization (WHO). For the operative analysis of MRI images, it's needed for segmentation of the tumor from MRI images then by doing augmentation that segmented tumor is augmented by different techniques. Furthermore, at last, we will classify the tumor by using fine-tuned CNN model.

8.4 System Development

The classification of tumor stages begins with a preprocessing method, followed by feature extraction and reduction and finally we use the deep learning algorithm for classifying in particular class.

Preprocessing
This preprocessing stage expands the quality of the brain tumour MR images which is making these images to get more fit for imminent processing by clinical experts. This is helping in enlightening parameters of MR images. The parameters include development in signal-to-noise, improvement in visual appearance of MR images, irrelevant noise removal with background of undesired parts, levelling regions of the inner part, preserving relevant edges.

Pre-processing of image before segmentation is grave for accurate detection of tumor. During this stage, we perform noise and artefacts reduction and perfecting of edges. There are minute chances of noise being present within the modern MRI images. Therefore, the most task of the preprocessing is to sharpen edges within the image. There are many imaging modalities like X-ray, ultrasonography, single-photon emission computerized tomography (SPECT) and MRI. we've specifically used MRI images for this study.

There are two sorts of noise we encountered once we were handling MRI images that are mainly Salt and Pepper noise (It seems like randomly sparse white, black or both pixels over the image) and Gaussian noise (This noise is caused by the arbitrary fluctuations within the signal) [1].

Resizing the Images into Small Size
The original MRI images are large enough to be analyzed manually by experts with high resolution and suitable size for human sensory system. In computer systems especially when it involves neural networks, processing large scale images may be a very costly process that needs huge material and software efforts. However, it's very clear that computer is different from biological brain system in image analysis. During a computing system it's enough to abstract the significant features of the image in any suitable size to try to the work. Thus, in neural networks the used images are generally resized to small sizes that are most difficult to be analyzed by humans. The resizing process applies an averaging algorithm that ensures the transfer of the features of every pixel within the original image to the new small image. Averaging is documented in mathematics because the mean of a group of values. It's considered as a brief description of multiple values and provides an honest idea about these values. In image processing, this process is 30 implemented to decrease the image complexity without losing any of its fundamental features [16, 17].

A moving window of suitable size is convolved with the first image to make a little version of the image. The moving window is applied both vertically and horizontally on the entire image pixels. All the features of the original image are included within the new image. Averaging algorithm is extremely constructive and useful with artificial neural network applications because it reduces the complexity of the studied network many times. The neural network will perform faster with less material requirements without losing its accuracy with small versions of images [7–9].

Convolution

Convolutional networks are enormously effective in everyday applications. The name 'convolutional neural network' designates that the network does a mathematical operation called convolution. It may be a specific quite linear operation. Convolutional networks are simply neural networks that use convolution instead of general matrix operation in a minimum of one among their layers. Computers read images as pixels, and it's expressed as a matrix (N × N × 3)(height by width by depth). The Convolutional Layer uses a group of learnable filters. This filter is employed to notice the occurrence of particular patterns or features present within the original image (Input).

This is typically stated as a matrix (M × M × 3), with a lesser dimension but an equivalent complexity because the input data. During the filter was convolved (slid) across the width and height of the input data, however it's scalar product is computed to offer an activation map [18, 19].

The basic diagram of the essential architecture CNN is shown in Fig. 8.7. The classification for CNN architecture is split into two stages they're training and testing stages. These images are separated into distinct categories by using classes or labels like normal and abnormal brain image and type of brain tumour. The steps performed in building a prediction model includes data pre-processing, feature extraction and classification with the utilization of appropriate loss function. Within the pre-processing, MRI images were resized to vary the dimension to form the dataset uniform. Finally, CNN is employed for automatic brain tumour classification.

The Pooling layer

At third step, we use a pooling function for switching the output of the layer further. This pooling function helps in replacing the output of internet at a particular location with a summary fact of the nearby outputs. For instance, the max-pooling operation recounts the utmost output within an oblong neighborhood. Other popular pooling functions include the typical of an oblong neighborhood, the L2 norm of an oblong neighborhood, or a weighted average supported a space from the central pixel.

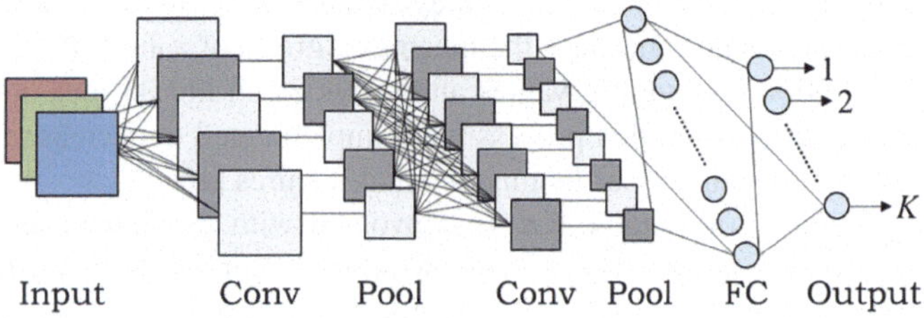

Fig. 8.7 CNN model architecture

It is often seen in between the convolution layers in CNN architecture. It helps in reducing the number of computation and parameters within the network. Pooling operation is completed for the only purpose of dropping the spatial size of the Image. It is completed independently on each depth dimension; therefore, the depth of the image remains unchanged. The foremost common sort of pooling layer generally applied is the max pooling [18].

This operation consists of taking the utmost feature (neuron) value over sub-windows within each feature map. It can be formalized as follows:

$$Hs,\ i,\ j\ =\ \max pZs,\ i\ +\ p,\ j\ +\ p \quad (1)$$

where p fixes the max pooling window size. The sub-windows are often overlapping or not. For shrining the dimensions of feature map, we use the max-pooling operation. This is often operated by the pooling size p and therefore the stride hyper-parameter, which corresponds to the horizontal and vertical increments at which pooling sub-windows are situated. Let S be the stride value and $Q \times Q$ be the form of the feature map before max-pooling.

We can define output for the max-pooling operation would be of size $D \times D$ where

$$D = (Qp)/S + 1 \quad (2)$$

Output layer

After various layers of Convolution and padding, we might require the output within the sort of a category. We can extract features and reduce the number of parameters from the first images with the help of convolution and pooling layers. However, to get the ultimate output, we have to use a totally connected layer to make an output adequate to the number of classes we'd like. This Convolution layers create 3D activation maps while we'd like the output on whether or not a picture belongs to a specific class. We will have the loss function like categorical cross-entropy at output layer, to compute the error in prediction. As the aerial is complete, it begins the back propagation to update the load and does the biases for error and loss reduction.

Activation functions

Activation functions are one among the most components of the neural networks. They're liable for making the choice to get suitable out-put for a given set of inputs. There are differing types of activation or transfer functions. Some transfer functions are on-off transfer functions which will either generate output or cancel it hooked into the input. Other transfer functions can generate different outputs proportional or as a mathematical function of the input sum.

The convolutional neural network makes use of nonlinear functions as activation functions which allow producing multifaceted mappings between the inputs and outputs for a network. This will allow stuffing of multiple layers during a string to create deep neural networks. Therefore we can understand that this series of layers in hidden layers of neurons are crucial for learning and modelling datasets with high

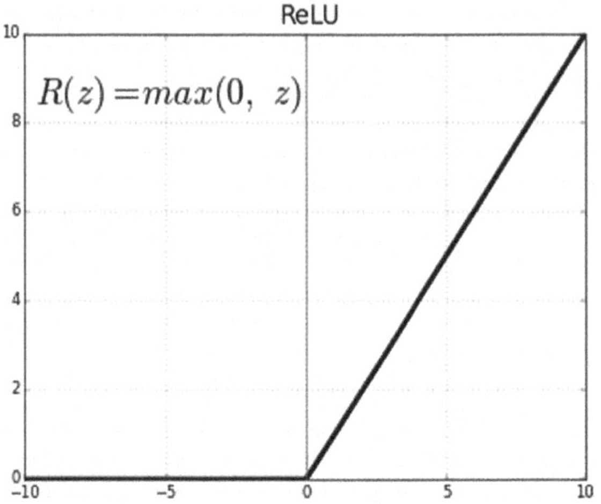

Fig. 8.8 Rectified linear unit (ReLU) [1, 20]

dimensionality and complexity. Using non-linear activation functions every overall operation might be executed during a neural network.

There are various alternatives for the non-linearity like softmax, sigmoid, hyperbolic, Rectified linear measure (ReLU), tangent, etc. In our work, ReLU and softmax activation function are used. ReLU are often mathematically defined as

$$y = \max(0, x)$$

ReLU activation function has a feature of derivative function which allows it for backpropagation and also it converges quickly. The Softmax activation function directs to a vector that is showing the probability distributions of a series of possible outcomes (Fig. 8.8).

The Softmax regression may be a sort of logistic regression which normalizes the input value into a vector of values and that is following a probability distribution whose total is equal to 1. Softmax is usually used for mapping the non-normalized output of a network with the probability distribution around a predicted output classes. Softmax is employed just for the output layer, for neural networks that require to classify inputs into multiple categories.

Data augmentation

Simply, the data augmentation is defined as the process of accelerating the quantity and variety of knowledge. High dimensionality and quality datasets are important for bringing assets into effective action of varied deep learning models. The main challenge in our work that we faced was lack of satisfactory data within the existing dataset to feed to the deep learning model and get good accuracy. Hence to achieve this good accuracy we extended the available data with the assistance of various augmentation techniques. we have performed the augmentation by rotation, skewness,

Table 8.1 Various parameters for data augmentation [21]

S. No.	Data augmentation technique	Parameters
1	Rotation (angle in degree)	−90°
		−45°
		45°
		90°
2	Flip	Top
		Bottom
		Right
		Left
3	Gaussian blur (sigma value)	0.25
		0.50
		1.0
		2.0
4	Sharpen (lightness value)	0.50
		1.00
		1.50
		2.0
5	Edges detection (alpha value)	0.25
		0.50
		0.75
		1.00
6	Emboss (strength value)	0.50
		1.00
		1.50
		2.0
7	Skew (tilt)	Left
		Right
		Forward
		Backward
8	Shear (axis and value)	X-axis 10°
		Y-axis 10°

flipping. We might use the parameters like embossing, edge detection, sharpening and Gaussian blur for the noise invariance [21] (Table 8.1).

VGG-16 CNN architecture

There is a research terminology called Transfer learning in machine learning that focuses on preserving knowledge acquired at the time of solving one problem and applying it to other relevant problem. For an instance, features learnt during problem of recognizing cars could be applied to recognizing that of trucks. We can use the pre-trained architectures and its optimized hyper parameters by making some changes to other models for some other relevant problem. Therefore, a pre-trained model is often defined as a model which is made by somebody else which was unraveled for an relevant problem. In another way, rather than constructing a model from scratch to unravel analogous relevant problem, we can use the model trained on other cases as a start line.

For a better understanding of the instance consider that you wish to shape a self-learning bus and so for which you have to indulge yourself for few years on building an image detection algorithm from scratch. On the contrary part you could have used foundation model which is nothing but as a pre-trained model from internet built upon ImageNet dataset. This is to be noted that a pre-trained model might not be 100% accurate for our application, but it saves an enormous amount of resources and time required to reinvent.

As per our research the use of pre-trained models has increased the accuracy that we obtained by our basic CNN model. This bound us to modify to the pre-trained models where we are not training the whole model, but we are training only a few of its layers. Therefore, we have used VGG16 model pre-trained on the ImageNet data and in association with the keras libraries.

In proposed methodology, fine-tuned VGG-16 CNN architecture is used for classifying the brain tumour. VGG-16 model constitutes of 16 weighted layers clearly as the name suggests VGG-16. Within these layers 13 layers are convolutional layers and leftover layers are fully connected or we can say it as dense layers as fully connected. Within the VGG-16 architecture, there are two convolutional layers which are followed by max-pooling layer. This will be clearly shown in Fig. 8.9 the mixture of convolutional layers followed by maxpooling can be observed [1].

Finally the 3 concluding layers called as fully connected. As already discussed, here we are employing a pre-trained model which can study the similarity and shapes within the data. Hence, we can alter the weights of only fully connected layers not of all layers.

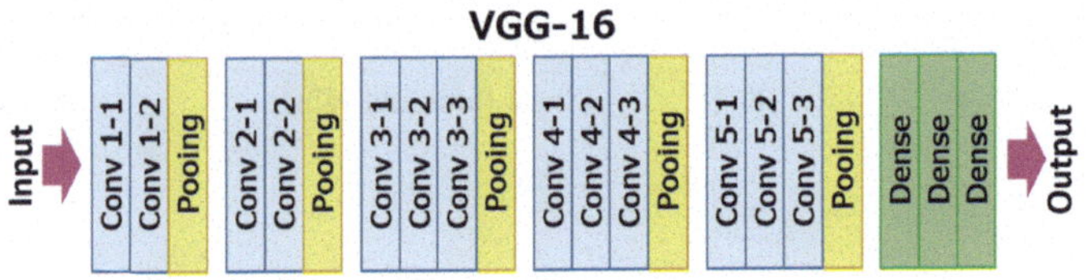

Fig. 8.9 Fine-tuned VGG-16 CNN architecture

8.5 Results

In this part, we have presented the experimental estimation for our intended model for classifying the brain tumor. Therefore, we have conducted experiments on two datasets, i.e. basic dataset and brain tumor dataset. We divided these datasets as 60, 20, and 20% for training, cross-validation, and testing sets. We know given datasets are too small, therefore, we are using data augmentation technique for increasing data by using different parameters. The statistics of both datasets before and after augmentation is tabulated (see Tables 8.2 and 8.3). The experiments we have assessed using Nvidia Quadro K2000 2 GB GDDR5 Graphics Card and deep learning.

Basic dataset

This Data Set consists of 235 MRI images which are further classified as two different categories (tumor present and tumor absent). We know the number of images in this dataset is too small; therefore, we have chosen the data augmentation technique for increasing this number. In deep learning for better understanding of the image, we need them in large numbers. Therefore, we have created a large number of images. The details of these newly created images are statistically tabulated in Table 8.2.

Brain tumor dataset

This dataset has 3704 T1-weighted contrast-enhanced MR images. The Resolution of these images was various pixel values, but by using the resizing algorithm, we have resized them to 512×512-pixel sizes. For this dataset also we have used data augmentation technique to get more images. The details of these newly created images are statistically tabulated in Table 8.3. We have performed a data augmentation because of which the number of images has increased from 3704 to 148,160.

Evaluation with other models

With this proposed system we can overextend to an image modality like ultrasound, CT, and Positron emission tomography (PET). Also, it is often extended to diagnose

Table 8.2 Statistics details of basic dataset (images)

Tumor (present/absent)	Images before augmentation	Images after augmentation
Present	135	5400
Absent	98	3920

Table 8.3 Statistics details of brain tumor dataset (images)

Type of Tumor	Images before augmentation	Images after augmentation
Meningioma	884	35,360
Glioma	1677	67,080
Pituitary tumor	1143	45,720

diseases associated with other tumors like cancer of the liver, prostatic adenocarcinoma and uterine cancers. In future, we'll expand our work for detecting the particular shape and size of the tumor with use of several deep learning models.

Theoretically, Sensitivity is the test's positives capability to appropriately identify the patient who has the condition. Mathematically it can be expressed here:

$$\text{Sensitivity} = \frac{\text{Number of true}}{\text{number of true positives} + \text{number of true negatives}}$$

Specificity gives the test's capability to correctly reject healthy patients without a condition. Mathematically it can be written as (Fig. 8.10):

$$\text{Specificity} = \frac{\text{Number of true negatives}}{\text{number of true positives} + \text{number of true negatives}}$$

In our proposed algorithm staggered the current techniques and obtained value of 95.71%, 83.28% and 93.37% for accuracy, sensitivity and specificity respectively (Table 8.4).

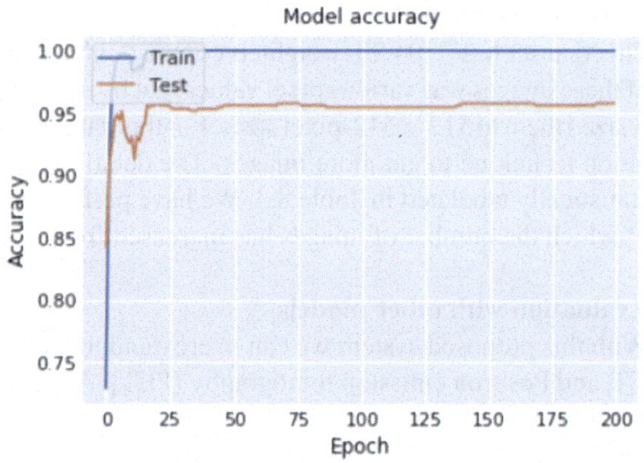

Fig. 8.10 Results of proposed fine-tuned VGG-16 CNN architecture for brain tumor dataset

Table 8.4 Comparison with other models for brain tumor classification [21, 22]

Model	Accuracy (%)	Sensitivity (%)	Specificity (%)
Cheng et al. (2015)	91.28	81	92
Muhammad Sajjad et al. (2019)	94.58	88.41	96.12
Proposed	**95.71**	**83.28**	**93.37**

8.6 Discussion

We have previously conferred above that, how several researchers are developing the instinctive brain image analysis methods for segmentation of brain and classification of tissues. Many of them use MRI (T1, T2, and FLAIR), because of its radiation-free nature and decent contrast. We have already deliberated, brain image analysis consists of image enhancement, image registration, features reduction, feature extraction and is not continually steady due to the possessions of noise and blurring due to organ actions. The performance of the medical data analysis highly depends on numerous factors such as transformation, image contents, modality, optimization of algorithm, similarity measures and implementation mechanism.

Gaussian (high-pass, low-pass) filter, histogram equalization, contrast starching is most normally used image improvement techniques for medical images. Huge amount of features are computationally expensive which is making a classification multifaceted. Consequently, genetic algorithm (GA), principal component analysis (PCA) and linear discriminant analysis (LDA) are the most popular methods for feature reduction. SVM, DT, naive Bayes classifier, Bayesian classifier, KNN, ANNs etc. are the most generally used ML methods for brain image classification and have grasped to high-level perfection in classification [23, 24, 20].

8.7 Conclusion

We have mainly focused to deliver state-of-the-art in brain tumour level, which comprises WHO rules for tumor classification, imaging modality, patho-physiology of cancer, key judgement methods and prevailing computer assisted systems for brain tumour classifications by means of deep learning techniques. It is already proved that many survives can be prevented if that cancer is marked with proper grade measured over quick and gainful analysis techniques. That's why, we need to create some fast, non-invasive and gainful diagnosis methods [3].

We have premeditated a unique deep learning algorithm for the categorization of brain tumor. We have performed this classification in this following way: Pre-processing, Augmentation of image dataset and lastly a fine-tuned VGG-16 CNN architecture. We have enhanced the correctness of categorizing the tumor by smearing deep learning models with the help of data augmentation techniques. We can use this research work as a part of the Computer-Aided Verdict tool. It is to be used by non-radiologist clinician/discussing doctors in the detection of tumor and its types [1].

In future, we will outspread our work for spotting the actual shape and size of the tumor with the help of different deep learning models.

References

1. Waghmare, V. K., & Kolekar, M. H. (2020). Convolutional neural network based automatic brain tumor detection. In *International Conference on Evolving Technologies for Computing, Communication and Smart World.*
2. McGuire, S. (2016). Health Organization, International Agency for Research on Cancer, World Cancer Report 2014. Geneva, Switzerland. *Advances in Nutrition, 7,* 418–419.
3. Mohsen, H., El-Dahshan, E.A., El-Horbaty, E. M., & Salem, A. M. (2017). Classification using deep learning neural networks for brain tumors. *Future Computing and Informatics Journal,* 1–4.
4. Bauer, S., May, C., Dionysiou, D., Stamatakos, G., Buchler, P., & Reyes, M. (2011). Multi-scale modeling for image analysis of brain tumor studies. *Transactions on Biomedical Engineering, 59*(1), 25–29.
5. Menze, B., Reyes, M., & Van Leemput, K. (2015). The multimodal brain tumor image segmentation benchmark (BRATS). *IEEE Transactions on Medical Imaging, 34,* 1993–2024.
6. Liu, J., Wang, J., Wu, F., Liu, T., & Pan, Y. (2014). A survey of MRI-based brain tumor segmentation methods. *Tsinghua Science and Technology, 19*(6), 578–595.
7. Dash, D. P., Kolekar, M. H., & Jha, K. (2019). Multi-channel EEG based automatic epileptic seizure detection using iterative filtering decomposition and Hidden Markov Model. *Computers in Biology and Medicine, 116,* 103571.
8. Kolekar, M. H., & Dash, D. P. A nonlinear feature based epileptic seizure detection using least square support vector machine classifier. In *TENCON 2015-2015, IEEE Region 10 Conference* (pp. 1–6).
9. Kolekar, M. H. (2011). Bayesian belief network based broadcast sports video indexing. *Multimedia Tools Application, 54*(1), 27–54.
10. Amit, B., Chinmay, C., Anand, K., & Debabrata, B. (2019). Emerging trends in IoT and big data analytics for biomedical and health care technologies. In *Handbook of Data Science Approaches for Biomedical Engineering* (pp. 121–152). Elsevier.
11. Kolekar, M. H., & Kumar, V. (2017). *Biomedical signal and image processing in patient care.* IGI Global Publisher.
12. Ching, T., Himmelstein, D. S., Beaulieu-Jones, B. K., et al. (2017). *Opportunities and obstacles for deep learning in biology and medicine.* bioRxiv 2017, 142760.
13. Greenspan, H., van Ginneken, B., & Summers, R. M. (2016). Guest editorial deep learning in medical imaging: Overview and future promise of an exciting new technique. *IEEE Transactions on Medical Imaging, 35*(5), 1153–1159.
14. Litjens, G., et al. (2017). *A survey on deep learning in medical image analysis.* [Online]. Available: https://arxiv.org/abs/1702.05747.
15. Pereira, S., Pinto, A., Alves, V., & Silva, C. (2016). Brain tumor segmentation using convolutional neural networks in MRI images. *IEEE Transactions on Medical Imaging, 35*(5), 1240–1251.
16. Ghosal, D., & Kolekar, M. H. (2018). Music genre recognition using deep neural networks and transfer learning. In *Proceedings of the Interspeech* (pp. 2087–2091), Hyderabad, India, Sept 2–6, 2018.
17. Bhatnagar, S., Ghosal, D., & Kolekar, M. H. (2017). Classification of fashion article images using convolutional neural networks. In *2017 Fourth International Conference on Image Information Processing (ICIIP)* (pp. 1–6). IEEE.
18. Havaei, M., Davy, A., Warde-Farley, D., Biard, A., Courville, A., Bengio, Y., et al. (2017). Brain tumor segmentation with deep neural networks. *Medical Image Analysis, 35,* 18–31.
19. Ari, A., & Hanbay, D. (2018). Deep learning based brain tumor classification and detection system. *Turkish Journal of Electrical Engineering & Computer Sciences, 26*(5), 2275–2286.
20. Kolekar, M. H., & Dash, D. P. (2016). Hidden Markov model based human activity recognition using shape and optical flow based features. In *Proceedings of IEEE Region 10 Conference* (pp. 393–397).

21. Sajjad, M., Khan, S., Muhammad, K., Wanqing, W., Ullah, A., & WookBaik, S. (2019). Multi-grade brain tumor classification using deep CNN with extensive data augmentation. *Journal of Computational Science, 30,* 174–182.
22. Cheng, J., Huang, W., Cao, S., Yang, R., Yang, W., & Yun, Z. (2015). Enhanced performance of brain tumor classification via tumor region augmentation and partition. *PloS one, 10,* e0144479.
23. Kolekar, M. H., & Sengupta, S. (2015). Bayesian network-based customized highlight generation for broadcast soccer videos. *IEEE Transactions on Broadcasting, 61*(2), 195–209.
24. Kolekar, M. H., & Dash, D. P. (2015). A nonlinear feature based epileptic seizure detection using least square support vector machine classifier. TENCON 2015 IEEE Region 10 Conference (pp. 1–6), Macao, China, Nov 2015.

Chapter 9
Early Detection of Dementia Disease Using Data Mining Techniques

M. Sucharitha, Chinmay Chakraborty, S. Srinivasa Rao, and V. S. K. Reddy

Abstract Brain imaging with data mining is rising in significance as it enables the provision of prognoses, treatments and a better comprehension of brain functioning. Data mining considers how it might utilize the data to uncover fresh knowledge and thereby improving decision-making processes. Though data mining is a mighty knowledge detecting method, there are limits in the way that it may be employed: it is application dependent. This chapter deals with the early detection of dementia disease with data mining techniques. Once the presence of the disease is detected, further diagnosis can be done so that the health of elderly people can be improved. Dementia is the loss of cognitive efficiency and disorder beyond natural aging that inhibits social and occupational performance. Typical clinical practice reveals that dementia's cognitive and functional losses lead to variations in behavior, but this is not a primary criterion as it lacks diagnostic specificity. Magnetic Resonance Imaging (MRI) detects dementia disease early before irreversible damage. Features are extracted from the segmented images using both Wavelet Packet Tree (WPT) and First-Order Histogram (FOH) method. Features are normalized and fused using the product rule fusion technique after computing Median Absolute Deviation (MAD) between two features. Classification accuracy is measured using both K-Nearest Neighbor (KNN) and Naïve Bayesian Classifier. Performance measures classification accuracy, average precision, average recall, and *F* Measure are evaluated. The overall classification accuracy achieved using the proposed feature fusion technique is 93.87%. The early detection of Alzheimer's helps caregivers in taking care of the patients. Once the abnormality is identified, the patient's condition is monitored using the wireless medium with the Internet of Things (IoT). It helps in creating a working environment for a patient at home by reducing health expenses and reduces burdens on health care professionals.

M. Sucharitha (✉) · S. Srinivasa Rao · V. S. K. Reddy
Department of Electronics and Communication Engineering, Malla Reddy College of Engineering and Technology, Hyderabad, India
e-mail: sucharitha_m2002@yahoo.co.in

C. Chakraborty
Department of Electronics and Communication Engineering, Birla Institute of Technology, Ranchi, Jharkhand, India

C. Chakraborty et al. (eds.), *Internet of Things for Healthcare Technologies*, Studies in Big Data 73, https://doi.org/10.1007/978-981-15-4112-4_9

Keywords Data mining · Dementia disease · Feature fusion · Classifier · Internet of Things

9.1 Introduction

Dementia is a neurodegenerative brain disease that tends to decline in cognitive abilities in a person, afflicted before that of natural aging. It is a syndrome that features disruption of many brain functions, such as memory, thought process, computation, learning ability, linguistic faculty, and so on. There is no loss of consciousness. The disruptions in cognitive functions are typically followed by and sometimes headed by loss of emotional control, social behavior or motivation [1]. Dementia affects millions globally in 2025, the number of people aged above 60 living was judged to be 35.6 million worldwide. Initial and precise diagnosis will reduce the costs related to care and arrangements because it allows patients to enter supportive therapy that assists in maintaining their independent state for a greater duration, thereby delaying hospitalization [2].

Initially, neuropsychological tests Mini-Mental State Examination (MMSE) or Folstein test is used to measure cognitive impairment in medicine and allied health to screen for dementia. MMSE relies on the verbal response which is difficult with language problems and is insensitive to the early changes of dementia [3]. Data mining came to be a tool for analyzing the data, however, the analysis and decision-making depends on the mood of the Psychologist. In addition to that, human error can be avoided. As decision-making is an important step it is overcome by data mining techniques. ID3 algorithm is put advancing by revising the ID3 algorithm of decision tree and the shortages of the ID3 algorithm [4]. An automated diagnostic system [5] is proposed for chronic wound status checking and is beneficial for the aging population. Segmentation is performed using the conventional fuzzy c-means clustering in combination with the standard computational learning schemes: Linear Discriminant Analysis (LDA), Decision Tree (DT), Naïve Bayesian (NB), and Random Forest (RF). The overall accuracy of 93.75% is achieved. Breast cancer is diagnosed using the data mining approach based on the mined tumor topographies [6]. Feature extraction and selection are critical to the quality of classifiers founded through data mining methods. A hybrid of k-means and support vector machine (K-SVM) algorithms is developed for extracting information to diagnose the tumor. K-means algorithm recognizes hidden patterns of the benign and malignant tumors separately. Machine learning methods such as neural networks, Multilayer Perceptron, Bagging, Decision tree, CANFIS, and Genetic algorithms are used for the classification of different stages of Alzheimer's disease [7]. Also, the data mining approach is used to classify various neurodegenerative disorders like Alzheimer's disease, vascular disease, and Parkinson's disease by considering the common risk factors. Electroencephalogram (EEG) and selected cognitive biomarkers are used instead of images to classify mild cognitive impairment (MCI), dementia and healthy subjects using a support vector machine classifier [8]. Better accuracy is achieved for each event from 73.4 to 89.8%

for three binary classes using the proposed method. Automated detection of brain atrophy patterns based on MRI for the prediction of Alzheimer's disease has been used in combination with support vector machine, Bayes statistics, and voting feature Interval to derive a quantitative index of pattern matching for the prediction of conversion from MCI to AD [9]. Cluster analysis of MR Imaging in Alzheimer's disease using decision tree refinement used a clustering algorithm to analyze the data and used a decision tree algorithm to model the level of importance of variants influencing the decision [10]. Neural networks are used which is trained to distinguish between normal and abnormal subjects of Alzheimer's disease [11]. PET can be a powerful tool for discriminating between normal and demented subjects. The highest ROC area of the PET-neural network combination achieved was 0.95. This classification can be used to either strongly confirm or rule out the presence of abnormalities.

Alzheimer's disease is a widely prevalent kind of dementia and probably contributed about 60–70% of all occurrences [12]. Certain medicines like cholinesterase inhibitors are capable of delaying the advancement of Alzheimer's disease. Also, Alzheimer's disease patients who begin the cholinesterase inhibitor therapy late show lesser benefits than those who began early. This observation had pushed research towards early diagnoses to judge the value of therapy. This chapter deals with the early detection of dementia disease using data mining techniques. Due to dementia disease, mortality and morbidity are more among elderly people. Hence health care is needed to reduce the scourge of this disease and this is achieved by early detection of disease using data mining techniques. The early detection of dementia makes the caregivers take care of the patients. For effective utilization of MRI images in machine learning approaches, features from the MRI image are extracted after localization of important features using segmentation techniques. The segmented sections are used to extract various features like energy coefficients, texture, color, histogram to name a few. The useful feature vector from the extracted features is selected and utilized to train the classifier.

9.2 Diagnosis of Dementia

The clinical diagnosis gives a context for evaluating current neuroimaging tools and anticipated progress in (1) diagnoses of incipient cases, (2) predicting incident cases, and (3) results of therapeutic trials. Currently, neuroimaging is incapable of telling us if a person has or does not have a cognitive disorder. This remains a clinical query. Neuroimaging with Computed Tomography (CT) or MRI has a major role in eliminating structural lesions of the brain in patients with dementia. Both modalities perform well in the detection of brain tumors, AD and hematomas. Precise diagnoses of dementia detecting the prodromal phase and MCI are major initial steps toward a cure and have been extensively researched in neuroimaging studies. Apart from neuropsychological exams, medical imaging is more frequently being utilized to assist in the diagnosis of dementia. Magnetic Resonance Imaging (MRI) is a neuroimaging technique utilized for visualizing brain anatomy and has a great level of spatial resolution and contrast among brain tissue kinds [13]. Among the recent classification techniques that have been built to permit individual class prediction, machine learning methods have been suggested for distinguishing MRIs between two sets of patients. The methods require training populations and testing populations for categorizing new entities into either class as demented or non-demented.

9.3 Methodology

9.3.1 *Feature Extraction*

The most significant information from the original data is obtained by feature extraction and represented in a lower dimensionality space. The input to an algorithm need not be too large. The performance of the decision learning system can be enhanced with a small set of relevant features that take less memory and computation time. Feature extraction should be done carefully from the input such that those data are enough for further processing instead of using the whole input. Feature extraction is designed for the representation of opinions and to reduce the dimension by removing noisy, irrelevant and redundant features. Features used in classifying images as demented or non-demented. In this chapter, two types of feature extraction techniques are developed, the extracted features are fused for better dementia classification. In this segmentation with a Gray-level co-occurrence matrix (GLCM) and Fuzzy Local Information C-Means (FLICM) is also performed for comparison [14]. Features are extracted using two different techniques as First-Order Histogram and Wavelet Packet Tree. It was proposed to fuse the extracted features from First-Order Histogram and Wavelet Packet Tree using the feature fusion rule.

9.3.1.1 First-Order Histogram

An image histogram is the representation of the distribution of pixels as a function of their intensity graphically [15]. Histograms are computed from images. Histogram's shape is a clue to an image's characteristics. Histogram-based [16] texture analysis depends on the intensity value concentrations on all or part of the histogram represented image. The random variable *I* represent an image region's gray levels. First-Order Histogram *P*(*I*) is defined as [17] seen in Eq. (9.1):

$$P(I) = \frac{\text{number of pixels with gray level } l}{\text{total number of pixels in the region}} \tag{9.1}$$

where the Mean m_1 and central moments μ_k of *I* is given by Eq. (9.2):

$$m_1 = E\left[I^1\right] = \sum_{I=0}^{N_g-1} I^1 P(I)$$

$$\mu_k = E\left[(I - E[I])^k\right] = \sum_{I=0}^{N_g-1} (I - m_1)^k P(I),$$

$$k = 2, 3, 4 \tag{9.2}$$

where is the number of gray levels.

Frequent central moments are Skewness, Variance, and Kurtosis depicted by μ_2, μ_3, and μ_4, respectively. Variance is histogram width measuring gray levels deviation from mean. Skewness measures histogram asymmetry around mean and kurtosis measures histogram sharpness. Standard deviation, average energy, mean, entropy, skewness, and kurtosis are the features derived [18]. The four features extracted using the First-Order Histogram for Dementia Classification is Mean-Variance, Skewness, and Kurtosis. First-order statistics-based features are translation and rotation invariant but capture only important information about gray levels and not the relative positions of gray levels within the image. Information is extracted from the gray-level co-occurrence matrix that measures second-order statistics.

9.3.1.2 Wavelet Packet Tree (WPT)

Wavelets refer to natural Fourier survey extension. A wavelet stands for a small wave with energy concentrated in time. Wavelet transform is flexible to time–frequency survey in earthquake engineering [19]. Wavelet transform is a mathematical device to transform data; it offers information on motions non-stationary time-dependent power regarding a specific interest frequency. Wavelets are mathematical functions that make the function of data simple to different frequency components and deal with the resolution matching the scale. Wavelets are zero mean oscillatory functions of finite energy, to get a process' time–frequency image [20]. Wavelet Transform (WT) is the mathematical tool for viewing an image or processing an image with multiple resolutions [21]. In general, the WPT is a classical wavelet transform, providing multi-resolution and time–frequency analysis. WPT is efficient for representing multi-resolution images and providing spatial and frequency characteristics.

A wavelet packet is represented as a function

$$\Psi^i_{j,k}(t) = 2^{-j/2}\Psi^i\left(2^{-j}t - k\right) \tag{9.3}$$

where i is the modulation parameter, j is the dilation parameter, and k is the translation parameter. $i = 1, 2, \ldots, j^n$, and n is the level of decomposition in the wavelet packet tree. The wavelet Ψ_i is obtained by the following recursive relationships,

$$\Psi^{2i} = \sqrt[1]{2}\sum_{-\alpha}^{\alpha} h(k)\Psi^{i}\left(\frac{t}{2} - k\right) \tag{9.4}$$

$$\Psi^{2i+1} = \sqrt[1]{2}\sum_{-\alpha}^{\alpha} g(k)\Psi^{i}\left(\frac{t}{2} - k\right) \tag{9.5}$$

Here, Ψ_i is the mother wavelet and discrete filters $h(k)$ and $g(k)$ are quadrature mirror filters associated with scaling function and mother wavelet function. The wavelet packet component at a particular node can be obtained as

$$f_j^i(t) = \sum_{k=-\alpha}^{\alpha} c_{j,k}^{i}\Psi_{j,k}^{i}(t)\mathrm{d}t \tag{9.6}$$

where $c_{j,k}^{i}$ corresponds to the wavelet packet coefficients. The depiction of the Wavelet Packet decomposition tree is shown in Fig. 9.1.

WPT technique ensures a different base family that represents a specific image. As research tries to reduce medical images, a good basis should reduce nonzero coefficients' in final transformed images. The best basis algorithm reduces transform coefficients entropy [22]. The algorithm uses a wavelet decomposition tree in the wavelet packets method. A decomposition tree node is assigned an entropy value. Entropy is a common method to calculate cost basis. The cost functions Shannon entropy [23] is used to measure signal complexity to wavelet coefficients generated by WPT also larger entropy results in higher process uncertainty and complexity. The Shannon entropy is defined as

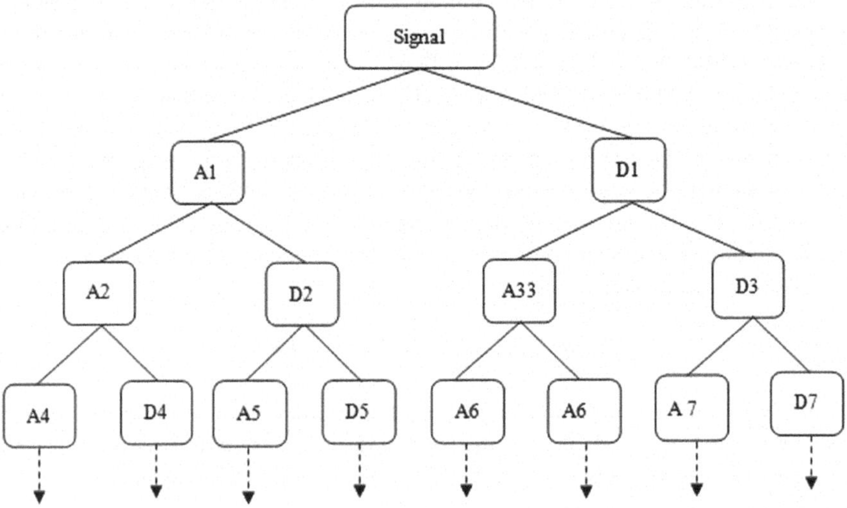

Fig. 9.1 Wavelet Packet decomposition tree

$$E(s) = -\sum_i I_i^2 \log I_i^2 \quad (9.7)$$

where I_i represents coefficients of image I in an orthonormal basis.

If entropy value >1, the information is more about the image so it should be decomposed more for obtaining a simple frequency component of the image which is useful for matching and selecting the best basis. Given the image, the best basis-based wavelet packet entropy is obtained by the following steps:

(a) A wavelet function W is selected and decomposition level L is specified.
(b) The sample means SM is calculated.
(c) SM is decomposed to a specified level with selected wavelet function, and a Wavelet Packet Tree T is returned. $B_{l,k}$ is the set of WPT basis vector, $0 \leq l < L$, $1 \leq k \leq 2^L - 1$.
(d) Energies $E_{l,k}$ is calculated for all subbands using (Eq. 9.7).
(e) Set the initial basis $B = \{B_{L-1,1}, B_{L-1,2}, \ldots, B_{l,k}, \ldots, B_{L-1,2}^{L-1}\}$ related to the subbands at the bottom level.
(f) The entropy of a parent node $E_{l,k}$ is compared with the sum of the entropy of two child nodes $(E_{l+1,2k-1} + E_{l+1,2k})$. If $E_{l,k} \leq (E_{l+1,2k-1} + E_{l+1,2k})$, then replace $B_{l+1,2k-1}$ and $B_{l+1,2k}$ by $B_{l,k}$ in B; else set $E_{l,k} = (E_{l+1,2k-1} + E_{l+1,2k})$, i.e., assign the sum of the children's entropy to the parent node.
(g) Repeat (f) for the next higher level until the root is reached.
(h) A sample is selected from the training set.
(i) The sample is decomposed to L using W.
(j) Wavelet coefficients are calculated with the corresponding best basis B.
(k) Max, Min, Mean and Standard deviation of the wavelet coefficients are calculated to form a 4-dimension feature.
(l) Repeat steps (h)–(k) for all samples.

The depiction of the Wavelet Packet tree with the best tree is shown above in Fig. 9.2. As wavelet transforms were fruitful in signal processing applications, a

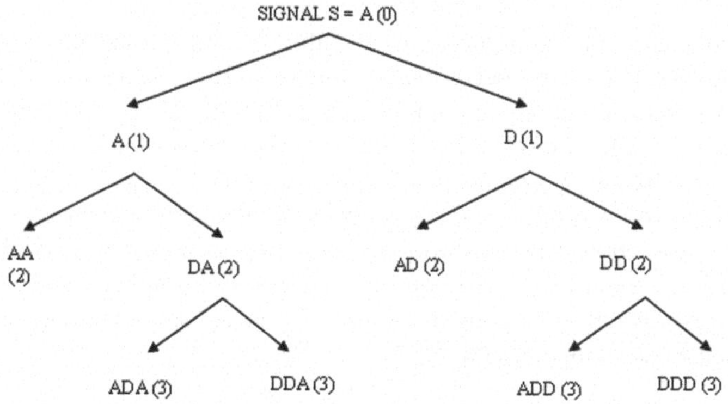

Fig. 9.2 Wavelet Packet Tree (Best tree)

continuous correlation linking $(i-1)$, i and $(i+1)$ feature sets are used as in the case of signals. The wavelet transform's localization property can extract spatial signal's finer details. These features are managed and estimated extracting information at all wavelet decomposition levels of a spatial signal. Discrete Wavelet Transform (DWT) was used in texture classification and image compression because of its multi-resolution decomposition property. N dimensions to lower dimension approximation generate approximation coefficients in the wavelet transform while error vectors generate corresponding detail coefficients [24]. Multi-resolution knowledge mining analyzes error vectors at various vector spaces V_k where $k < N$ for representing stable knowledge. In dimensionality reduction, it searches for appropriate error vector e_k in lowest K dimensional space where $K < N$ that holds optimum or enough detail for a classifier and extracts error vectors expressed knowledge at different dimensions.

9.3.2 Fusion of Features

Fusing WPT features and First-Order Histogram was suggested. Features extracted using First-Order Histogram and WPT are first normalized. The product rule fusion technique fuses normalized features after securing Median Absolute Deviation (MAD) between two features [25]. In MAD, the median of all values is computed and the difference of each from the median value is calculated. A positive value is a difference between value and median and the median of that difference set is MAD. The MAD is the average of the absolute deviations from the median. It measures how the data points vary or spread out from the median, $\bar{x}$

To find the MAD

1. Find the median
2. Find the distance of each data point from the median by subtracting the median from the data point $x - \bar{x}$
3. Since distance is always positive, find the absolute value $|x - \bar{x}|$
4. The MAD is the median of all the absolute value.

The combination of two or more images information for a specified application is image fusion. For fusion performance, Intensity, Hue, Saturation (IHS) transform, PCA statistical/arithmetic combination and multiscale fusion were resorted to in the past. Wavelet transform is a popular multiscale transform. Image fusion is undertaken in a frequency domain where contourlet transform is used. Compared to other multiscale transforms, it is more condensed, directional and ensures information at every resolution. The transform focuses on representing point discontinuities and conserving an image's time/frequency details [26]. Simplicity and being able to uphold image details with point discontinuities make contourlet transform-based fusion scheme suit change detection.

The image fusion steps are as follows:

Step 1: WPT and MAD are taken.
Step 2: Fusion rule is applied on approximate, diagonal, horizontal, and vertical coefficients of both images.
Step 3: Perform MAD for a fused image

9.3.3 Classifiers

Supervised machine learning like Naive Bayes, KNN, and Decision List algorithm are used for analyzing the data sets of heart patients [27]. The extracted features from FOH and WPT are fused and are then classified as dementia or non-dementia. The classification is undergone by using two classifiers, KNN Classifier, and Naïve Bayesian Classifier.

9.3.3.1 KNN Classifier

K-Nearest Neighbor (KNN) is a simple pattern recognition algorithm, it is a traditional nonparametric supervised classifier to ensure optimal values for K [28]. Current methods used KNN for brain image classification as normal or tumorous. KNN Classifier is used to compute the distance between the training samples and test samples in the nearest neighbors. Vector X is allotted to the class to which the majority of that K-nearest neighbors belong. Finally, the samples are classified with the majority vote on the classes of its K-nearest neighbors. Data points are assigned in a training phase in n-dimensional space. Training data points have associated labels that designate their class. A wavelet transform-based KNN algorithm exploits important information hidden in transform coefficients reducing computational complexity. KNN has a slow running time.

9.3.3.2 Naive Bayesian Classifier

Due to the poor run-time performance in KNN, another classifier chosen for dementia classification is the Naive Bayesian Classifier. Singh and Chetty [29] proposed a Naive Bayesian Classifier to detect brain abnormalities by assuming independent features. A selected kernel function maps attribute vectors to feature space (having higher dimensions), linearly/nonlinearly. Naive Bayes is a probabilistic classifier which applies Bayes' theorem (Baye's rule) with independence (Naive) assumptions. Bayes rule for multiple pieces of evidence is represented mathematically as in Eq. (9.8):

$$P(H|E_1, E_2, \ldots, E_n) = \frac{P(E_1, E_2, \ldots, E_n|H) \times P(H)}{P(E_1, \ldots, E_n)} \tag{9.8}$$

where $P(H|E_1, E_2, \ldots, E_n)$ is the posterior probability, $P(H)$ is the priori probability of H and $P(H|E_1, E_2, \ldots, E_n)$ be the priori probability. After feature extraction and feature fusion, Naïve Bayesian Classifier is used in order to classify whether the image corresponds to the normal image or dementia image. In the present work, the samples are categorized as healthy subjects or subjects suffering from dementia diseases class by KNN Classifier.

9.3.4 IoT for Patient Monitoring

Data mining techniques are used to detect whether the patient is suffering from dementia disease or not. Once the abnormalities are identified using the computer-aided diagnosis method, further caregiver is essential to take care of the patients. In this chapter, the remote monitoring of dementia disease in elderly people using the IoT has been presented. The IoT is a physical device that is used for the exchange of data, patient monitoring, treatment progress observation, and the housing of vaccines. It can improve the interaction of doctors and patients for the effective and approachable treatment processes. Telemedicine with artificial intelligence technique in robotics healthcare, the advancement of telerobotic surgery and Internet of Robotic Things (IoRT) described. Details on wearable devices already available targeting the biomedical and healthcare applications that are capable of collecting, analyzing by standard protocols by machine intelligence for predictions of health-related issues are described [30]. Electronic healthcare makes a distance between the patient and a doctor irrelevant. The concept of the Internet of Things (IoT) driven healthcare and health monitoring is further enhancing the growth of the electronic healthcare sector. In an IoT driven healthcare setup, the data collected originates from various things deployed for facilitating the proper diagnosis [31]. Implementation of IoT in the healthcare sector besides solving many issues is resulting in analysis or even predictions of patients' health status. As the IoT ensures linkage between virtual and real-world entities and thus enables anytime connectivity of anything [32]. Hence, the IoT approach in healthcare is proving valuable in assuring compliance with some of the right principles in healthcare. IoT results in improved communication between medical staff and patients to solve problems more effectively. This is because in the IoT approach the ubiquitous sensors and connected systems can provide the valuable and right information at the right time for better healthcare delivery. Hence, Internet of Things paves way for new opportunities for the right care, another important paradigm for proper healthcare [33]. The healthcare solutions based on IoT technology are gaining popularity due to the continuous monitoring, cost-effectiveness and scalability characteristics. IoT enabled smooth homes are not only aiming to provide an environment for supported living but are also enabling regular monitoring of elderly people in a modest manner. Sensors could be placed in areas to detect movement and vital signs. In this proposed method, the activities of the patient life-like temperature, heart rate, and pulse are computed using sensors. Depending on the value of the sensors, the notification will be sent to the doctor's mobile. Based on the notification, the doctor can give the suggestion immediately to the patient as well as to the caregiver for further immediate action. A smartphone application is to be designed to help patients to avoid medicine administration errors. It represents a novel attempt to integrate healthcare support with mobile computing which helps the patient to remember the events. This is achieved by sending reminders to the patient and the function to be performed are alerting by issuing medicine in-take reminders, provide medicine identification and in-take directions and also maintain the medicine in-take records.

9.4 Results and Discussion

Images are acquired from OASIS database and the evaluation of dementia classification is undergone by considering 68 dementia images and 144 normal images. Figure 9.3 shows the first-order histogram achieved for the sample images 1 and 2 respectively.

The sample of the image after applying wavelet decomposition with the best basis for dementia and non-dementia is shown in Fig. 9.4. Then a WPT post-ordered search is undertaken where a best basis decision compares the node's quantitative values to a node's descendant branch's cumulative effects. The performance indices like classification accuracy, average precision, average recall, and *F* measure are evaluated for dementia disease classification.

1. Classification Accuracy

   The percent of correct classification (PCC) is used as the measure for evaluating the performance of Dementia Classification.

$$\text{CA} = \frac{\text{No. of Dementia images correctly classified}}{\text{Total No. of Normal images correctly classified}} \times 100$$

2. Average Precision

$$\text{Precision} = \frac{\text{Number of relevant images retrieved}}{\text{Total number of images retrieved}}$$

3. Average Recall

$$\text{Recall} = \frac{\text{Number of relevant images retrieved}}{\text{Total number of relevant images in database}}$$

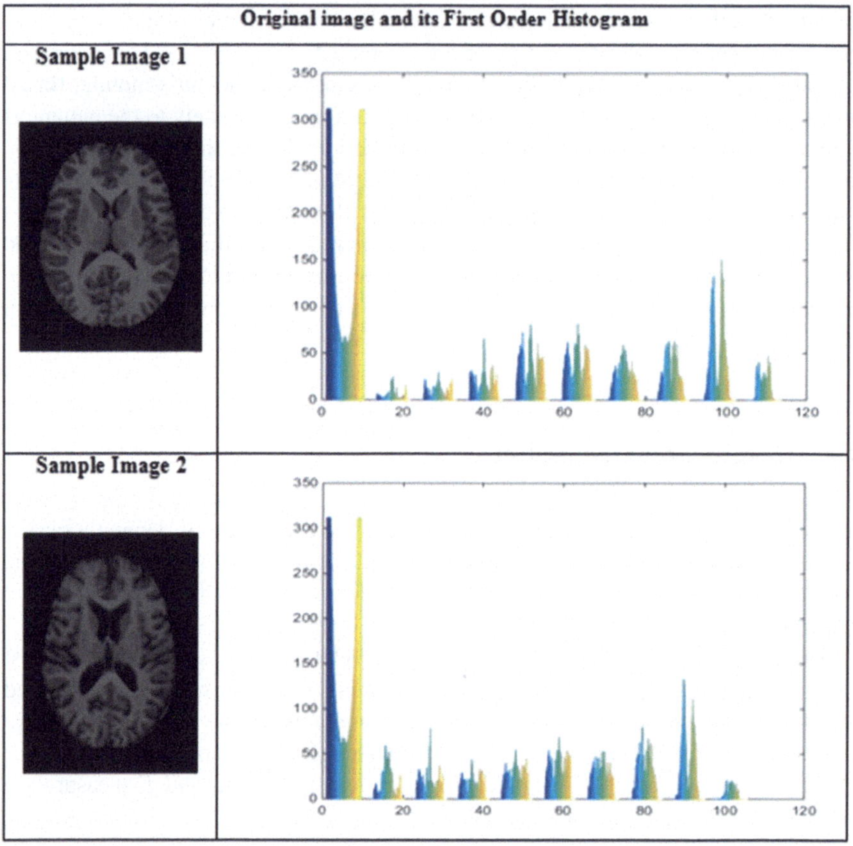

Fig. 9.3 First-Order Histogram

4. *F* Measure

$$F \text{ measure} = \frac{2 * \text{precision} * \text{recall}}{\text{precision} + \text{recall}}$$

The performance of the classification accuracy, average precision, average recall, and average *F* measure has been evaluated using the following methods:

First-Order Histogram and KNN Classifier,
First-Order Histogram and Naïve Bayes Classifier,
WPT and KNN Classifier,
WPT and Naïve Bayes Classifier,
Fused features and KNN Classifier, and
Fused features and Naïve Bayes Classifier

The above methods are compared with GLCM and FLICM segmentation.

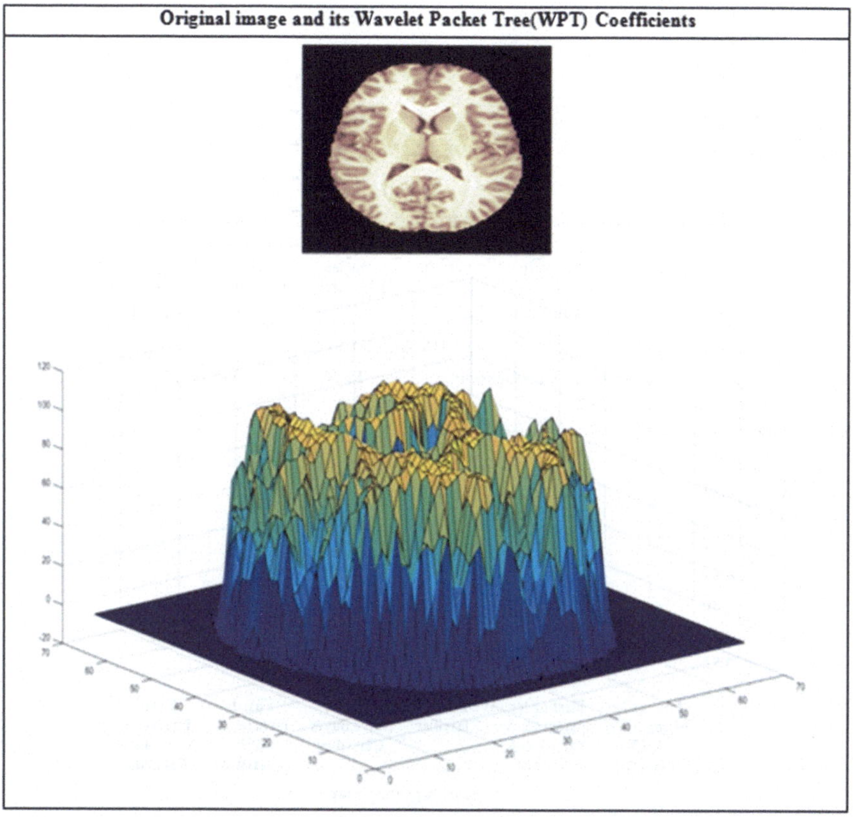

Fig. 9.4 Wavelet Packet Tree

From Fig. 9.5, it is observed that the performance of the proposed fused method with FLICM segmentation improved the average classification accuracy by 1.12% when compared with GLCM segmentation methods. It is observed that fused features and Naïve Bayes classifiers using FLICM segmentation achieve a classification accuracy of 93.87% which is better than the fused features and KNN Classifier.

From Fig. 9.6, it is detected that the performance of the proposed fused method with FLICM segmentation increased the average precision by 1.12% when compared with GLCM segmentation methods.

From Fig. 9.7, it is detected that the performance of the proposed fused method with FLICM segmentation improved the average recall by 1.64% when compared with GLCM segmentation methods.

From Fig. 9.8, the performance of the proposed fused method is observed as FLICM segmentation increased the average *F* measure by 1.28% when compared with GLCM segmentation methods. Table 9.1 shows the comparison of dementia classification and it is observed that 63 dementia images are correctly classified using the fused features and Naïve Bayes Classifier.

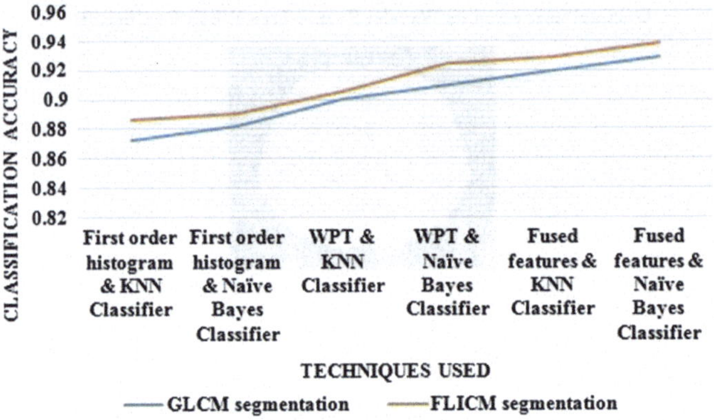

Fig. 9.5 Classification accuracy for fused features

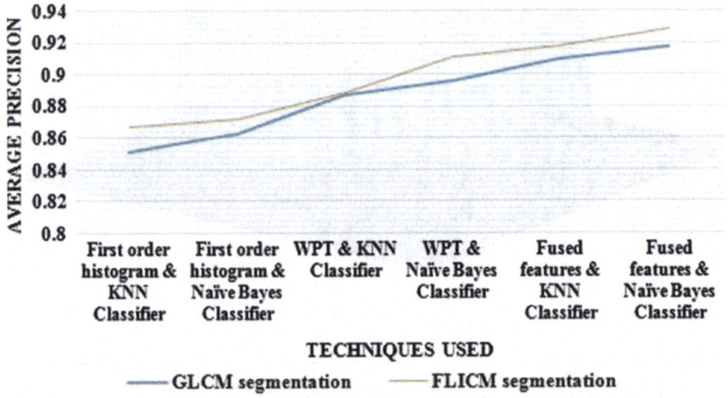

Fig. 9.6 Average precision for fused features

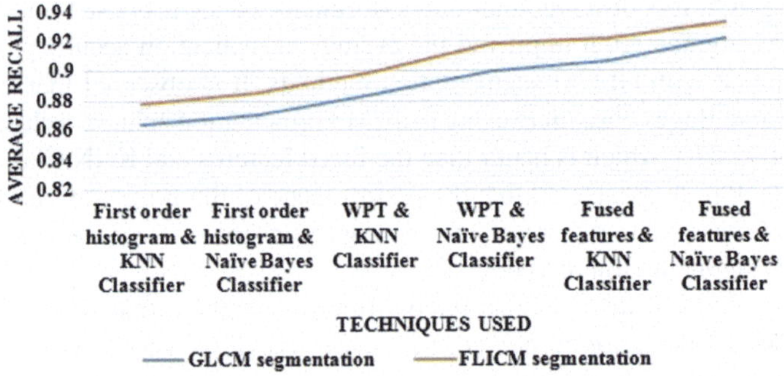

Fig. 9.7 Average recall for fused features

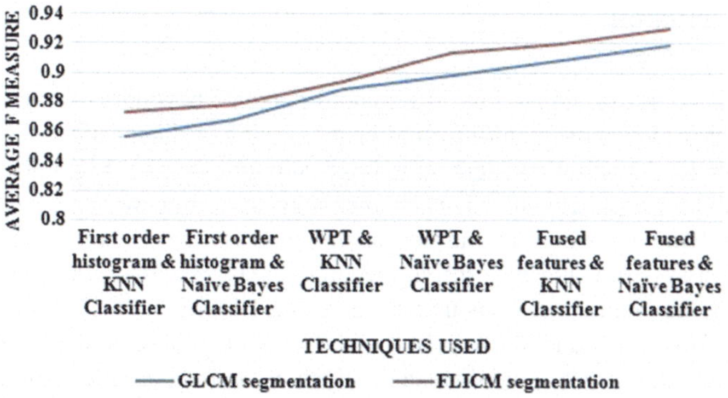

Fig. 9.8 Average *F* measure for fused features

Table 9.1 Number of dementia correctly classified for fused features

Techniques used	GLCM segmentation	FLICM segmentation
First-Order Histogram and KNN Classifier	57	59
First-Order Histogram and Naïve Bayes Classifier	59	59
WPT & KNN Classifier	60	60
WPT & Naïve Bayes Classifier	60	61
Fused features and KNN Classifier	60	62
Fused features and Naïve Bayes Classifier	61	63

From Fig. 9.9, the performance of the proposed method increased the number of dementia correctly classified by 1.94% when compared with GLCM segmentation methods is observed.

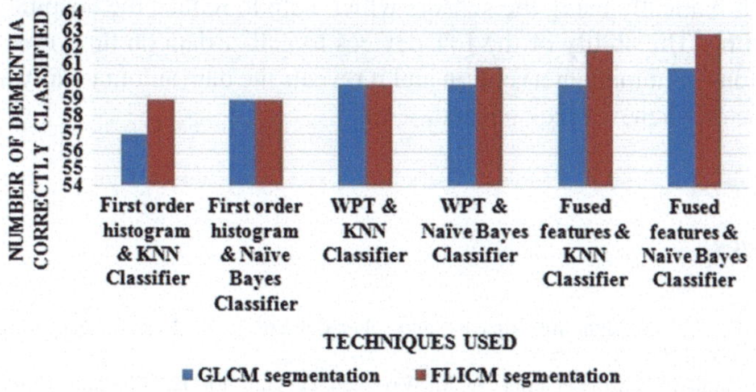

Fig. 9.9 Number of dementia correctly classified for fused features

9.5 Conclusion

Dementia is cognitive ability loss in impaired persons, beyond usual aging. Brain aging results in slow movement/information processing. A diagnostic tool MRI evaluates dementia. An automatic dementia diagnostic tool is needed as it afflicts more than 36 million people globally. This chapter suggests a framework to classify MRI images for dementia using data mining techniques. The work presents a dementia classification system using data mining techniques. OASIS data set images evaluated the scheme. Segmentation is undergone using GLCM and FLICM techniques. First-Order Histogram and WPT features are fused and are classified by KNN and Naïve Bayes Algorithms. Performance analysis is undergone after feature fusion using both GLCM segmentation and FLICM segmentation. Classification accuracy is better for fused features with Naïve Bayes Classifier than the fused features with KNN Classifier. The overall classification accuracy achieved using the proposed feature fusion technique is 93.87%. Results prove that the new method achieved better accuracy, precision, recall and *F* measure for fused features and Naïve Bayes Classifier. The proposed method was successfully applied to MR image acquired from OASIS database for dementia identification. This proposed system using data mining techniques can provide an important assistant to physicians, thus to make their decisions on their patients. The results including classification accuracy, precision, and recall and *F* measure showed that the proposed system can effectively identify possible dementia patients from the healthy. In future, accuracy can be improved further by including a suitable feature selection technique after the features are extracted with the present mechanisms.

A monitoring system based on the Internet of Things devices helps to monitor and analyze the physical activities of Alzheimer's disease patients. This method aims in helping the patients to improve their life quality and carry out their routine activities while providing the caregiver with a mechanism to follow the patient's activities round-the-clock from their own location itself. The patient monitoring and control system frequently checks the pulse rate, heartbeat rate, the temperature of the patients automatically using the sensors which help to reduce the hospital visit and also save time. The ability of the IoT devices to gather data on their own removes the limitations of human intervention and it reveals the data automatically and sends it to the doctor whenever they needed.

References

1. Duthey, B. (2013). Alzheimer disease and other dementias. In *A public health approach to innovation* (pp. 1–74).
2. Bron, E., Smits, M., van der Flier, W. M., Vrenken, H., Barkhof, F., Scheltens, P., et al. (2015). Standardized evaluation of algorithms for computer-aided diagnosis of dementia based on structural MRI: The CAD Dementia challenge. *NeuroImage, 111,* 562–579.
3. David, P., & Mark, W. (2010). Neuropsychological Assessment of Dementia: Access NIH public, PubMed central, US National Library of Medicine National Institutes of Health.

4. Hu, R. (2011). Medical data mining based on decision tree algorithm. *Canadian Center of Science and Education, 5,* 14–19.
5. Chakraborty, C. (2019). Computational approach for chronic wound tissue characterization. *Informatics in Medicine Unlocked, 17,* 1–10.
6. Zheng, B., Yoon, S. W., & Sarah, S. (2014). Breast cancer diagnosis based on feature extraction using a hybrid of k-means and support vector machine algorithms. *Expert Systems with Applications, 41,* 1476–1482.
7. Joshi, S., Bhagya Shree, S. R., & Sheshadri, H. S. (2010). Classification of neurodegenerative disorders based on major risk factors employing machine learning techniques. *International Journal of Engineering and Technology, 2,* 350–355.
8. Sharma, N., Kolekar, M. H., Jha, K., & Kumar, Y. (2019). EEG and cognitive biomarkers based mild cognitive impairment diagnosis. *IRBM, 2,* 113–121.
9. Plant, C., Teipel, S. J., & Ewers, M. (2010). Automated detection of brain atrophy patterns based on MRI for the prediction of Alzheimer's disease. *NeuroImage, 50,* 162–174.
10. Hamou, A., Simmons, A., Bauer, M., Lewden, B., et al. (2011). Cluster analysis of MR imaging in Alzheimer's disease using decision tree refinement. *International Journal of Artificial Intelligence, 16,* 1–10.
11. Shane Kippenhan, J., Barker, W. W., Nagel, J., Grady, C., & Duara, R. (1994). Neural network classification of normal and alzheimer's disease subjects using high-resolution and low resolution PET cameras. *Journal of Nuclear Medicine, 35,* 7–15.
12. Matsuda, H. (2007). Role of neuroimaging in Alzheimer's disease with emphasis on brain perfusion SPECT. *Journal of Nuclear Medicine, 48,* 1289–1300.
13. Natarajan, S., Joshi, S., Saha, B. N., Edwards, A., Khot, T., Moody, E., Maldjian, J. A., et al. (2012). A machine learning pipeline for three-way classification of Alzheimer patients from structural magnetic resonance images of the brain. In *11th International Conference on Machine Learning and Applications (ICMLA)* (Vol. 1, pp. 203–208).
14. Sucharitha, M., & Parimala Geetha, K. (2015). Brain tissue segmentation using Fuzzy clustering techniques. *Technology and Health Care, 23,* 571–580.
15. Kaur, M., Jain, K., & Lather, V. (2013). Study of image enhancement techniques: A review. *International Journal of Advanced Research in Computer Science and Software Engineering, 3.*
16. Selvarajah, S., & Kodituwakku, S. R. (2011). Analysis and comparison of texture features for content based image retrieval. *International Journal of Latest Trends in Computing, 21.*
17. Aggarwal, N., & Agrawal, R. K. (2012). First and second order statistics features for classification of magnetic resonance brain images. *Journal of Signal and Information Processing, 3,* 146–153.
18. Srinivasan, G. N., & Shobha, G. (2008). Statistical texture analysis. In *Proceedings of World Academy of Science: Engineering and Technology* (p. 48).
19. Amiri, G. G., & Asadi, A. (2009). Comparison of different methods of wavelet and wavelet packet transform in processing ground motion records. *International Journal of Civil Engineering, 7,* 248–257.
20. Mokji, M. M., & Abu Bakar, S. R. (2007). Gray level co-occurrence matrix computation based on Haar wavelet. In *Computer Graphics, Imaging and Visualization* (pp. 273–279).
21. Kim, S., Kang, W., Lee, E., & Paik, J. (2010). Wavelet-domain color image enhancement using filtered directional bases and frequency-adaptive shrinkage. *IEEE Transactions on Consumer Electronics, 56,* 1063–1070.
22. Preda, R. O., & Vizireanu, N. D. (2011). Quantization based video watermarking in the wavelet domain with spatial and temporal redundancy. *International Journal of Electronics, 98,* 393–405.
23. Shannon, C. E. (1948). A mathematical theory of communication. *Bell System Technical Journal, 27,* 379–423.
24. Abramovich, F., Bailey, T. C., & Sapatinas, T. (2000). Wavelet analysis and its statistical applications. *Journal of the Royal Statistical Society: Series D (The Statistician), 49,* 1–29.

25. Polikar, R., Tilley, C., Hillis, B., & Clark, C. M. (2010). Multimodal EEG, MRI and PET data fusion for Alzheimer's disease diagnosis. In *Annual International Conference of Engineering in Medicine and Biology Society (EMBC)* (pp. 6058–6061).
26. Venkateswaran, K., Kasthuri, N., Arathy, C., Haran, V., Jeni, D. D., et al. (2013). A survey on unsupervised change detection algorithms. In *International Conference on Circuits, Power and Computing Technologies* (pp. 897–903).
27. Jyothi Soni, J., Ansari, U., Sharm, D., Soni, S., et al. (2011). Predictive data mining for medical diagnosis: An overview of heart disease prediction. *International Journal of Computer Applications, 17,* 43–48.
28. Sivaramakrishnan, A., & Karnan, M. A. (2013). Novel based approach for extraction of brain tumor in MRI images using soft computing techniques. *International Journal of Advanced Research in Computer and Communication Engineering, 24.*
29. Singh, L., & Chetty, G. (2012). A comparative study of MRI data using various machine learning and pattern recognition algorithms to detect brain abnormalities. In *Proceedings of the Tenth Australasian Data Mining Conference* (Vol. 134, pp. 157–165). Australian Computer Society.
30. Amit, B., Chinmay, C., Anand, K., & Debabrata, B. (2019). Emerging trends in IoT and big data analytics for biomedical and health care technologies. In *Handbook of data science approaches for biomedical engineering* (Vol. 5, pp. 121–152). Elsevier.
31. Mersini, P., Evangelos, S., Efrosini, S., & Athanasios, T. (2013). Health internet of things: Metrics and methods for efficient data transfer. *Simulation Modelling Practice and Theory, 34,* 186–199.
32. Boyi, X., Xu, L., Hongming, C., Cheng, X., Jingyuan, H., & Fenglin, B. (2014). Ubiquitous data accessing method in IoT-based information system for emergency medical services. *IEEE Transactions on Industrial Informatics, 10,* 3131–3143.
33. Parah, S. A., Sheikh, J. A., Ahad, F., Loan, N. A., & Bhat, G. M. (2015). Information hiding in medical images: A robust medical image watermarking system for E-healthcare. *Multimedia Tools and Applications.*

Chapter 10
Social, Medical, and Educational Applications of IoT to Assist Visually Impaired People

Soham Sharma and M. Umme Salma

Abstract General daily tasks have always been a problem for visually impaired people. Identification of daily objects becomes a hectic task. Traditional methods such as a walking stick and a guide dog have been helpful to the visually impaired for basic navigation. Such, methods have a lot of limitations and often fail under varied situations. Technologies such as Computer Vision and Pattern Recognition (CVPR), Image Processing (IP) Internet of Things (IoT), etc. have made a major contribution to overcoming the limitations. IoT brings a lot of technical and automated solutions to assist the visually impaired people. Data science and analytics are a major part of the process. Data accumulated via various sensors can be processed and used to identify obstacles and enhance basic navigation using haptic and voice feedback. Raw data goes through a series of analysis and refinement. This is then processed into a form which is understandable to the system and can be directly interpreted to perform various components of an application. These applications involve education, navigation, entertainment, security, consumer, etc. These applications are across various verticals of technologies differing in terms of hardware, software, and protocols. Various economically feasible and accurate solutions are now available. While, optimization remains an issue. These devices have generally been very helpful to ease the lives of visually impaired people. The main aim of this article is to provide essential details related to real-world applications of IoT in the field of education, healthcare, entertainment, security, navigation, and solutions to address the daily challenges faced by visually impaired people. The structure of the article includes introduction to IoT, applications of IoT in modern era is dealt in detail in Sect. 10.1. Followed by hardware device and communication technologies in Sect. 10.2. Section 10.3 deals with state of art which focus majorly on research contributions related to applications of IoT and smart devices benefiting the lives of visually impaired. Section 10.4 incorporates the future scope and concludes with a summary in Sect. 10.5. The article covers more than 30 research contributions in the

S. Sharma · M. Umme Salma (✉)
Department of Computer Science, CHRIST (Deemed to be University), Bengaluru, India
e-mail: ummesalma.m@christuniversity.in

C. Chakraborty et al. (eds.), *Internet of Things for Healthcare Technologies*, Studies in Big Data 73, https://doi.org/10.1007/978-981-15-4112-4_10

past ten years which includes journal papers, conference papers and patents which provide a detailed and clear view on the research being carried out in the field of IoT to help the visually impaired.

Keywords IoT · Sensors · Wearable sensors · Sensor applications · Machine learning · Arduino · Smart devices

10.1 Introduction

IoT is an advanced technology finding its applications in all walks of life targeting our day to day activities, providing ease and automation in all the fields. "*IoT, in modern times is an interconnection of various devices such as microcontrollers, sensors,* etc. *which exchange, process and analyze data to perform certain decision-based operations.*" IoT in its earliest form has been around us without any coined terminology. It can be commonly seen in general day to day devices in our vicinity. In modern times, IoT is substantially targeting the interests of automation and human strenuous tasks, providing smart and optimized solutions. In 2018, Microsoft announced another round of $5 Billion investment over the next few years focusing on cloud services and other IoT analytics. Sonos, the leading smart speaker's manufacturer launched its IPO to the public. Rockwell Automation also announced $1 billion investments for its future IoT R&D. 5G networks also saw a rise, while it was introduced in late 2018 to 4 cities of the USA. According to a recent survey, it has been revealed that China is the top investor in IoT followed by Korea and India, respectively. It also predicted by Morgan Stanley that, "There will be more than 75 billion IoT devices by 2020". 23% of global businesses are utilizing IoT solutions in their operations. This has given a substantial rise to the global wearable technology market.

10.1.1 Applications of IoT in Modern Era

IoT has been around us for many years in different forms and it was only recently that terminology was coined for it. It gained immense popularity after the introduction of Arduino. Arduino was developed in 2003 by IDII in Italy. It is an open-source hardware and software company manufacturing single-board microcontrollers and kits for building digital components. These microcontrollers are programmed using C & C++ languages. These devices also support an IDE, which is written using JAVA. IoT has a myriad of applications from the production of large-scale industrial products to individual care systems. Today, IoT is one of the most important and widely popular technology in the market. It is being incorporated in various general day to day devices to ease our efforts and work more efficiently. There exist myriad applications

Table 10.1 Challenges faced by visually impaired people

S. No.	Challenge	Category
1	Navigation	Personal
2	Sensing and dealing with sudden weather changes	Environmental
3	Communicating with others	Social
4	Using technology	Technological
5	Inability to read completely or partially	Educational

of IoT influencing all walks life including consumer applications, agricultural applications, social applications, engineering applications, financial applications, health applications and many more. These applications range out from individual scale to large industrial scale and have their own importance. One such important application of IoT is individual care. In an individual care application, more importance is given to smooth and safe running of individuals' life. It deals with smart assistance, strong navigation system, personal care, and security of an individual. The individual may be a healthy person or an individual who requires special care such as children, senior citizens, patients suffering from ailments and diseases, or specially-abled people.

Specially-abled people are the people who aren't different from other people but they are the ones challenged with physical and/or mental challenges. Dumb, deaf, visually impaired people are the people who are considered as specially-abled people. Specially-abled people especially visually impaired people face a lot of challenges in their day to day life. The major problem is navigation and apart from this there are many other problems faced by them. Some of the important challenges faced by visually impaired people are given below (refer Table 10.1).

Table 10.1 clearly indicates the major challenges fall in six main categories namely personal, environmental, social, technological, and Educational. In this article, we aim to discuss the application of IoT to address the above-mentioned problems.

It is believed that a dog and a cane are the best friends for a visually impaired person. But, science technology especially IoT has emerged as an unseen ally befriending them and answering all the needs and necessities of the visually impaired persons. At ACIC-Santa Catarina Association for the Blind Integration, the very first e-cane prototype was showcased during the year 2009 [44]. Some of the applications of IoT befriending visually impaired people are listed below (refer to Table 10.2).

Table 10.2 specifies some of the real-world IoT applications used worldwide to solve the day to day problems faced by visually impaired people. Making more such applications is the aim of the researchers. In this research article, the main focus is to provide detailed information regarding such applications of IoT in making the lives of visually impaired people much easier. The survey paper covers more than 30 articles collected from various peer-reviewed journals and conferences. The focus is to facilitate the readers with updated information on recent trends in IoT solving various challenges faced by visually impaired people. The mainly dealt challenges are safety, navigation, recognition, and health monitoring.

Table 10.2 Applications of IoT for specially-abled people

S. No.	Application type	Example
1	Consumer application	Amazon Echo [4] DOT Watch [23] Blitab [11]
2	Healthcare	Omron Thermometers [42] Prodigy Diabetic Supplies [47] A&D Medical Talking Blood Pressure Monitor [39]
3	Security	V.Alrt [52]
4	Navigation	Dr Odin Smart Stick [24] We Walk Smart Stick [54] Bawa Cane Stick [10]
5	Education	Feelif [27] SMART Brailler Thinker Bell Labs [51]
6	Entertainment	B-Touch Mobile Phone [2] 3D PhotoWorks [45]

After the Introduction in Sect. 10.1, Sect. 10.2 provides the information regarding the most widely used hardware devices and communication technologies to solve day to day problems faced by specially-abled people in general and visually impaired people in specific. With the knowledge of technologies and devices, we further head to cover the recent advancements in research related to IoT-based technologies and devices have been produced by various researchers to solve blind people's issues. Apart from this, many software-based models have been discussed in Sect. 10.3 to provide more insight into the related topics. Section 10.4 sheds light on the future scope of the same and finally, in Sect. 10.5 an overall summary of the survey is being projected followed by the conclusion.

10.2 Hardware Devices and Communication Technologies

Depending upon the application IoT makes use of a variety of hardware devices and technologies. This section deals with some of the major and widely used hardware devices and communication technologies specifically meant to solve the problems related to blind people.

10.2.1 Communication Technologies

Communication between IoT devices stands as the backbone for data exchange and analysis. This is implemented using various technologies which are commonly seen

Table 10.3 Communication Technologies used to build IoT applications

S. No.	Technology	Standard	Frequency	Range	Data rates
1	Bluetooth	Bluetooth 4.2	2.4 Ghz ISM	50–150 m	1 Mbps
2	Zigbee	Zigbee 3.0	2.4 Ghz	10–100 m	250 kbps
3	Z-Wave	Z-Wave Alliance ZAD12837	900 MHz ISM	30 m	9.6/40/100 kbit/s
4	6LowPan	RFC6282	Adapted from Bluetooth or ZigBee	N/A	N/A
5	Thread	Thread	2.4 Ghz ISM	N/A	N/A
6	Wi-Fi	802.11n	2.4–5 Ghz	50 m	600 Mbps Max
7	Cellular	GSM/GPRS/EDGE (2G), UMTS/HSPA (3G), LTE (4G)	900/1800/1900/2100 MHz	GSM: 35 km Max HSPA: 200 km Max	35–170 kps (GPRS), 120–384 kbps (EDGE), 384 Kbps–2 Mbps (UMTS), 600 kbps–10 Mbps (HSPA), 3–10 Mbps (LTE)
8	NFC	ISO/IEC 18000-3	13.56 MHz ISM	10 cm	100–420 kbps
9	Sigfox	Sigfox	900 MHz	Rural: 30–50 km Urban: 3–10 km	10–1000 bps
10	Neul	Neul	900 MHz ISM	10 km	100 kbps Max
11	LoRaWAN	LoRaWAN	Various	Urban: 2–5 km Sub Urban: 15 km	0.3–50 kbps

in our daily drivers (refer Table 10.3) [19]. Bluetooth is one of the most popular data exchange implementations which has evolved over the years to become a solid justification of security and enhanced connectivity rates.

Even though there are many technologies that can be exploited for making real-world assistive applications for visually impaired people majority of them are built using NFC, ZigBee, and LOWPAN as they can be supported by many hardware devices. Details related to major hardware devices used in IoT are given in section B.

10.2.2 Hardware Devices

Hardware devices incorporate a set of microcontrollers, sensors, power and memory devices (refer Table 10.4). These are essential to establish physical connections between two endpoints communicating with each other. As mentioned in Sect. 10.1,

Arduino is one of the most popular microcontrollers due to its ease of availability and high compatibility levels.

Some of the sensors specifically used to design the applications related to assistance of visually impaired people are schematically represented in Fig. 10.1.

Table 10.4 Hardware devices used to build IoT applications

S. No.	Device	Type	Description
1	Arduino Uno Rev3	Microcontroller	It is the most popular and most widely used Arduino board. It is based on the ATmega 328P Datasheet
2	Arduino Nano	Microcontroller	Arduino Nano is the small and compact board by Arduino which is similar to the Arduino Uno Board and also based on ATmega328P Datasheet
3	Node MCU ESP8266	Microcontroller	It is a fully TCP/IP stack compatible microchip by Espressif Systems. It has a 32-bit microcontroller and 16 GPIO pins
4	Raspberry Pi 3B+	Microcontroller	It is a 3rd generation single-board computer by Raspberry Pi Foundation. It has a 1.4 Ghz 64-bit quad-core processor
5	Arduino Mega 2560 Rev3	Microcontroller	It is a microcontroller by Arduino based on ATmega2560. It is widely used for its ability to support 54 digital input and output pins
6	Mobile	Communication device	A mobile phone is a compact and handheld communication device which can be used to make phone calls and send short messages
7	Neo-6 M	Navigation device	Neo-6 M is a widely popular global positioning system compatible with Arduino. It can be used to acquire position, speed and time data while the position is changed

(continued)

Table 10.4 (continued)

S. No.	Device	Type	Description
8	Camera	Capturing device	A camera is a capturing device that can be used to record the visual images of the surroundings. It varies in terms of quality and sizes, ranging from small micro cameras compatible with Arduino to full-frame digital single-lens reflex cameras
9	5 V battery	Energy device	A battery is an energy device consisting of one or more cells. These cells have chemicals which are later converted into electrical energy on usage
10	HC-SR04	Sensor	HC-SR04 is a very popular and common ultrasonic sensor compatible with Arduino. It can be used to detect objects in 2–400 cm range
11	Microphone	I/O device	Microphone is a voice capturing device that is used to convert sound waves into electrical variations. These variations can be stored, transmitted or altered
12	Buzzer	I/O device	A buzzer is an audio output device which can be used for signaling by producing a buzzing noise
13	RFID Reader	I/O device	Radiofrequency identification reader is a device that is used to read radio frequency information from the tags. This transmission of information occurs through radio waves

(continued)

Table 10.4 (continued)

S. No.	Device	Type	Description
14	RFID Tag	I/O device	Radiofrequency identification tags are devices which store information. This information can be read using a reader through radio waves
15	Vibration module	I/O device	It is a haptic feedback device which can be used to generate vibrations using an electric motor
16	Barcode reader	I/O device	It is a scanner which can be used to scan barcodes using optics
17	Barcode	I/O device	A visual and machine-readable method of data representation
18	HC-05	I/O device	A Bluetooth module designed to provide wireless communication using serial port protocol
19	LED	I/O device	Light-emitting diode is a source of light when current flows through it
20	DHT11	Sensor	It is a digital humidity and temperature sensor
21	MQ-2	Sensor	It is a gas sensor which can detect LPG, Propane, and Hydrogen
22	IR Infrared flame detector	Sensor	A flame detector has a resistor, capacitor, potentiometer, IR receiver, and comparator

10.3 Literature Survey

The first application of IoT related to solving problems of visually impaired people was proposed by [25] where the engineers proposed a model for testing parts for their precision. A sound gauge was developed which had an amplifier connected along with cable. The parts are measured for their thickness and corresponding audio feedback as well as visual feedback is given through the device.

Later, with the improvement in science and technology many improved and sophisticated research contributions to assist visually impaired people were put forth

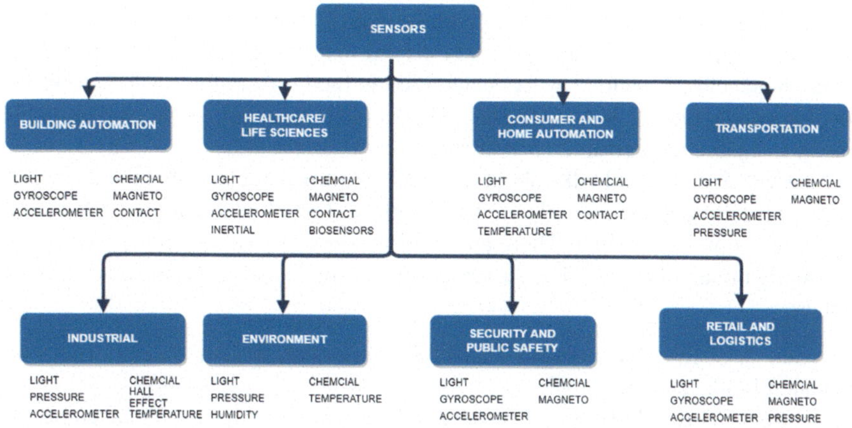

Fig. 10.1 Sensors in IoT

by various researchers. Some of the important contributions related to the same is discussed in this section.

In this section, the state of the art is divided into six subsections as listed in Table 10.2. Under each subsection, the related research contributions are discussed in detail.

10.3.1 Consumer Applications

A system to assist the visually impaired to effectively use the city bus system is proposed by [53]. An interactive wireless solution is developed to reduce the difficulties of the visually impaired. The system has two modules namely bus module and user module which are connected to each other. The user is required to make an input of 4 digits, this sends a notification to the corresponding bus module where and audio feedback is made along with an LED flash. The success rate is claimed to be 100% in certain situations. This is a low-cost assistance device for the visually impaired to board a specific bus.

A smart system to assist the visually impaired people is developed by [46]. This method has various modules. Text to speech module is a combination of image and speech processing. This module is used to analyze the 3d image of the environment and convert it into text and later use Google's application interface to convert it to audio output. The other modules are object and image recognition. These are used to identify general objects in a person's daily life such as books, pens, etc. Face recognition analyses various aspects of a face such as the jawline, eyes, nose, etc. These are then compared with the images in the database for recognition.

Wearing glasses and a walking assistant developed by [55]. Technologies such as cloud computing and ZigBee has been used for device communication. The walking assistant and the glasses have ultrasonic sensors and GPS module embedded on them. These are used to collect data, which is passed onto the GSM module embedded on the handheld assistant. The collected data is then transmitted to the cloud for governmental database and processing. The whole system has a solar rechargeable battery to ensure uninterrupted power supply.

A survey done by [26] talks about the WHO reports that claim that there are 285 million visually impaired people around the globe. Out of which around 39 million people are completely blind. There are multiple systems to assist in the navigation of visually impaired people. The survey covers wearable and carry-on smart devices such as:

- Visual Assistive Technology: Vision Enhancement, Vision Substitution, and Vision Replacement.
- Electronic Travel Aids: Set of sensors and hardware devices used to accumulate data and provide the processed output to the user.
- Electronic Orientation Aids: Pedestrian navigational aids.
- Position Locator Devices: GPS-based navigation and obstacle detection devices.

A modification of an existing smart backpack is proposed by [20]. It incorporates photoelectric sensors, RFID and ZigBee technology to assist visually impaired people. The photoelectric sensor emits light which is blocked when obstructed by an obstacle. RFID technology is used to detect unique objects by scanning the RFID tags. Audio feedback is provided to the user about the current location and the distance between them using text to speech libraries. An application needs to be installed in the smartphone for the system to work. The assistance device is claimed to be accurate in most of the test cases.

10.3.2 Healthcare

A survey on the personal healthcare system by [5] describes the role of RFID technology in association with IoT to accumulate and process data using multiple channels. This data is generally temperature, humidity, and other factors in a human environment. The processed data is compared with human behavior. The survey also discussed the scope and future trends in personal healthcare-based research.

An IoT Architecture to monitor the health of medically challenged and aged people by [1] is a set of six cloud-based modules. It has physical sensors for the collection of user information, a circuit for interfacing, a positioning system for outdoors, a microcontroller which is not very resource-intensive, a cloud-based server and a transceiver. The authors claim it to be a low-cost solution for implementing cloud-based wearable sensors for healthcare devices.

A patent by [49] demonstrates a medicine organizer for visually impaired people. It can hold multiple veils of medicines. Each veil has openings to dispense the medicine. With seven openings, each opening represents a unique day of the week. Each veil is marked in Braille to make it easy for the user to understand.

Biomedical data serves as primary data for monitoring the health conditions of individuals. An IoT-based system for managing and acquiring biodata data was proposed by [6] where the authors mainly focused on monitoring the heart rate and blood pressure of elderly people. The biomedical data was collected by establishing the communication between the system and electronic sphygmomanometer through blue tooth. The collected data is compared with the standard healthy readings based upon age and gender and the results are notified to the individuals as well as their caretakers. In case of emergency, the notification is also given to the doctor so that quick help can be provided. For the individuals who are visually impaired a special module called text to speech conversion is activated where the information is automatically converted to audio message. The system was designed to focus mainly on monitoring the individuals affected by obesity, hypertension, and diabetes. However, as future work, it was directed to be expanded towards other diseases and disorders.

Independent and free locomotion is possible only when all the psychomotor and sensor organs co-ordinate and perform well. But in the case of visually impaired persons movement is always been a problem due to lack of vision. In [48] the authors discuss various IoT-based approaches to solve the locomotive problem specifically for visually impaired individuals. The authors explain different approaches involving tactile auditory, software-based, smartphones based and other sophisticated devices based warnings to help in safe movement. The article not only focuses on finding the obstacle below the waistline but also those above the waistline. Some specialized canes such as UltracaneTM and Bat-KTMSonar which work purely on Ultrasound and sonar waves have been discussed. More elaborate information is provided in Sect. 10.3.4 where the point of discussion is entirely focused on navigation.

Authors in [15] have performed a detailed analysis on body area network of sensors. This can be used to monitor the patient remotely in emergency scenarios or general monitoring. Highly scalable architecture to provide real-time data has also been presented. It is a combination of both internal and external sensors. Various low-cost and less resource-intensive designing aspects have been discussed. Major focus is to prevent the hazardous effects of using WBAN and the radiation associated with it.

The same author has also suggested a remote monitoring system [16] for chronic wounds using smartphones. The system is claimed to be highly reliable and fast. The major aim is targeted to develop a tele-wound technology network (TWTN) system to inexpensively access the patient information remotely.

An analysis of emerging trends in biomedical data analytics has been performed by [9]. The author has discussed the workflow of big data in image analytics, artificial intelligence and its role in healthcare, smart wearable (IoT), and advancement in biotechnology. Based on the analysis it is concluded that the future of healthcare heavily depends on the various technologies and methodologies which are being developed and researched upon. These advancements are advantageous and gaining mass popularity and funding for the same.

10.3.3 Security

A situational awareness system to assist the visually impaired people proposed by [28] had a significant contribution to avoid accidents. A crowdsourced localization system is developed which provides audio feedback based on the location of a user in a 3D mapped environment. The system is based on various wearable and social sensors to analyze the environment. This system permits the user to participate in activities that align with his point of interest and also prevent accidents.

A currency reader for visually impaired by [36] uses a camera-based approach to identify the value of the currency. Real-time processing is done on the high-quality images captured by mobile cameras. An Ada-boost framework is used to train the currency reader for efficient ground subtraction and correction of the perspective. It is supported by major operating systems such as Windows and Symbian and can easily process 10 frames/s.

Authors in [21] claim that in near future artificial retina made up of IoT and Artificial Intelligence (AI) based system will be able to capture the images send it to the smartphone connected to the server process the data and identifies the images captured. This application can be used to identify the faces of the people and orient the information to visually impaired people.

The real-time analysis [18] of incoming data in unforeseen scenarios and the corresponding action taken to tackle those scenarios are a very important characteristic of an application. Such applications resemble human tendencies. Such applications are very complex to put into production, but also ensure proper security. Such scenarios can be effectively tackled with the help of IoT systems, one such system is the Automatic Product Security system where an entity can be used to provide derived security while the interaction is happening between cyberspace and individual/system. The best example for such IoT-based system is a QR code with an embedded link that can be used for fetching the relevant information.

A sophisticated IoT system mainly designed considering security and privacy issues was formulated by [55]. Here, the authors proposed a prototype where a special type of wearing glass and walking assistant was designed in such a way that the components effectively communicated with the system without compromising the security. The main reason behind the top security was that the entire system was built on ZigBee communication fully surrounded by secured communication protocols. The prototype also reveals that an embedded GPRS module with full-fledged 3G, 4G ID pin was attached in order to communicate with cloud computing center which facilitates high speed.

10.3.4 Navigation

The development of a navigation aid for the visually impaired people was proposed by [13]. This system involves the usage of ultrasonic sensors and vibration modules attached to a microcontroller. These sensors are integrated on a person's shoulder as well as the cane stick. The ultrasonic sensors detect obstacles within six meters forward distance and the microcontroller sends out output to the vibration modules which produce haptic feedback. Based upon the intensity of the vibration the blind person senses the obstacle is on his way and thereby changes his path before it approaches him.

The same author [14] produced another device with two different modules. One module used to detect obstacles using an ultrasonic sensor and to notify the user using haptic feedback. The other module is a navigational aid that is used to track and record the routes of a user by manual decision inputs using buttons. This recorded route can be later played using audio feedback during future commute. The system stores multiple routes that can be switched based upon an index.

A voice-based navigational aid for the visually impaired people developed by [41]. A smart cane is developed which has ultrasonic sensors embedded on it. These ultrasonic sensors are used to identify obstacles and sudden changes in the environment based on certain distance-based threshold values. The device can detect potholes as well as obstacles as close as 4 cm. An MP3 module is used to provide an audio output based on the ultrasonic sensor readings. This system works effectively in both the indoor and outdoor environments.

The assistive aids for the visually impaired people are talked about by [29]. It proposes a navigational assistance device which is economically feasible. It incorporates a camera and infrared sensors and is based on the Kinect's infrared capabilities. The obstacles are identified using a corner and depth detection method. The system is claimed to be reliable while identifying hurdles and suggest a secure route. The system prompts the user to turn in the direction accordingly.

An application for assisting the visually impaired people in [43] campus navigation. The system uses a GPS module to find the shortest path and guide the user. The system also has mounted sensors such as ultrasonic sensors to detect obstacles. These sensors transmit the information over Bluetooth to the android application which in turn provides an audio notification. The system uses 8051 microcontrollers to perform various operations.

A hurdle detection and navigational solution for visually impaired people is proposed by [3]. This system works in a designated area where it has been implemented. It has three modules. The first module determined the position of a user in the area. The second module detects various obstacles using ultrasonic sensors and mapping techniques. And the third module involves a user interface which makes it possible for the user to navigate.

An alternative to the cane stick used by the visually impaired to navigate is introduced by [7]. This device has various sensors mounted on it such as ultrasonic, IR, water, fire and LDR sensors. These are connected to the Arduino Uno R3 for processing. The output is given to the user through the buzzers, vibrator and voice alarms connected to the microcontroller. It also proposes a GPS navigation system through a mobile phone and earphones to prove audio navigational information.

A model that provides an electronic aid by [37] developing a gadget, i.e., a guiding stick which has a GPS module embedded in it. Paired with a Bluetooth headset, this device can be used to navigate around the environment. The GPS module helps to determine the location of the user and the system gives audio feedback to the user. The ultrasonic sensors emit waves that are used to calculate the distance between the object and the user. Based on which the intensity of the vibration module increases or decreases.

Various researchers talk about the problems faced by the visually impaired people they also talk about the unexpected environmental hurdles and the risks involved with it. Hence, [35] proposes a mobile-based guidance system. It provides a navigational route from the initial to the final point. It works with or without internet connectivity. The application is used to capture the image of the surrounding which is later processed at the backend. A neural network algorithm in the backend recognizes objects and hurdles and sends an output to the user. The efficiency of the system is 60%, while it is used to detect objects.

An electronic travel aid for visually impaired people proposed by [8]. This system has a combination of various sensors working together to detect obstacles. This system effectively uses ultrasonic sensors and depth-sensing techniques to detect obstacles. Auditory feedback is given to the user based on the detection. It also has integrated an augmented reality technique to benefit the partially visually impaired people. The AR glasses along with depth-sensing mechanism are used to make effective navigational decisions.

A navigational device to assist visually impaired people is developed by [12]. It proposes a device which provides varied pitch according to the proximity of the obstacles from the user. The system was tested on eight blindfolded users with the device and 12 blindfolded users without the device to complete a Hebb–Williams Maze. The set of users with the devices completed the maze faster than others in most of the trials. The rate of errors was less in the group with the device. The device not only serves as a navigational tool for direct paths but also provided an accurate means to traverse crossroads.

A navigational system to assist the visually impaired to commute to their point of interest and to identify their location while using the public transport system is introduced by [34]. The user is required to have a smartphone with GPS. The system updates the existing routes with new routes and downloads them from the backend. The GPS signal is refreshed every 5 s. Multiple applications are developed to assist blind pedestrians to walk and use public transport systems effectively.

10.3.5 Education

An enhanced adaptive utility device was introduced by [33] for visually impaired people. A digital sign system is developed, where various digitally encoded signs are distributed across the building. The user has a handheld reader which consists of infrared camera, image recognition techniques and a map with audio output. This system was tested on four different sets of users, resulting in an output that deemed it to be reliable for identifying various points of interests and routes.

A patent by [22] demonstrated a painting kit for visually impaired. This kit has a set of scented paints which can be identified by braille. It also has a work board with matching patterns on a sheet. A tactile indication can be provided by a shape. A vocal output is also provided when pressure is applied against a specific shape.

A writing device based on braille notation developed by [38] can be used as an alternative device for visually impaired students and teachers. It is designed with a concise brain cell which is single character in nature and a microcontroller that has an advanced tactile system. A modified neuron-based technology has been used to analyze this study. The system is limited to develop words up to three characters only. This system is also connected to mobile applications using Wi-Fi module.

A TTL serial camera with audio support is proposed by [50]. Instead of the traditional Braille system, this system captures the data in JPEG format and transmits it to the mobile device using Wi-Fi. An OCR application is used to convert the image into text. The text is further converted into audio using text to speech and is also stored in a cloud environment for future reference.

The authors in [17] claim that with the help of a combination made up of Augmented Reality (AR) an IoT system embedded with different sensors visually impaired people can be given the feel of different objects and materials along with the detailed explanation over voice. Using this the visually impaired people learn about different allows materials their characteristic, behavior, nature, changes w.r.t to surrounding, etc. through their other sensory organs specifically through touch.

10.3.6 Entertainment

Three different methods to assist the visually impaired people were proposed by [32]. The applications are location-based and can be used with modern-day smartphones. The first application Swipe and Scan Your Surroundings can be used to identify the various points of interest in the environment. The application uses swipe gestures to search the environment, and a text to speech service provides audio navigational output to the user. The second application Talking Transit is used to enhance the commute of visually impaired people in Tokyo. This provides services to search the timetable for the public transit and permits bookmarking, automated notifications and real-time status of railways. The third application Smart Building is used to monitor the status of the room and can be used to automate the controls of a room such as the lights, air conditioner, etc. A user is also notified if they are within 2 meters of a door. The notification consists of the information of the room such as A302 classroom.

A smart home solution has been proposed by [30]. The system has three layers in its stack.

1. Physical Layer: Raspberry Pi 3 Model B, Amazon Echo.
2. Application Layer: Alexa Skills Kit, Amazon Web Services.
3. Programming Layer: Python, Node.JS.

Raspberry Pi is used to drive power to the non-smart home components. Voice commands trigger subroutines in the Raspberry Pi to drive power to the various appliances. This system is highly extensible and is a low-cost alternative to smart home devices currently available in the market.

The author [40] analyzes 42 smart platforms based on their architecture and adaptiveness towards third party systems. The analysis infers that most of the smart systems are placed in a user's home and are not in regular contact with third party services and there are very limited cloud-based platforms available in the market. He also stresses on the importance of studying smart living concepts to understand platforms in a much better way.

Shopping for many has become a luxury or entertainment. The authors in [31] came up with a new system that entirely changed the way of shopping especially for the visually impaired. The system entitled Ambient Assisted Living Environments using RFID worked in five phases. Phase-1 online registration. Phase-2 RFID tag assignment where two tags are given to blind as wearable device one for finding item and another for getting navigation details. Phase-3 shopping, whenever the blind person picks an item and keeps in basket the information is sent to server and billing starts, phase-4 Direction category. Phase-4 is getting item details with the help of item RFID tag and phase-5 getting help for directions using direction RFID tag. The help is in the form of an audio message. Other applications related to helping the blind people to shop on their own are smart grocery shopping application where a portable RFID or Barcode reader is given to blind which scans the grocery item and sends the information in audio format via Bluetooth. The main advantages of using RFID over barcode are no line-of-sight issues and the ability to store more information. ShopTalk, Grazi, and Trinetra are some more examples of IoT-based applications assisting the visually impaired to be better shoppers [21].

The comparative details related to the articles discussed in these articles are provided (refer Table 10.5) in which the information related to articles covered in journals and conferences based on the applications is clearly specified.

Table 10.5 Distribution of articles

S. No.	Application	No. of articles from journals	No. of articles from conference
1	Consumer	4	1
2	Healthcare	6	2
3	Security	3	2
4	Navigation	8	4
5	Education	4	1
6	Entertainment	4	1

10.4 Future Scope

IoT is a revolutionary advancement in the field of computer science. It can help to support people with different abilities. This can significantly improve their quality of life. Visually impaired people face many challenges in their daily commute. There has been a lot of research on the same, but there has not been any single widely accepted solution till now. These solutions are unable to satisfy their needs completely. With the introduction of IoT in medical science, there has been a growth in blind related research. Conventional solutions such as a stick or a dog are generally preferred over an electronic aid. A reliable and relatively low-cost solution needs to be developed for the differently-abled. It is also essential to figure out a plan to improve the acceptance of such solutions. These solutions can significantly help the blind to commute and make smart decisions based on the environmental situations around them. The literature also reveals that strong research can be carried out in designing health-related devices. Such devices can be used to monitor the health of the user remotely and notify the concerned person or paramedics regarding any alarming situations or any emergency. Major focus can be given to design smart homes specially customized for blind people. This will bring more accessibility and ease to accommodate when a visually impaired person changes his location or moves to a new place.

10.5 Summary and Conclusion

During the survey, it was analyzed that IoT is becoming widely popular among the current technological trends. IoT has its applications in all the major domains related to both individual and large-scale applications. The most interesting and challenging research at the individual level is carried out in developing IoT-based applications for the assistance of visually impaired people. The IoT-based devices can be very helpful for assisting the visually impaired people in smoothly carrying out their day to day life activities. IoT research focuses on targeting the health needs, personal care, security, and other customized requirements, however, navigation is the widely explored area of application. There are quite an ample number of articles available on navigation-related research and communication technologies explored for the same. Among a list of myriad sensors, some majorly used sensors are Ultrasonic, Heat, Smoke, DHT, Haptic, GSM, GPS, RFID which are used along with microcontrollers such as ZigBee, Arduino Uno, Arduino Mega, Raspberry Pi, etc. to facilitate the visually impaired people taking smart decisions and warn them in emergency situations such as an obstacle or an accident. These devices can be attached to make a range of devices such as a smart stick, glasses, backpack, etc. Machine learning techniques and social sensors can be used to analyze the environment and notify the user about it. IoT along with SDN and data science techniques can create a big network profiting the blind and helping them to be a lot more independent.

It was also analyzed that most of the applications target the navigational ease of visually impaired people. The basic idea of the early set of papers evolves around the smart stick concept which has been enhanced over the years. The introduction of economically feasible and sophisticated sensors in the market used in a union with machine learning techniques has widely improved the success rates of the devices assembled in recent years.

These devices have evolved over time, but they are yet to reach high accuracy levels in detecting the environment around the visually impaired user and notifying him/her. They have high chances of failing and wrong judgements in terms of sudden occurrence of an obstacle. They have not been tested to perform in situations such as natural calamities. 360° detection of obstacles remains an issue due to the information overload and confusion between the sensors.

The incorporation of IoT-based technology in the day to day activities of a visually impaired people has been significantly beneficial. It has also been inferred that most of the research has been done in the fields of navigation and consumer applications for visually impaired. Future research is suggested to be directed toward healthcare and entertainment. It is very exciting to see the future of the same and how it gets even better.

References

1. Abdelgawad, A., Yelamarthi, K., & Khattab, A. (2016). IoT-based health monitoring system for active and assisted living. In *International Conference on Smart Objects and Technologies for Social Good* (pp. 11–20). Berlin: Springer.
2. abledata.acl.gov. (2019). able data. https://abledata.acl.gov/product/b-touch-mobile-phone. Accessed November 23, 2019.
3. Aladrn, A., Lpez-Nicols, G., Puig, L., & Guerrero, J. J. (2016). Navigation assistance for the visually impaired using RGB-D sensor with range expansion. *IEEE Systems Journal, 10*(3), 922–932. https://doi.org/10.1109/JSYST.2014.2320639.
4. Amazon. (2019). Amazon echo. https://www.amazon.in/Amazon-Echo-Smart-speaker-Powered/dp/B0725W7Q38. Accessed November 23, 2019.
5. Amendola, S., Lodato, R., Manzari, S., Occhiuzzi, C., & Marrocco, G. (2014). Rfid technology for IoT-based personal healthcare in smart spaces. *IEEE Internet of Things journal, 1*(2), 144–152.
6. Antonovici, D. A., Chiuchisan, I., Geman, O., & Tomegea, A. (2014). Acquisition and management of biomedical data using internet of things concepts. In *2014 International Symposium on Fundamentals of Electrical Engineering (ISFEE)* (pp. 1–4). IEEE.
7. Anwar, A., & Aljahdali, S. (2017). A smart stick for assisting blind people. *Journal of Computer Engineering, 19*(3), 86–90.
8. Bai, J., Lian, S., Liu, Z., Wang, K., & Liu, D. (2017). Smart guiding glasses for visually impaired people in indoor environment. *IEEE Transactions on Consumer Electronics, 63*(3), 258–266.
9. Banerjee, A., Chakraborty, C., Kumar, A., & Biswas, D. (2020). Emerging trends in IoT and big data analytics for biomedical and health care technologies. In *Handbook of data science approaches for biomedical engineering* (pp. 121–152). Academic Press.
10. bawa. (2019). bawa. https://www.bawa.tech/. Accessed November 23, 2019.
11. Blitab. (2019). Blitab. https://blitab.com/. Accessed November 23, 2019.
12. Botzer, A., Shvalb, N., et al. (2018). Using sound feedback to help blind people navigate. In *Proceedings of the 36th European Conference on Cognitive Ergonomics* (p. 23). ACM.

13. Bousbia-Salah, M., & Fezari, M. (2007). A navigation tool for blind people. In *Innovations and advanced techniques in computer and information sciences and engineering* (pp. 333–337). Berlin: Springer.
14. Bousbia-Salah, M., Redjati, A., Fezari, M., & Bettayeb, M. (2007). An ultrasonic navigation system for blind people. In *2007 IEEE International Conference on Signal Processing and Communications* (pp. 1003–1006). IEEE.
15. Chakraborty, C., Gupta, B., & Ghosh, S. K. (2013). A review on telemedicine-based WBAN framework for patient monitoring. *Telemedicine and e-Health, 19*(8), 619–626.
16. Chakraborty, C., Gupta, B., & Ghosh, S. K. (2020). Mobile telemedicine systems for remote patient's chronic wound monitoring. In *Virtual and mobile healthcare: Breakthroughs in research and practice* (pp. 977–1003). IGI Global.
17. Chien-Yu, L., Chao, J. T., Wei, H. S. (2010). Augmented reality-based assistive technology for handicapped children. In *2010 International Symposium on Computer, Communication, Control and Automation (3CA)* (Vol. 1, pp. 61–64). IEEE.
18. Coetzee, L., & Olivrin, G. (2012). Inclusion through the internet of things. In *Assistive Technologies*. IntechOpen.
19. CommTech. (2019). Commtech. https://www.rsonline.com/designspark/eleven-internet-of-things-iot-protocols-you-need-to-know-about. Accessed November 21, 2019.
20. Cruz, F., Yumang, A., Mañalac, J., Cañete, K., Milambiling, J.: Smart backpack for the blind with light sensors, ZigBee, RFid for grid-based selection. In *AIP Conference Proceedings* (vol. 2045, p. 020054). AIP Publishing.
21. Domingo, M. C. (2012). An overview of the internet of things for people with disabilities. *Journal of Network and Computer Applications, 35*(2), 584–596.
22. Donovan, K. R. (1993). Painting kit for the visually impaired. US Patent 5,217,378.
23. Dotincorp. (2019). Dot watch. https://www.dotincorp.com/. Accessed November 23, 2019.
24. drodin.in. (2019). Smart walking. https://drodin.in/product/smart-walking-stick-with-fm-radio-09a/. Accessed November 23, 2019.
25. Electrical Engineering. (2019). Electronic sound gauge helps blind to test production parts. https://ieeexplore.ieee.org/document/6442409. Accessed November 21, 2019.
26. Elmannai, W., & Elleithy, K. (2017). Sensor-based assistive devices for visually-impaired people: Current status, challenges, and future directions. *Sensors, 17*(3), 565.
27. feelif.com. (2019). feelif. https://www.feelif.com/. Accessed November 23, 2019.
28. Joseph, S. L., Xiao, J., Chawda, B., Narang, K., & Janarthanam, P. (2014). A blind user-centered navigation system with crowdsourced situation awareness. In *The 4th Annual IEEE International Conference on Cyber Technology in Automation, Control and Intelligent* (pp. 186–191). IEEE.
29. Kanwal, N., Bostanci, E., Currie, K., & Clark, A. F. (2015). A navigation system for the visually impaired: A fusion of vision and depth sensor. In *Applied bionics and biomechanics 2015*.
30. Kaundinya, A. S., Atreyas, N. S., Srinivas, S., Kehav, V., & Kumar, N. (2017). Voice enabled home automation using amazon echo. *International Research Journal of Engineering and Technology, 4*, 682–684.
31. Kesh, S., et al. (2017). Shopping by blind people: Detection of interactions in ambient assisted living environments using RFid. *International Journal of Wireless Communications and Networking Technologies*, 6(2).
32. Kim, J., Bessho, M., Koshizuka, N., & Sakamura, K. (2014). Mobile applications for assisting mobility for the visually impaired using IoT infrastructure. In *Proceedings of 2014 TRON Symposium (TRONSHOW)* (pp. 1–6).
33. Legge, G. E., Beckmann, P. J., Tjan, B. S., Havey, G., Kramer, K., Rolkosky, D., et al. (2013). Indoor navigation by people with visual impairment using a digital sign system. *PloS One, 8*(10), e76783.
34. Lima, A., Mendes, D., & Paiva, S. (2018). Outdoor navigation systems to promote urban mobility to aid visually impaired people. *Journal of Information Systems Engineering & Management, 3*(2), 14.

35. Lin, B. S., Lee, C. C., & Chiang, P. Y. (2017). Simple smartphone-based guiding system for visually impaired people. *Sensors, 17*(6), 1371.
36. Liu, X. (2008). A camera phone based currency reader for the visually impaired. In *Proceedings of the 10th International ACM SIGACCESS Conference on Computers and Accessibility* (pp. 305–306). ACM.
37. Mala, N. S., Thushara, S. S., Subbiah, S. (2017). Navigation gadget for visually impaired based on IoT. In *2017 2nd International Conference on Computing and Communications Technologies (ICCCT)* (pp. 334–338). IEEE.
38. Martillano, D. A., Chowdhury, A. F. D., Dellosa, J. C. M., Murcia, A. A., Mangoma, R. J. P. (2018). Pindots: An assistive six-dot braille cell keying device on basic notation writing for visually impaired students with IoT technology. In *Proceedings of the 2018 2nd International Conference on Education and E-Learning, ICEEL 2018* (pp. 41–47). New York, NY, USA: ACM. https://doi.org/10.1145/3291078.3291106. http://doi.acm.org/10.1145/3291078.3291106.
39. Medical and Online. (2019). Bp checking device. https://medical.andonline.com/product/premium-blood-pressure-monitor-verbal-assistance/ua-1030t?commerce_product=14. Accessed November 23, 2019.
40. Nikayin, F., & De Reuver, M. (2013). Opening up the smart home: A classification of smart living serviceplatforms. *International Journal of E-Services and Mobile Applications (IJESMA), 5*(2), 37–53.
41. Noorithaya, A., Kumar, M. K., & Sreedevi, A. (2014). Voice assisted navigation system for the blind. In *International Conference on Circuits, Communication, Control and Computing* (pp. 177–181). IEEE.
42. Omron (2019). Omron thermometers. https://www.omronhealthcare-ap.com/in/category/10-temperature-measurement. Accessed November 23, 2019.
43. Pawar, M., & Najawan, R. (2016). Route finding application for blind people. *IJEDR, 4*.
44. perkins.org. (2019). Smart Brailler. https://www.perkins.org/services/smart-brailler/. Accessed November 23, 2019.
45. photoworks.com. (2019). Photoworks. https://www.3dphotoworks.com/. Accessed November 23, 2019.
46. Priya, U., Thakare, K., Ankit, P., Ajinkya, R., & Om, S. (2017). Smart assistance system for the visually impaired. *IJSRP, 7*(12).
47. prodigymeter.com. (2019). Prodigy meter. http://www.prodigymeter.com/consumers/diabetic-supplies/. Accessed November 23, 2019.
48. Ramirez, A. R. G., González-Carrasco, I., Jasper, G. H., Lopez, A. L., Lopez-Cuadrado, J. L., & García-Crespo, A. (2017). Towards human smart cities: Internet of things for sensory impaired individuals. *Computing, 99*(1), 107–126.
49. Siegler, K. R. (1999). Medicine organizer. US Patent 5,941,394.
50. Sruthi, M., Rajasekaran, R. (2018). Reading assistance for visually impaired people using TTL serial camera with voice. In *Contemporary applications of mobile computing in healthcare settings* (pp. 170–180). IGI Global.
51. thinkerbelllabs.com. (2019). Thinker bell lab. https://www.thinkerbelllabs.com/. Accessed November 23, 2019.
52. VSNmobile.com. (2019). Vsn mobile. https://vsnmobil.com/products/v-alrt/. Accessed November 23, 2019.
53. Wang, H. L., Chen, Y. P., Rau, C. L., & Yu, C. H. (2014). An interactive wireless communication system for visually impaired people using city bus transport. *International Journal of Environmental Research and Public Health, 11*(5), 4560–4571.
54. wewalk.in. (2019). Walking stick. https://wewalk.io/en/. Accessed November 23, 2019.
55. Zhou, M., Li, W., & Zhou, B. (2017). An IoT system design for blind. In *2017 14th Web Information Systems and Applications Conference (WISA)* (pp. 90–92). IEEE.

Chapter 11
Design of an Embedded System for Remote Monitoring of Malnutrition for People Living in Rural Areas

Bikash Dey

Abstract Malnutrition is caused by the disparity between the amount of food nutrients that a body needs and the amount that the body receives via food. People who are living in remote areas or in rural areas are observed to suffer from malnutrition. Malnutrition is the case of the people living in rural areas and is a major concern for the overall health of the people. Malnutrition develops very slowly over the years. Changes at the cellular level begin to happen after a prolonged period of malnutrition. As a result of the malnutrition, the body loses its ability to fight against infections. For a prolonged period of time, many symptoms of the disease start emerging like anemia, edema, and goiter, so proper diagnosis and information collection are very necessary to find a remedy for this health problem. Internet of things (IoT) can play a great role in conjunction with an embedded system that will be used to collect data from those remote areas and be used to make a detailed analysis of the diseases caused by malnutrition. In this chapter, the detection and monitoring of nutrition levels with the help of proper embedded systems and IoT will be discussed. The design of proper embedded systems and the required interfacing programs for this purpose is a major issue. The proposed embedded system should work with Internet-connected devices [smartphone, other embedded devices] to be chosen very carefully with properties like low power consummation, low cost, and with the advanced interface for IoT. The embedded system should also be capable of exchanging data and commands via GPRS in the case where GSM networks are available or via Bluetooth transmission. The embedded system to be discussed also is having an interface with an android app for data exchange/control via smartphone.

Keywords Malnutrition · Embedded systems · Bluetooth · GPRS · Android

B. Dey (✉)
JIS College of Engineering, Kalyani, West Bengal, India
e-mail: bikash.dey@jiscollege.ac.in

C. Chakraborty et al. (eds.), *Internet of Things for Healthcare Technologies*, Studies in Big Data 73, https://doi.org/10.1007/978-981-15-4112-4_11

11.1 Introduction

Malnutrition is a problem for people who are living in rural areas and not getting proper food nutrients due to various reasons. The problem can be worse if we don't have to have a system to store the data regarding those people properly. The proper care and necessary medical aids can only be provided if there is an efficient embedded system available that can store a large amount of data for the people with a very easy interface to operate. To retrieve the information needed about the malnutrition status either for a single person or for a large number of people living on that rural area, embedded systems can play a very important role. Then only as a whole a complete medical picture can be drawn for those people and proper reason can be known, and proper medical remedy can be found out for those mass people.

The design challenges for such embedded system are as follows.

(1) The system should be easily integrable.
(2) The system should be of low cost.
(3) It should consume less power.
(4) Should have very easy user interface.
(5) Design should be modular in hardware and in software also.
(6) The system should have the capability to upgrade easily when there is a need to incorporate more people.
(7) Should be cable of using with smartphones as smartphones are most frequently used now days.
8) The hardware and its interface should have real-time event handling capability.
(9) Effective interaction with outside world through easy interface via SMS/Wi-Fi data exchange or via GPRS.

11.1.1 Problem Statement

Malnutrition is a growing problem in the rural areas which is caused mainly due to the disparity between the amount of food nutrients that a body needs and the amount it receives. This imbalance is most frequent in the rural areas as well as for the people who are under poverty level. Many diseases which generally observed among those people are mainly caused due to this malnutrition (especially due to under nutrition). Overnutrition may also be the cause of many diseases. This kind of malnutrition develops very slowly over months or years. The body's immunity level get hampered severally as the over the time the nutrition level of the body get decreased. Variety of diseases may be caused due to this malnutrition. The problem to manage those large amounts of data using some reliable, efficient, easy to use embedded system is a design challenge for embedded system designers. Once the data for a large number of people logged and properly maintained then proper medical treatment as well as making of future policies are possible for reducing the malnutrition.

IoT plays a vital role in addition to the design of embedded systems for advanced data storage and access. The problem of handling a large amount of data with the limited random storage capability of the embedded systems and making the logged nutrition test data and analysis data available throughout the world from any place and any time is to be solved with the help of IoT and advanced interface design for the embedded systems for IoT.

11.2 Literature Review

11.2.1 Issues of Nutrition

For any country, economic growth can be sustained if the mass population of the country is having good health and does not suffer from malnutrition. Nutrition-free countries will be possible when there is a diverse diet, including staple foods, vegetables, fruits, animal source foods when and where needed. The label of nutrition is affected due to many causes such as sanitation, safe drinking water, and disease. In addition to that, education can play a key role in improving nutritional intake and balance. Food insecure populations have a very high impact on society. Food vulnerable populations are, in general, characterized by a high or very high level of undernutrition or acute malnutrition. For example, low weight for height is a very important factor which may limit the development of an individual, and the effect can be over all the society. The malnutrition related to children is a very important issue for countries of Asia. Nutrition at early childhood plays a key role in their cognitive achievement, learning capacity, and as well as household welfare. General studies have been shown that low birth weight, protein–energy malnutrition in childhood, iron deficiency iodine deficiency, etc., all result to nutrition-related deficiencies, and this creates a lot of problems for the child who is ready to go to school for their primary education. When a significant proportion of the population is under malnutrition, the GDP growth rates will suffer. For adults, body mass index (BMI—defined as the ratio of body weight in kilograms to the square of height in meters) is an important parameter to be measured. Low stature and low BMI are associated with lower involvement in the labor force—not only do people with lower stature or BMIs earn less, but they are less likely to be able to earn wages at all. All the above problems are undernutrition, but the other end, there is malnutrition spectrum who is leading to overweight and obesity is called overnutrition. Obesity is a problem which is increasing in developed countries, has not given much attention in developing countries because undernutrition is the main issue in those developing countries. Overnutrition is a result of the diets that are characterized by dense energy nutrients, foods that are high in fat, sugar, and salt. This type of malnutrition is a major contributor to heart disease, stroke, diabetes, and cancer.

11.2.2 Biomedical Applications and Embedded Systems

The embedded system plays an important role in many biomedical applications for clinical analysis as well as for patient monitoring. The design of the autonomous, customized embedded system is an expensive task. There is an increasing demand for computing and communication in the embedded system, while it is to be used for the biomedical field. Many applications such as biochemical operations, chemical analysis, DNA analysis, proteomic analysis, and real-time pervasive patient monitoring are the fields where the embedded system communication and computing have been used very effectively. Portability and computing power are the key factors that lead to the integration of wireless devices on embedded systems in order to communicate with the world. The embedded systems must have good computing power and, on the other hand, must be easily integrable with the other systems along with the reliability and security issues properly implemented. Embedded system technology has various roles to play not only for biomedical applications but applications in various fields like industrial, telecommunication [1], etc. Embedded systems used in a wide range of diagnostic devices for biomedical applications that range from different handheld devices to biomedical instrumentation. For example, blood glucose monitors, blood pressure monitors, test detection of various diseases like dengue malaria, portable ECG, digital thermometer, digital flow sensors, and much more. Wireless technology incorporated with embedded systems helps for self-management and self-testing of various physical parameters such as blood pressure, blood glucose, and body temperature. Embedded systems equipped with wireless technology are more beneficial to patients and doctors, especially for monitoring purposes in a large environment [2]. Telemedicine is another field where an embedded system can also be used to diagnose prognosis and manage many patients. It also helps the physicians and the patients to access important information in real time [2, 5]. With the help of Internet-connected devices and web services, it is possible to create a community database of wound images for pressure, diabetic, arterial, and venous ulcer and its annotation with the supporting metadata through the telemedicine platform. Using a smartphone, it also becomes a possible acquisition of the data and has an interaction between the patient and doctor remotely [6]. The IoT and big data can play a crucial role in the analysis of the vast medical image database from various medical sources and in combination with AI [7]. With the advent of IoT, it is possible to have a smart healthcare system to improve the diagnosis and treatment of patients, access to advanced and emergency medical services [8].

11.3 A Brief Overview of Necessary Nutrition Tests

11.3.1 Albumin Blood Test

This test is used to measure the amount of albumin that is present in a person's blood [1]. Albumin is generally produced by the liver, and this helps to keep fluid in the bloodstream. So it does not leak into other tissues. It also carries various substances like hormones, vitamins enzymes to different parts of the body. Low albumin levels indicate a problem with the liver or kidney of humans. In a broad sense, this is basically a liver function test, and this helps to find out the different levels of enzymes and proteins that are present in the liver, including albumin. This test also helps to find out different substances present in the blood like electrolytes, glucose, proteins such as albumin. So in the case of rural areas, the diseases for which this test can be effective are jaundice, fatigue, weight loss, appetite loss, dark-colored urine, etc. Lower albumin labels than normal may result in liver disease, kidney disease, malnutrition, infection, inflammatory bowel disease, or maybe thyroid disease. If the album levels are higher than the normal levels, dehydration or diarrhea may result. Results are in grams per deciliter (g/dL). A normal albumin range is 3.4–5.4 g/dL. Lower albumin level results are due to malnutrition. Lower albumin level also results due to liver disease or an inflammatory disease. Higher albumin levels may result acute infections, burns, and stress from surgery or a heart attack.

11.3.2 Lipid Profile

Lipid panel or lipid profile is a total cholesterol check, calculating the amount of good and bad cholesterol and triglycerides found in the blood (which is a type of fat). Too much cholesterol may cause heart disease, stroke, and blockage of arteries.

A cholesterol test in general does the following.

(1) Total cholesterol: which is the total amount of cholesterol present in the blood
(2) Low-density lipoprotein (LDL) type of cholesterol: This is the bad cholesterol, if more amount of this is present then it increases the risk of heart attack.
(3) High-density lipoprotein (HDL) cholesterol: which is referred to as good cholesterol because it helps to reduce the LDL.
(4) Triglycerides: stored in the fat cells because of extra calories which are not needed by body. People who are overweight and diabetic and generally consumes too much sweets, drink too much alcohol may have this kind of triglyceride levels.

The results of this test are measured in milligrams (mg) of cholesterol per deciliter (dL) of blood.

Ideal results are given for an adult man.

- LDL: 70–130 mg/dL (the lower the number, the better)
- HDL: more than 40–60 mg/dL (the higher the number, the better)
- total cholesterol: less than 200 mg/dL (the lower the number, the better)
- triglycerides: 10–150 mg/dL (the lower the number, the better)

If the cholesterol numbers are outside of the normal range stated above, then there may be a higher risk of heart disease, stroke, etc.

11.3.3 CMP Test

CMP test or comprehensive metabolic panel test is a blood test that gives information about the person's fluid balance levels of electrolytic like potassium, sodium, etc. This test also gives information about the working condition of the liver and kidneys of the respective person. This test can also find out the type of glucose used by the body for energy. The high glucose levels may end up with diabetics. The electrolytes, like calcium, sodium potassium, and chlorides, play an important role for the body and have a balance between them that information can also be revealed from this test. Normal levels of these electrolytes are required for the proper functioning of cells present in the body. This test also reveals the levels of albumin and total protein. Having a lower level of these proteins may be due to kidney disease or liver disease or due to the nutritional problems. In general, a CMP test can give information about the kidney and liver working functions, blood glucose levels, electrolyte levels, and how much protein is in the blood. The results' range is the standards for individual tests like glucose, calcium, protein, albumin, total protein, electrolytes, sodium, potassium, CO_2 (carbon dioxide, bicarbonate), and chloride test.

11.3.4 CBC Test

This is a complete blood count test, and it is used to evaluate the overall health condition. This test can also detect a wide range of disorders, which include anemia, infection, leukemia, etc. Different components of blood cells its features can be revealed by this test. The information about red blood cells, white blood cells, hemoglobin, and hematocrit can also be found for this type of test. This test can also be prescribed by a doctor for overall health monitoring to diagnose a medical condition or to monitor medical conditions. Table 11.1 shows the standard ranges for this test. Table 11.1 is normal complete blood count results for adults.

Table 11.1 Normal complete blood count results for adults

Red blood cell count		Hemoglobin		Hematocrit		White blood cell count	Platelet count	
Male	Female	Male	Female	Male	Female		Male	Female
4.35–5.65 trillion cells/L[a],(4.32–5.72 million cells/mcL[b])	3.92–5.13 trillion cells/L (3.90–5.03 million cells/mcL)	13.2–16.6 grams/dL[c] (132–166 grams/L)	11.6–15 grams/dL (116–150 grams/L)	38.3–48.6%	35.5–44.9%	3.4–9.6 billion cells/L (3400–9600 cells/mcL)	135–317 billion/L (135,000–317,000/mcL)	157–371 billion/L,(157,000-371,000/mcL)

[a]L = liter, [b]mcL = microliter, [c]dL = deciliter

11.3.5 Total Protein Test

Proteins are essential for cells and tissues as well as an essential part of the growth, development, and health of the body. Blood contains albumin and globulin, which are the major providers of the proteins for a body. Albumin prevents fluid from letting out of the blood vessels where is globulin protein having an important role in the immune system. This test is to measure the total amount of albumin and globulin that is present in the body. This test is very important for the routine checkup of health. This kind of test can be advised by the doctor when there is unexpected weight loss, symptoms of kidney or liver disease. This test specifically looks for the amount of albumin and globulin present in the blood and whether they are a normal level or not. This also reveals the albumin and globulin ratio (*A*/*G* ratio) in the blood first. The normal range is between 6 and 8.3 grams per deciliter (g/dL) for total protein. This range may vary slightly from laboratory to laboratory. The *A*/*G* ratio (albumin to globulin) is usually slightly above 1. If the ratio is too low or too high, the source and condition need to be established through additional testing. If the ratio is small, it may suggest: inflammatory disorder, multiple myeloma, cirrhosis, kidney disease. A high ratio of *A*/*G* can signify hereditary or leukemia deficiencies.

11.4 Design of the Embedded System

11.4.1 Parts Required for the System Design

The core or heart of our system is an Arduino board (Arduino UNO). There are specific reasons for choosing this kind of embedded systems board with an onboard ATmega328P microcontroller. The Arduino board hardware and software are very easy to use for beginners as well as very flexible for advanced level embedded system designers. The software needed for the Arduino board runs on a variety of operating systems like MAC, Linux, windows. For low-cost implementation, this is the first choice for the engineers. This board has a simplified interface to work with its onboard ATmega328P microcontroller. The board is inexpensive in comparison with other microcontroller development boards. The software used to design and program Arduino is cross-platform software, which helps the developers of different platforms to work with this board very easily. The IDE of the software also has a very clean programming environment. The software and hardware both are open source, which helps a large community to enrich the resources by their own work and integrate it with the existing one.

11.4.1.1 Arduino UNO Board

The basic components of the Arduino UNO board are microcontroller (ATmega328P), memory, I/O pins, etc. The recommended supply voltage is 7–12 V. There are 14 digital input–output pins, six analog input pin, 32 kb of programming memory, among which 5 K used by the bootloader. The amount of SRAM that is available in the system is 2 KB.1 KB of EEPROM, and clock speed is 16 MHz. The weight of the system is as low as 25 g. There is also a 3.3 V supply voltage generator by the onboard regulator, which can be very effective for supplying the power to the devices/modules connected to this board. The board also having the serial interface for supporting SPI communication, using the SPI library which is provided by the open-source software of the Arduino (Fig. 11.1).

Power Supply
Arduino UNO board can be powered by the USB from PC or via external power supply. External power supply can come from AC to DC adaptor or DC battery, and the range is 7–12 V as per recommendation.

ATmega328P
This microcontroller is the heart of the Arduino board. This microcontroller is having 32 KB of program memory, 6 PWM channels, 10-bit resolution ADC.2K SRAM,

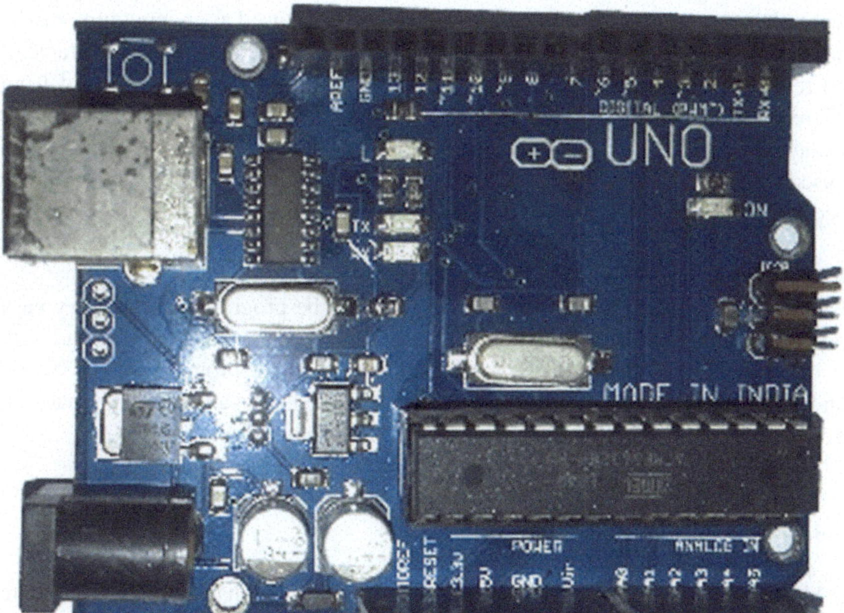

Fig. 11.1 Arduiono UNO board

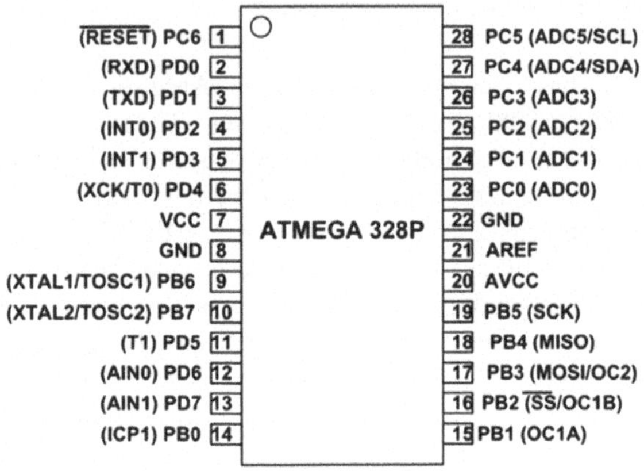

Fig. 11.2 ATmega328 IC

1K EEPROM. This is also having a programmable serial USART, master/slave SPI serial interface, I2C interface, on-chip analog comparator, etc.

Memory

The system has 2 kilobytes of static RAM and one kilobyte of EEPROM (Fig. 11.2).

I/O Pins

There are 14 digital pins on the UNO board, which can be used as an input or output. These pins are configurable and can be configured to be used as an input pin or to be used as an output pin. Some of the pins are having specialized functions like transmit and receiver, which can be used for transmitting and receiving data to and from different serial transmission devices, for example, Bluetooth device, GSM device, or maybe Wi-Fi device. There are few other pins also available in the board which is used for analog-to-digital conversion and supplying the power at 3.3 V or can be used for generating the PWM signal.

Device Programming

Using the Arduino IDE software, the Arduino can be programmed in a very easy and convenient way. Open-source software can be used for this purpose, and with the help of a preloaded bootloader at the Arduino board, the program file (HEX file) can be downloaded to the Arduino UNO board. There is also a facility to bypass the bootloader and program the device via the ICSP interface also.

11.4.1.2 GSM Shield

GSM shield is a module that can be integrated very easily with the Arduino system to achieve Internet connectivity as well as the connectivity with GSM for voice calling and SMS (Fig. 11.3). Internet connectivity can be provided via the GPRS of this shield. To work properly with this module, there is already existed a *GSM library*

Fig. 11.3 GSM shield

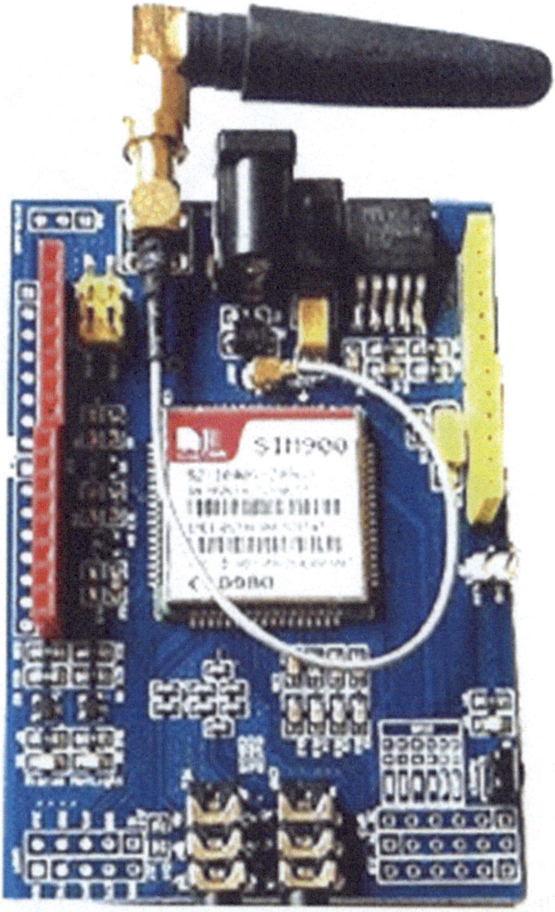

provided with the Arduino IDE. For proper operation of the GSM shield, there is a need for the SIM card and after that the device can be programmed to interact with the GSM shield. To communicate with the Arduino board, the TX and RX pins can be used.

11.4.1.3 Wi-Fi Module (ESP 8266)

Figure 11.4 is a simple Wi-Fi microchip with a full TCP IP stack. This Wi-Fi module allows Arduino to be connected with Wi-Fi whenever there is a Wi-Fi network available around the Arduino board. This device requires 3.3–3.6 V to operate properly. This 3.3 V can easily be supplied from the Arduino board. RX and TX pins are used to transmit and receive data from the Arduino board to and from this module. The ESP8266 has a 32 bit RISC CPU, 64 KiB of instruction RAM, 96 KiB of data RAM,

Fig. 11.4 Wi-Fi module

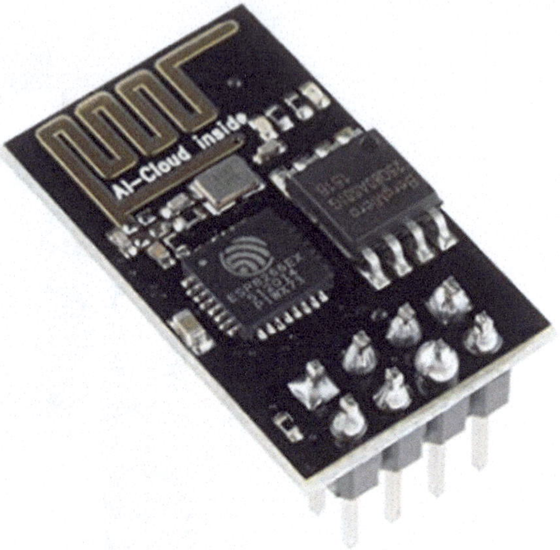

IEEE 802.11 b/g/n Wi-Fi. This module is also capable of transmitting and receiving data via the SPI, I2C interface. This module performs UART on dedicated pins and is also having a 10 bit ADC.

11.4.1.4 Bluetooth Module (HC-05)

The communication with the Arduino board via Bluetooth is possible with the help of the HC 05 module, which is used for Bluetooth communication. Arduino communicates with this device with its serial port, and the transmission and reception take place through the TX and RX pins of the Arduino board. For proper working of the device, this board requires a power 3.3–6 V and that device can easily be powered by the 3.3 V of Arduino board (Fig. 11.5).

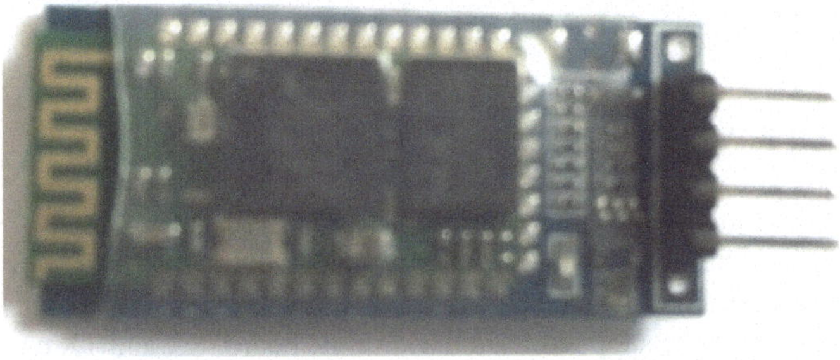

Fig. 11.5 Bluetooth module (HC-05)

11.4.1.5 SD Card Module

The SD/MMC card module allows Arduino to communicate with the Arduino for reading and writing to the SD/MMC card (Fig. 11.6). For the programming purpose, the SD library is used. This library gets installed with the installation of the Arduino IDE by default.

11.4.2 Structure of the System

The embedded system is composed of the Arduino-based embedded hardware board and the required hardware modules along with the software modules running in the hardware (Fig. 11.7). The required android app software components are also shown,

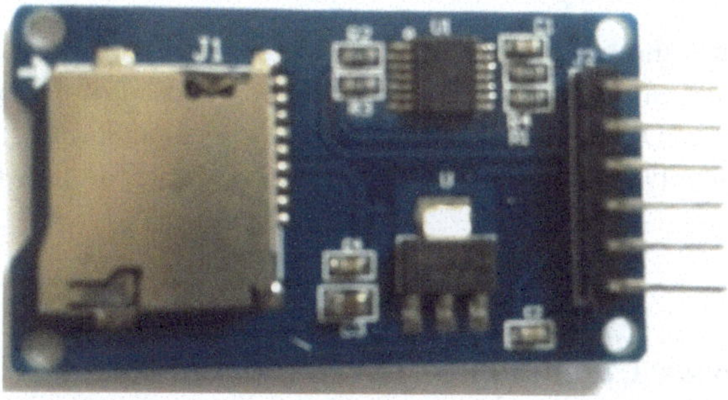

Fig. 11.6 SD/MMC card module

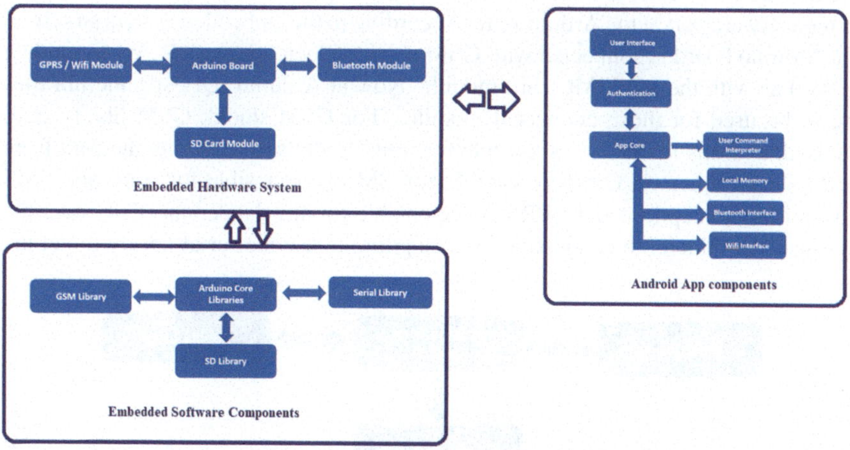

Fig. 11.7 Overall structure of the complete system (embedded hardware, software and the Android app)

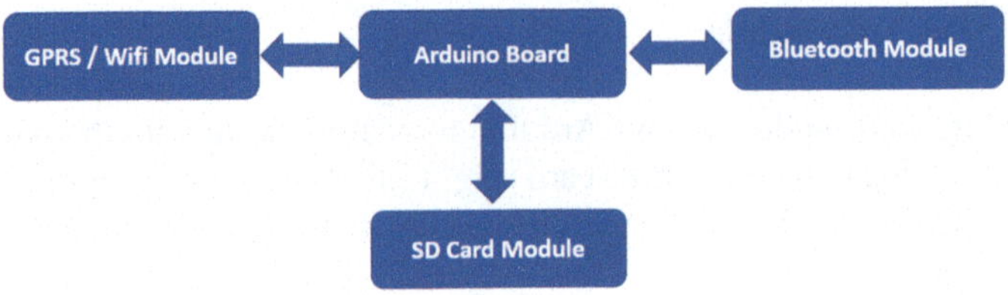

Fig. 11.8 Block diagram of the hardware components

which will interact with the hardware system via the Bluetooth channel or via the Wi-Fi link based on the policy of operation and access of the embedded system.

11.4.3 Embedded System Hardware Components

Figure 11.8 shows the basic block diagram of the embedded system that will be present in the medical test center. The system is composed of the Arduino board, Bluetooth module, SD card module, and GPRS or Wi-Fi module, or both. This system can very conveniently store nutrition data for all the people for the whole village or a few villages.

11.4.4 Software Components (for Development)

These are the software components for the development purpose of the Arduino board (Fig. 11.9). Here are all libraries that are going to be used for the development of the software part at the Arduino site. According to the embedded system structure, the Arduino board is connected with GSM shield, Bluetooth module, Wi-Fi module as well as with the SD/MMC card module. Now at Arduino IDE, specific libraries are to be used for those connected modules. For GSM shield, GSM library is to be used, and this library is responsible for transferring and receiving the data from GSM shield either via GPRS or via GSM. GSM is responsible for voice and SMS transmission/reception, and GPRS is responsible for any data connectivity over the Internet. For Bluetooth connection, we are going to use the serial library to get the

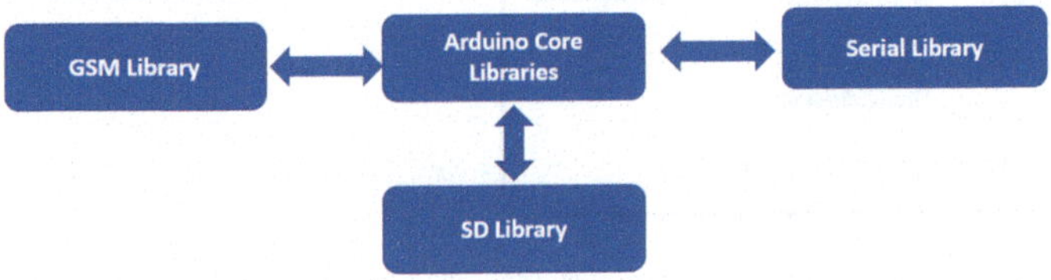

Fig. 11.9 Software components of the system (at Arduino side)

data and send the data via a Bluetooth link. The same serial library can be used for Wi-Fi connection also to transmit and receive data. For saving and retrieving data from the SD/MMC card, SD card library is to be used.

11.5 Operation of the Embedded System

11.5.1 Initial Nutrition Test Data Logging

The medical nutrition-related test laboratory should have an operator with his personal smartphone, which is very common now. The hardware will be at the medical nutrition test center. This is the main hardware, and all the data recording and processing will be at this hardware (Arduino-based hardware mentioned above). This hardware system can be accessed by any person having a proper level of authorization via Internet/Wi-Fi/Bluetooth. The overall working of the system is as follows. The operator at the medical test center will feed the test data to the system via the mobile app and utilizing the Bluetooth link. The app will then interact with the local hardware, and the data will be updated at the local hardware/system. The data storage of the embedded system may use the SD card (as SD cards of high capacity are available nowadays). As a rough estimate, 128 GB SD/MMC card may store data for 1–1.2 crore people according to the data scheme that will be mentioned in the following section.

11.5.2 An Overview of the People Coverage for a Rural Area Using the System

The amount of data that can be stored to the system decides how many people's data can be accommodated with the designed device, for example, if it is considered that a person has undergone 50 nutrition-related medical tests and each test result comprises 50 digit number and 128 GB is SD/MMC card being used, then 1–1.2 crore people's data can be stored which may cover one or several rural villages. So that is the amount of data that can be stored/recorded because nowadays 128 GB SD/MMC card is available, and the cost is affordable. The following discussion reveals the above-mentioned fact. Here, it is considered that each person test data contains a maximum 50 tests and some basic personal information, and each test data result is of a maximum 50 digit number (maximum). From Arduino's point of view character type of data takes 1 byte, and the numeric digit type of data takes 2 bytes.

Sample format for per person test data:

Person name: 100 bytes [say 100 character]

Address: 100 bytes

So basic information took 200 bytes.

Test name: 100 bytes

Test data: 200 bytes say (50 digit number takes 2 × 50 bytes + test data unit allowed to take another 100 bytes) [Maximum]

So single test data takes 300 bytes [Maximum]

If 50 such test data then 50 × 200 bytes = 10,000 bytes ~10 K

Total data size for a person = 10,000 bytes + 200 bytes (personal data) = 10,200 bytes = 10.2 KB

Now 128 GB SD card = 128,000 MB = 128,000,000 KB

So can store data for ~12,549,019 people.

So can store data for 1 crore to 1.2 crore people.

*The Arduino serial library may restrict this number to 2 GB storage only, but better library can be designed also to access all 128 GB storage.

11.5.3 Initial Setup at the Nutrition Medical Test Center

For the initial setup, the medical test center should be equipped with the hardware and smartphone (Android OS) to the operator who is going to insert the different nutrition test results for a particular person to the hardware with the help of the mobile app. The mobile app is going to store the information to the hardware via the Bluetooth link. The mobile app and the device communicates via Bluetooth, and when a proper command is issued from the operator side, the details of the results of the nutrition test will be stored to SD/MMC card with the help of the Arduino board. This is the initial setup that has to be performed at the nutrition test center. For malnutrition detection and record purpose, the diagnostic test center should be capable of performing tests like the lipid profile test, the CMP test, the CBC test, the albumin test, total protein, and maybe more than that. The designed embedded system can accomplish the recording of 50 such tests (maximum) (Fig. 11.10).

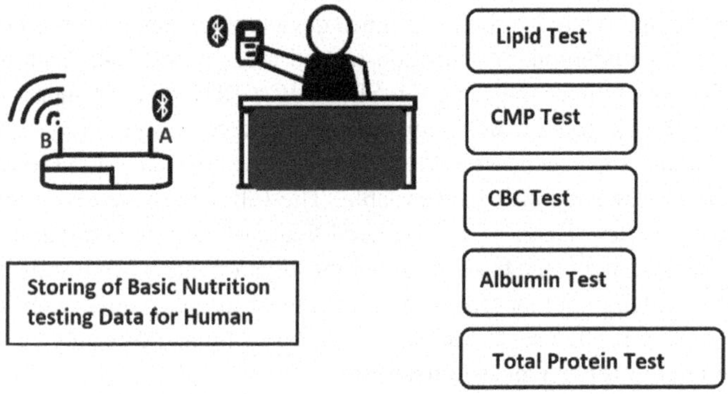

Fig. 11.10 Initial setup at the nutrition medical test center

11.6 Program Development and the Device Programming

11.6.1 Arduino IDE

Arduino's Integrated Software Development Environment (IDE) is open-source software which is used for the development of Arduino-based programs. This software allows the users to write the sketches (i.e., programs) to the host environment for different Arduino boards. The language that is used for programming is similar to C language. There are plenty of libraries available for the development of programs for the Arduino boards, and once the program development is done, then this IDE can also be used for programming the device by writing the hex codes to the program memory of the board via the USB port (Fig. 11.11).

The structure of an Arduino program is straightforward. It can have a minimum of two blocks, the first one is the preparation block, and the second one is the execution block. Setup() is the preparation block, and the loop() is the name of the execution block. When the program starts, the setup function is the first one to be executed. The statements that are written inside the setup block are called only once. For this reason, the setup functions or blocks is said to be used as an initialization purpose like starting of serial communication, etc. Execution block runs after the setup function or setup block execution is over. Execution block uses different host statements like reading the inputs and outputs checking conditions, etc.

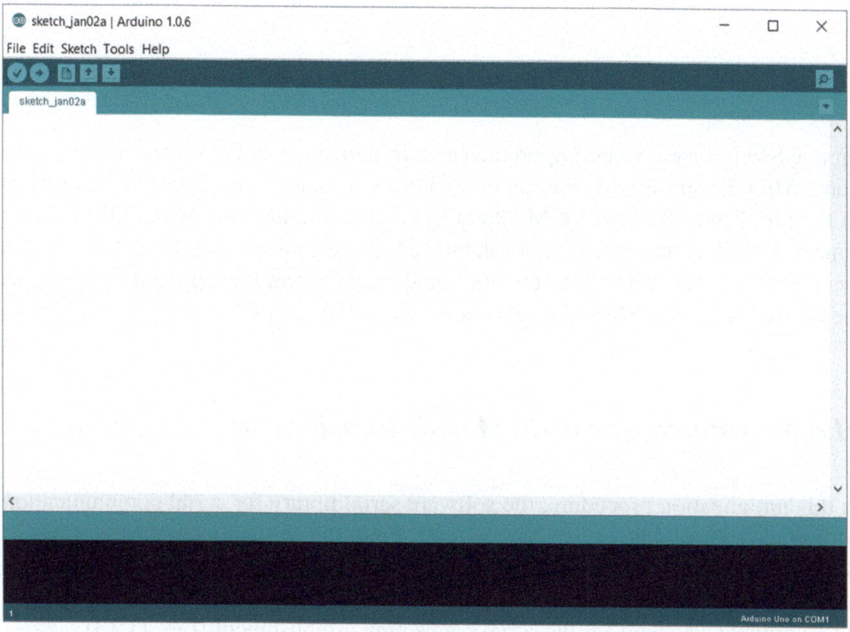

Fig. 11.11 Arduino IDE

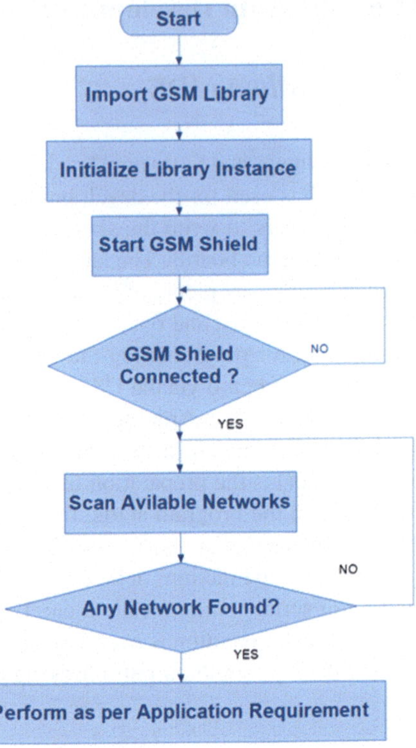

Fig. 11.12 Flowchart to initialize GSM shield

11.6.2 Arduino and GSM Shield Initialization Flowchart

First, GSM library is to be imported. Then, initialization of library instance is to be done. After the successful creation of the library instance, serial communication has to be initialized after that GSM shield to be started and wait for the GSM shield connection. Once the connection established, the scanning procedure starts for the available networks. When the network found, then the required application performs the desired task like (SMS, data exchange, etc.) (Fig. 11.12).

11.6.3 Arduino and Wi-Fi Module Initialization

In this initialization procedure, the software serial library for serial communication with the Wi-Fi module (ESP8266) is used. First, the software serial library has to be initialized. Then Arduino will wait for the connection with the Wi-Fi module, if connection established, then we perform the necessary data exchange tasks via the Wi-Fi module else wait for the serial connection establishment (Fig. 11.13).

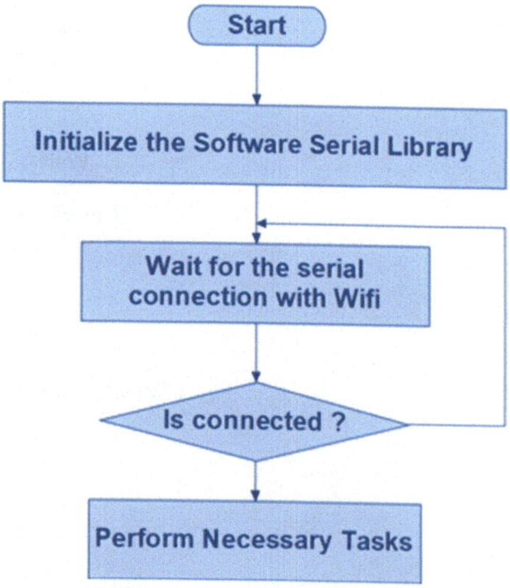

Fig. 11.13 Flowchart for Arduino and Wi-Fi module initialization

11.6.4 Flowchart for the Arduino Program for the Proposed Embedded System

This is the program that is going to run on the Arduino board's microcontroller (ATmega328P), and this is the basic programming flowchart. Initially, Arduino will be waiting for the command from the android app, and once proper command is issued from android app, then it will check for the type of command received, whether it is the command to store the nutrition data for a person or it is a search to find the nutrition data for a particular person or it is something like retrieving overall nutrition status for all the people whose data were saved on the storage device. After executing the command, proper subroutines/functions are going to run, and the result will be sent via a wireless link (Bluetooth/Wi-Fi) to the app and again wait for the command from the app. This basic flowchart, which is for the program running on the Arduino, is a very oversimplified flowchart of the overall process. More details about different parts of the flowchart and the communication between the app and the Arduino board will be discussed in the subsequent sections (Fig. 11.14).

11.6.5 Special Data Packet Format

Basic data packet format for serial transmission (Arduino to SD/MMC card as well for mobile to Arduino) is shown in Fig. 11.15.

In the SD/MMC card, the data are written as a file using the SD library of Arduino. The data packet format for serial data transmission from the app to Arduino is very important because Arduino UNO is having a very less amount of static memory (SRAM), which is of the order of 2 KB and the nutrition test result data which

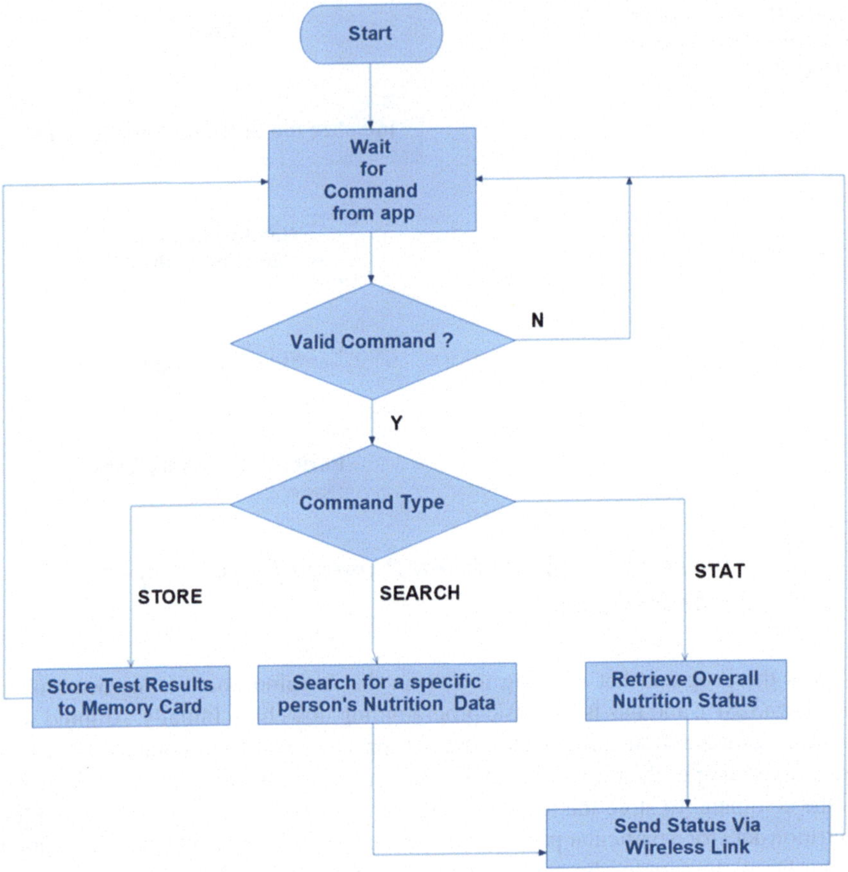

Fig. 11.14 Basic programming flowchart for Arduino

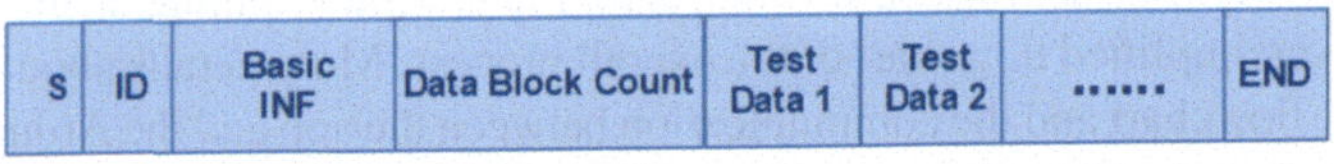

Fig. 11.15 Data packet structure for serial transmission of data to storage device (SD/MMC card)

maybe 10 k or more. Those data of length 10 K or more cannot be stored directly to the Arduino and then to SD/MMC card. So, for this reason, we need to create the packet in a proper format so that the data can transmit from the app to Arduino via a serial link without making any stress on the memory. The serial data packet starts with a START byte (denoted by S in the figure), after that there is a unique person ID, then some basic information about the person (limited to 100 bytes) and then nutrition test data block count and testing data appears serially one after another. At last, there is an optional END Byte. The start may be of 1 byte long, the person's

ID is a maximum of 4 bytes. ID and basic information data blocks may have some prefixed data length, and that data block size has to be decided before writing the software program for the Arduino program. This data size is based on the fact that the amount of data storage (SD/MMC) card is available with the system. The START field (Specified as S in figure) is 8 bit long, ID field is 32 bit long(maximum), basic INF field is of 800 bits, test data size is 10 K(according to the nutrition tests mentioned in this chapter), and the END filed ID of 2 bit long.

11.6.6 Flowchart for Writing to SD Card from Arduino Board

To view the nutrition data to PC/laptops in addition to the app in a smartphone, data is to be stored using SD card's file system implemented by the SD library of Arduino. This algorithm is very important because of the limitation of static RAM of Arduino board and the size of the nutrition test data. The memory of Arduino is 2 K, so more than 2 K data cannot be handled at a time. In general, to be on the safe side, not more than 1 K data should be handled at a time by the Arduino program. But our nutrition test data may take as much as 10 K based on the nutrition test type and according to the proposed data scheme. So the data that is coming from the app and getting saved to the SD/MMC card by the Arduino board must go through proper synchronization. This is a flowchart for store operation in the Arduino board and will be active when from the android app STORE command issued. First, there will be the initialization of serial port for communication with the MMC or SD card and also initialize the Bluetooth module, which is HC-05 (used to communicate with the android app). The medical test data will be coming from the app via the medical test operator. The situation is like that, the operator will be using his smartphone where the designed android app is installed. For storing the data to SD/MMC card by the Arduino board. Now once Arduino initialized its serial port as well as the Bluetooth module, then it will wait for the app to initiate data transfer of the packets. First, the ID packet received from the app, then the Arduino board sends a signal to the app via the Bluetooth channel to hold on, now based on the ID received, the Arduino board creates a file with (using serial port). The file name will be the same as that of the ID it just received by the Bluetooth channel from the app. Once the was the new file created in the SD/MMC card then Arduino will signal the app to send a packet count data, now as the packet count data is received, then Arduino will set up a counter and continuously received that amount of consecutive nutrition test data packs and writes that to the file in a serial fashion to the SD/MMC card. Then, Arduino checks if the count is 0 or not, if the count is 0 then it closes the file, and if the count is not zero, in then again, go and receive the data and decrease the count by one. Once the file is closed, then it goes back to the wait state and again waits for app to initiate another data packet transfer for another person. Please note this algorithm is actually initiated when the app first issued a store command then this algorithm runs in the Arduino board (Fig. 11.16).

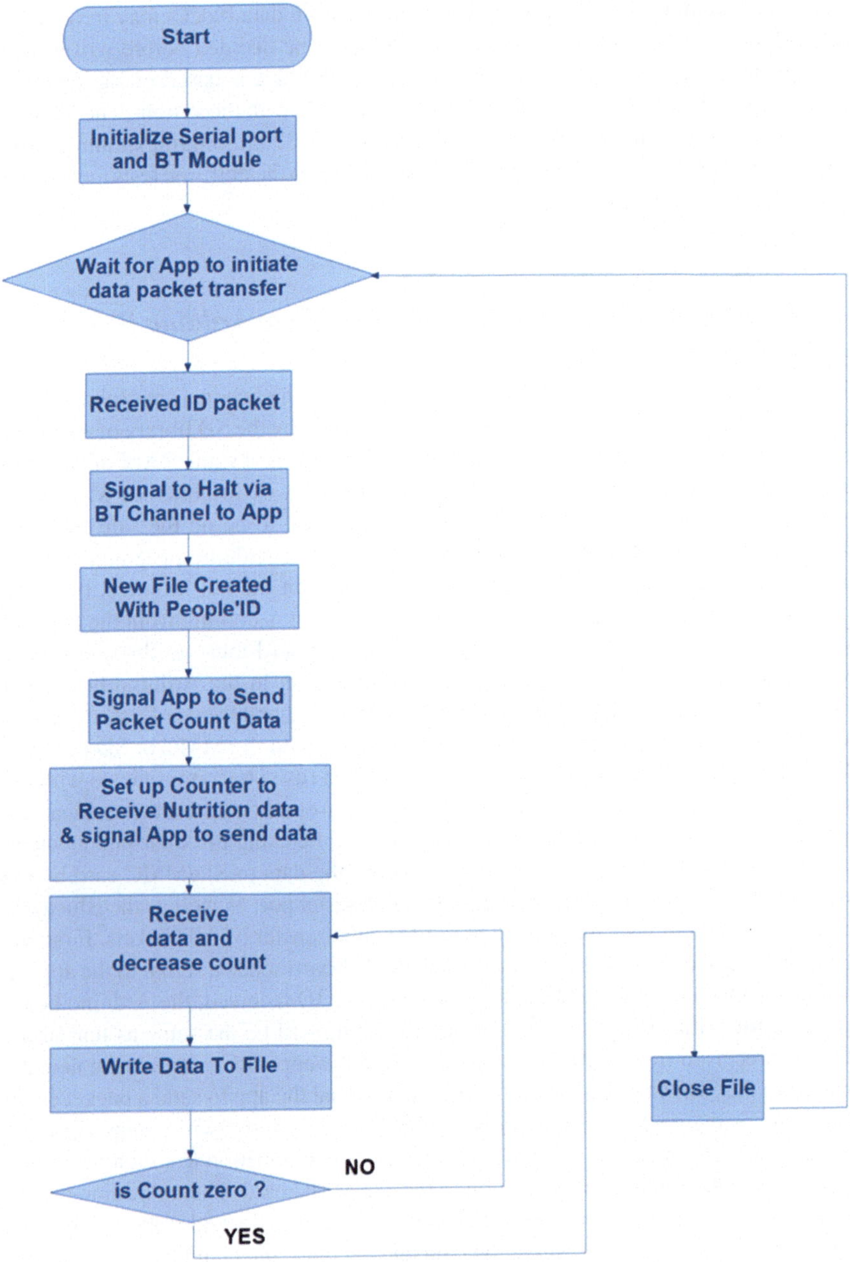

Fig. 11.16 Flowchart for algorithm of writing to SD/MMC card from Arduino board

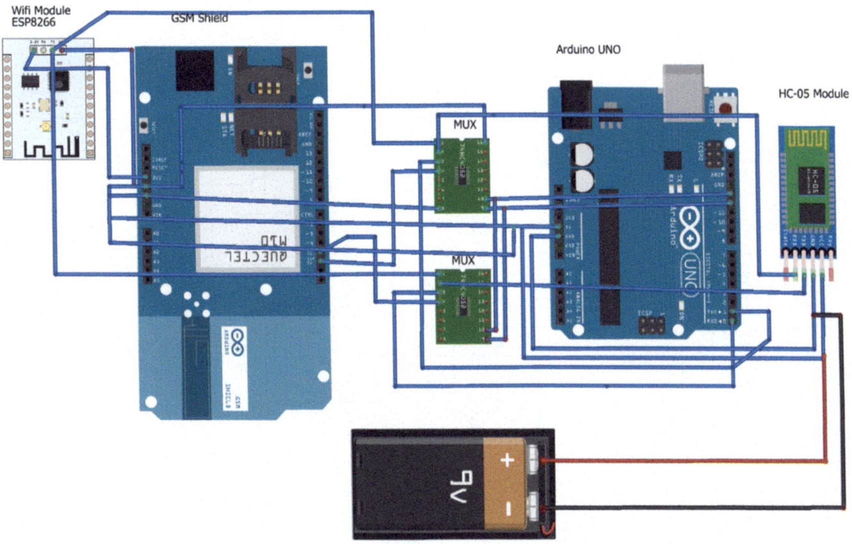

Fig. 11.17 Hardware connection diagram

11.6.7 Connection Diagram for the Hardware System

The embedded system comprises Arduino UNO, GSM shield, HC-05 (Bluetooth Module) and Wi-Fi Module ESP8266, and MUX IC. The Arduino board is connected to the battery for the power supply, and the other modules like Bluetooth module, Wi-Fi module, GSM shield, and SD/MMC card module are also being powered up from a 9 V battery. The multiplexers are connected to multiplex the TX and RX data from GSM shield, Wi-Fi module, and the Bluetooth module. Few pins in the Arduino are dedicatedly used for the multiplexer control (Fig. 11.17).

11.6.8 Schematic Diagram for the Hardware

See Fig. 11.18.

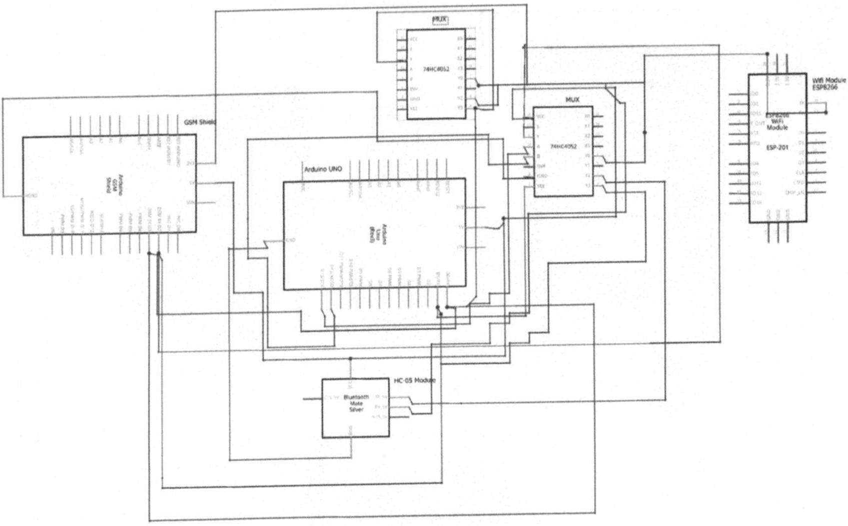

Fig. 11.18 Schematic diagram of the embedded system that is been discussed

11.7 Development of the Android App Supporting the Proposed Embedded System

11.7.1 Internal Component Architecture of App

See Fig. 11.19.

11.7.2 Details of Software Components Used in App

11.7.2.1 Bluetooth Interface

Bluetooth stack, which is present in the Android, helps to exchange data wirelessly with other devices or Bluetooth-enabled devices. There are very helpful Bluetooth API's available with the Android, with the help of them the Bluetooth functionalities are being provided. API allows the application to wirelessly connect other Bluetooth devices and enable point to point and multipoint communication wireless link. With the help of Bluetooth API, the following functionalities can be achieved. The steps to communicate via the Bluetooth protocol are scan and query for other Bluetooth devices, RFCOMM channel establishment, utilization of service discovery to connect with other devices, transfer of data either point to point or multipoint, and multiple connection management. To communicate via Bluetooth channel, the responsible devices must form a channel between them, which is called the pairing process.

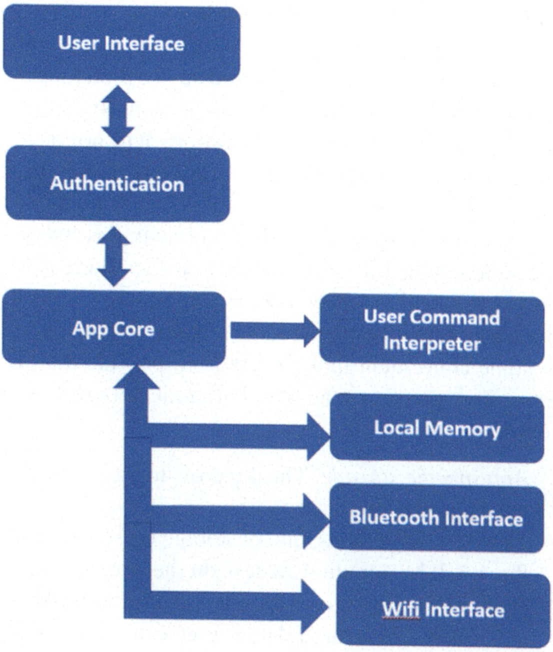

Fig. 11.19 Internal component architecture of the app

One discoverable device must handle the request for incoming connection, while the other device finds the discoverable device using the service discovery process. Discoverable devices must accept the pairing request, and then, the two devices create a bond between them through which they exchange the security keys. Once the pairing and bonding process of successful, the devices may exchange data. The channel may be released after the session is complete. The channel between the devices still remains for the future connection so that they can reconnect automatically when it is required and when they are in the range of Bluetooth and as long as the device does not delete the bond.

11.7.2.2 Wi-Fi Module

Wi-Fi is being provided by the Wi-Fi manager class of Android. This class contains all API required for Wi-Fi connectivity and data exchange. With the help of Wi-Fi manager provided by the Android API, list of configured networks can be updated, viewed, and also, individual entries can be modified. It can detect the currently active Wi-Fi network, state of the network can also be queried, and connectivity can be established or be disconnected. Access point scanning is also possible and retrieving enough information to decide the access point to be connected to. This API is very useful for Wi-Fi specific operations.

11.7.2.3 Local Memory Module

The internal storage of the Android device used for private data on the device memory, saving, and loading files in the file system to the internal storage are dependent on the application, and other applications will not have access to these files. Android file system is responsible for storing and retrieving data from the Android device via the file system API. There are different methods available for file system class which can help to perform different activities like storing and retrieving data from file, deleting the file, and creating new file. There is very easy and safe way to handle data at the local memory and they are safe to use multiple concurrent threads. When the file system is being used, the reading writing, etc. all can be done asynchronously in some convenient manner. Android provide the file system similar to disk based file system on other platform. Different storage types used to save the app data is as follows.

App specific storage: This kind of storage is only for app and other apps does not have permission to access this.
Shared storage: This kind of storage is used to be shared with other apps whenever there will be a mutual Access on the storage data.
Preferences: Private or primitive data stored like a key value pair.
Databases: Structured data source can be stored in a private database.

11.7.2.4 User Command Interpreter

This is a custom layer/interface which is useful for interpreting the commands The command will be provided by the user for performing basic steps like storing the nutrition test data, retrieving the person specific data and searching for the data and getting mass nutrition status. All those commands will finally be interpreted at the Arduino device after the initial processing done by the app and send via the Bluetooth (BT) channel to the Arduino device.

11.7.2.5 User Interface

This is the interface via which the user is going to interact with the app core. This interface is responsible for taking the commands from the user and passes it to the underlying layers such as command interpreter. The command interpreter then transmits the command to the Bluetooth or Wi-Fi channel based on the availability of the connection type. The data may temporarily be saved at the local storage for temporary processing.

11.7.2.6 Authentication Interface

This is also a custom interface which is mainly used for the authentication purpose of the operator who is going to enter the nutrition test data to the system via Bluetooth link. This layer or interface can also provide some authentication for the person who will be accessing the hardware remotely via the Internet link for the searching of nutrition data for a person as well as to know the mass nutrition status of the people living in particular rural areas.

11.7.3 Overall Working of the System

The user interface is the first part of the app that the user is going to interact with for accessing the app. There are two types of users for this app. User type 1, who is the nutrition test data entry operator, is responsible for adding the nutrition test data (CBC, protein test, etc.) to the Arduino-based system, which is situated at the local test center. This communication is done via Bluetooth only from the android app to Arduino. There is another type of user (User 2) who want to get only the information about the nutrition status of a particular person or want to get the overall nutrition status of a remote area people (whose data are already stored in the Arduino device by the operator). User type 2 person should choose the Wi-Fi option and the proper command to retrieve the specific person's nutrition data or the overall nutrition status data for a rural area. For User type 1, use Bluetooth connection to store the data at the local system. This local system would be accessed by the user of type 2 via the Internet connection from a remote place.

11.7.4 Internal Component Architecture of the App

The app is designed for Android mobile, and the Java code may be used for designing the app. The app components are shown in Fig. 11.19. There are two other components with which the app is going to interact. First, there will be a user interface, and the user interface is responsible for taking the data as well as commands from the user. Then, there is a user command interpreter block. This interpreter block is responsible for interpreting the type of command the user has issued. The possible commands maybe the search operation, store operation, or knowing the mass nutrition status. There can be a local memory module that is responsible for storing the data temporarily at the app. Though all the data has to be stored in the hardware, local storage at the app side is necessary for the temporary storage of data for that purpose, whatever memory available in the mobile is sufficient. There is a Bluetooth interface, also. The Bluetooth interface is responsible for storing the data to the hardware as well as issuing different commands to the hardware by the mobile phone app. There is a Wi-Fi interface, also. This Wi-Fi interface is responsible for accessing the hardware (Arduino board) remotely when an active Wi-Fi hotspot is present. For example, if one user wants to know the status of a particular person's nutrition data, and there is some Wi-Fi facility available near the hardware, then user can extract the data via the Wi-Fi interface. So this is some extra provision that is made based on the fact whether Internet facility in the form of Wi-Fi hotspot is available or not.

11.7.5 Flowchart for in Android App Program

See Fig. 11.20.

Description of Android app program flowchart:
The first Android app initializes the Bluetooth interface and then waits for task choice by the user. Then, if the command by the user is to store data, then the data will be taken from the user as input and it will create the proper data packet for serial transmission to the Arduino board. Then, the app will send a start signal to the Arduino, send start byte of the packet, then wait for the signal from Arduino as an acceptance of the start byte and ID. Then, the app will send nutrition test data to the Arduino board serially. After completing the data sending to Arduino, the android app again will wait for the command from the user. Next, is the user chose to search person-specific nutrition data, then it will take the search ID (unique ID that identifies the person) from the user and send it to the Arduino, then wait for Arduino signal to know when the data is ready from Arduino side, and get serial data from the Arduino and display data on the screen of android mobile. After the display, app control again goes back to the wait state for the command from the user. When the user chooses to get the mass nutrition data, the specific command will be sent to the Arduino board. Then, the Arduino board calculates the mass nutrition score considering all the nutrition test data from all the persons present in that specific rural area whose nutrition medical test data is stored in the system. The details of the algorithmic flow chart to find out the mass nutrition score by the Arduino hardware is shown in the next section.

11.7.6 Flowchart for the Function to Get the Mass Nutrition Score

This is the function to be executed when the command is to get the mass nutrition status. From the local EEPROM storage of the Arduino, the basic test types are loaded. Then memory initialized with the standard normal sets of nutrition data for those types of tests. Then the SD/MMC card is contacted for the number of saved nutrition data for all the people (whose nutrition test information is present). Then a counter initialized with the total number of people. From the SD/MMC card, the test data extracted and compared with the standard data for that nutrition test. This way,

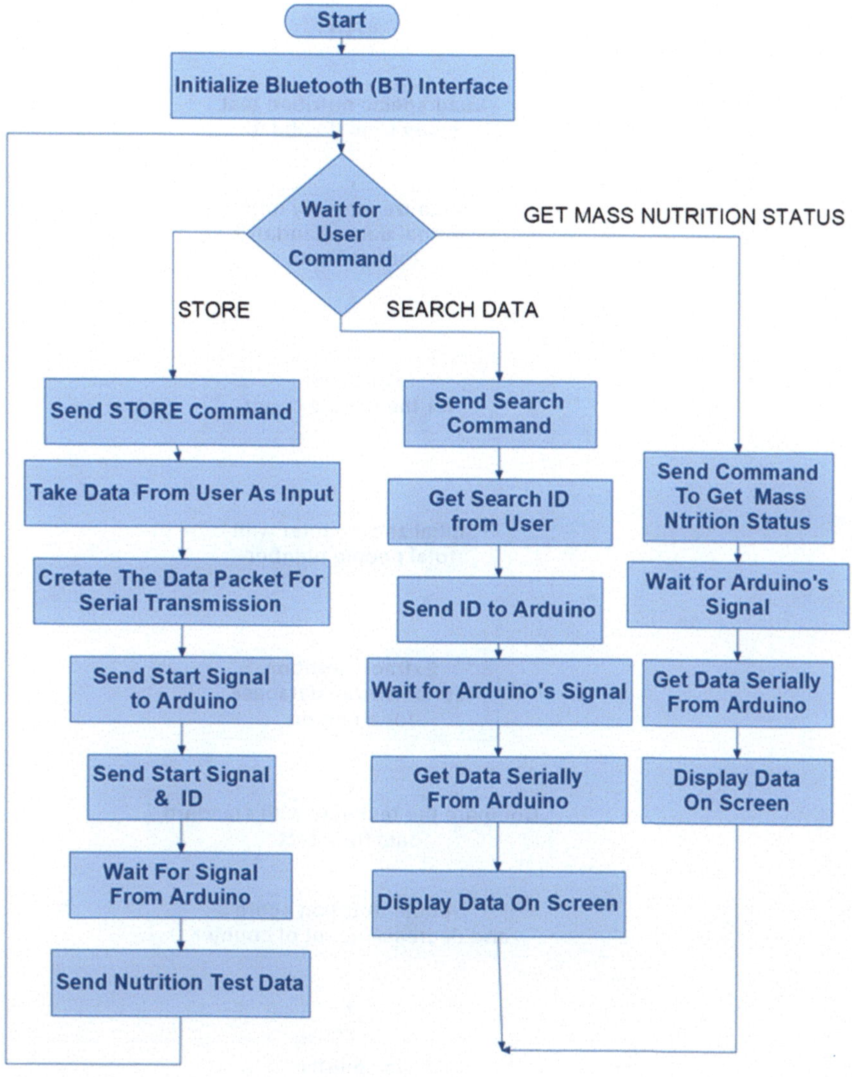

Fig. 11.20 Overall flowchart of app program for android mobile

for a person, all the test data taken from the SD/MMC card and then compared with the corresponding standard normal range, and based on the comparison, a nutrition score calculated. The same procedure repeated for all the persons present in the SD/MMC card, and finally, when no more data is present, then the final nutrition status is returned (Fig. 11.21).

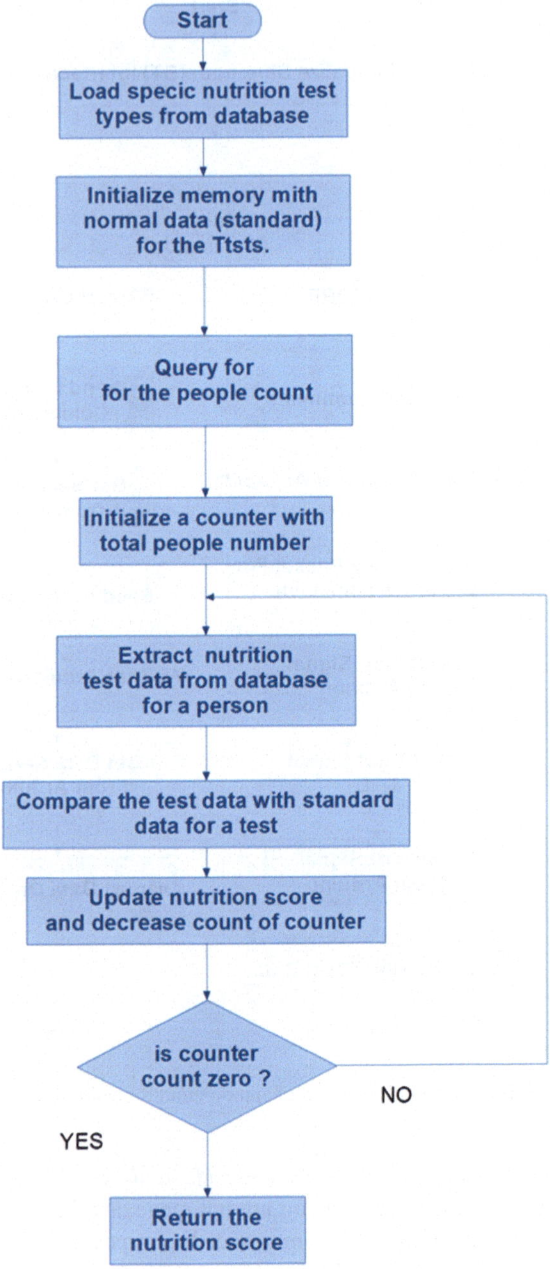

Fig. 11.21 Flowchart of the function to get the mass nutrition score

11.8 Conclusion

This chapter presents the details of the design of the embedded system for the recording/logging, remote monitoring of the malnutrition data over a rural area with advanced detailing of the hardware as well as the detailed description of the software components required for the hardware. The software components required for the android app also presented in this chapter. The algorithms are also described decomposing them into several small functions (tasks) as well as the algorithmic flowchart for the development of the android app also been discussed. The advantage of such a system is that it can monitor the overall health of the people living in a rural area in a large scale. The system is cost-effective as well as power consumption is also very less. With the help of the system described in this chapter, it is possible to record the nutrition data for a large number of people as well as the overall nutrition status can be found. Once the total status is available, the necessary medical steps can easily be taken for the remedy of the malnutrition issue.

11.9 Future Scope

The future scope of the project can be diverse in nature. On the one hand, the whole design of the embedded system and the related IoT interface (GPRS, GSM, Wi-Fi) can be implemented using the single-chip VLSI architecture. The needed algorithms and the necessary protocols can be implemented using FPGA by using VHDL/Verilog language. On the other hand, the same kind of design and algorithms can be used for different types of medical data logging and access purpose and can faithfully be used with IoT interface.

References

1. Sousa, L., Piedade, M., Germano, J., Almeida, T., Lopes, P., Cardoso, F., et al. (2007). *Embedded system design: techniques and trends* (Vol. 231, pp. 353–362). Boston: Springer.
2. Bamidis, P. D., & Pallikarakis, N. (2010). Application of embedded system for sightless with diabetes. *IFMBE Proceedings, MEDICON, 29,* 871–874.
3. Martinak, L., & Penhaker, M. (2010). Application of embedded system for sightless with diabetes. *MEDICON 2010 IFMBE Proceedings, 29,* 871–874.
4. Panneerselvam, P. (2014). Application of embedded system for a genetic disease, sickle cell anemia. In *International Conference on Advances in Electrical Engineering (ICAEE).* https://doi.org/10.1109/icaee.2014.6838446.
5. Wang, J., Zhao, J., & Yan, B. (2010). Realtime and embedded system testing for biomedical applications. *Journal of Software, 5,* 1060–1067.
6. Chakraborty, C., Gupta, B., & Ghosh, S. K. (2014). Mobile metadata assisted community database of chronic wound. *International Journal of Wound Medicine, 6,* 34–42. ISSN: 2213-9095.

7. Amit, B., Chinmay, C., Anand, K., & Debabrata, B. (2019). *Handbook of Data Science Approaches for Biomedical Engineering: Emerging trends in IoT and big data analytics for biomedical and health care technologies* (Ch. 5, 121–152). Amsterdam: Elsevier. ISBN: 9780128183182.
8. Akash, G., Chinmay, C., & Bharat, G. (2019). Sensing and monitoring of epileptical seizure under IoT platform, IGI. In *Smart medical data sensing and IoT systems design in healthcare* (pp. 201–223). https://doi.org/10.4018/978-1-7998-0261-7.ch009.

Chapter 12
A Review on Security and Privacy Concern in IoT Health Care

Joy Chatterjee, Manab Kumar Das, Sayon Ghosh, Atanu Das, and Rajib Bag

Abstract Internet of things (IoT) is one of the most optimistic technologies that have remarkably changed the concept of the healthcare industry which offers a huge added value in the identification of diseases and monitoring the patient remotely. The research community and the public sector are very much focused on this application domain to develop various e-health regulations and policies. However, IoT-based healthcare systems suffer from several security issues that are varied from other domains in terms of methodologies, motivations, and consequences, due to the complexity of the environment and the nature of the deployed devices. The expansion of healthcare IoT devices, along with the absence of network segmentation, inadequate access controls, and dependency on legacy systems has widen attack area for cybercriminals to exploit or steal personally identifiable information (PII) and protected health information (PHI) without interrupting healthcare information transmission processes. Predicting attacks quantitatively may reduce the risk of fraudulent data; different approaches were noticed to identify and predict the IoT intrusions such as network metric based and machine learning approach. This work will review the related security models to identify the approaches of intrusion detection and prediction related to IoT devices as well as software connected in healthcare systems. This provides an overview of the most recent threats and security issues for IoT-based healthcare systems that may affect the efficient and effective functioning of such infrastructures.

Keywords IoT health care · Personally identifiable information (PII) · Protected health information (PHI) · Network segmentation · Vulnerabilities · Cryptography · Steganography · IoT security · Body sensor network (BSN)

J. Chatterjee (✉) · M. K. Das · S. Ghosh · R. Bag
Supreme Knowledge Foundation Group of Institutions, Hooghly, India
e-mail: joy.chatterjee@skf.edu.in

A. Das
Netaji Subhash Engineering College, Kolkata, India

C. Chakraborty et al. (eds.), *Internet of Things for Healthcare Technologies*, Studies in Big Data 73, https://doi.org/10.1007/978-981-15-4112-4_12

12.1 Introduction

The applications of IoT are very blooming and have become a rising subject to nurture nowadays in the domain of information and communication technology. The idea of IoT opens a new door of invasion for the researcher. In this area, different types of IoT-enabled devices are connecting through the Internet for communicating to each other. Our daily life becomes more comfortable through the rapid development of IoT in the field of smart automation systems [1]. There are varieties of applications in IoT, although most popular applications can be reflected in healthcare sector, transportation, retail sector, industrial application, etc. It is very challenging for the companies how the concept of IoT can be incorporated for their end product to create value for their customers along with a vast market place.

The overall growth of a country depends on the economy but in most of the cases, the economic growth can be stagnant due to the bad health condition of individuals of a particular nation. A reliable and secure healthcare system makes a nation more powerful. Most of the people in our country belong to rural area and it is a very complex task to assemble health information [2]. As per the 2011 census report, 68.84% of the total population in India locates in remote areas or villages who are not benefited from modern medical treatment. The modern medical facility cannot reach them and fulfill their basic requirements [3]. Recent day's IoT can be implemented to resolve the different types of healthcare-related issues. In this domain of IoT, variety of healthcare-related data such as level of glucose, body temperature, blood pressure (BP), and concentration of insulin are sense with different type of IoT healthcare sensor devices and also this huge amount of data store in a cloud server for continues monitoring of the health situation of a person which is shown in Fig. 12.1. IoT healthcare application provides different facilities for medical patients or older

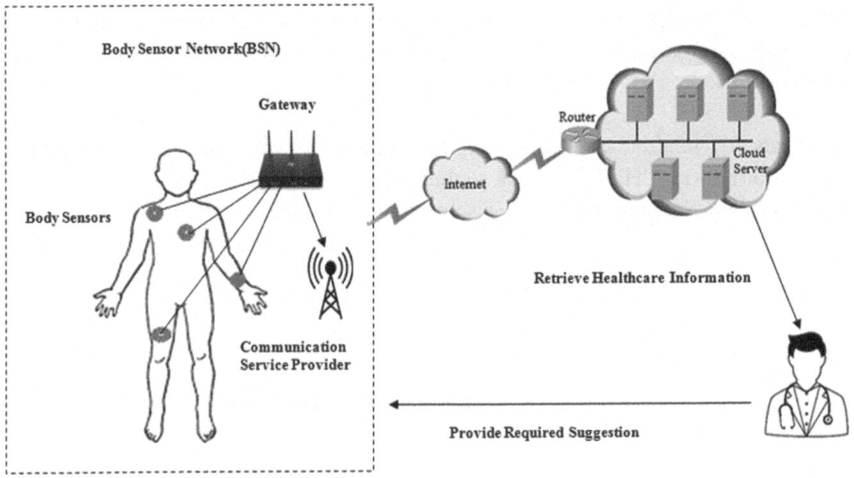

Fig. 12.1 General framework of IoT healthcare system

persons who belong to an interior location or single. Nowadays, a huge amount of aged persons suffering at list one chronic disease as why most of them are not able to take care of themselves [4]. In these situations, IoT health care plays an important key role to solve the problems and provide the suggestions for better treatment [5]. Some of healthcare-related problems can be easily identified and others are unknown to the doctors. For these unidentified situations required some information to know the proper treatment. To resolve such type of unknown situation, a new area of IoT can be introduced known as Ontology [6]. Quality-based IoT healthcare applications provide better medical service to disabled patients with low cost. In this field, different types of methodology can be helpful for medical innovation for new researchers.

12.2 Overview of IoT-Enabled Technologies and Services in the Field of Health Care

Yang et al. [7] developed a system that monitors a patient remotely. Network architecture was developed consisting of three layers of medical intelligent service, management of medical equipments, and collection of data from variety of sensors. iMedBox, iMedPack, and Bio-Patch are the three main blocks involved in this system. These give strength to interoperability and network connectivity and also provide a solution for dispensing actual medicine on time according to the remotely prescribed prescription and remind the user.

Jara et al. [8] suggested a framework for health monitoring through mobile on IoT. This strengthens the health monitoring system of patients as well as general people by continuous supervision of different parameters and data collected by the different devices. It offers a device for continuous transmission of vital signs via 6LoWPAN and identification of specific patient via RFID.

A minimum charge e-health was adapted by Castillejo et al. [9]. A Bluetooth-enabled device was implemented to increase efficiency and accuracy. The key feature of this application is that it provides a service of data aggregation method from actual sensors of the actual nodes. This can be termed as sensor virtualization by the person who is using this system.

Architecture for analyzing data gathered from various sensors on the cloud was proposed by Doukas and Maglogiannis [10]. They mentioned different cloud-based services of data storing from sensor such as iDigi, ThingSpeak, Nimbits, and Pachube. They also highlighted various cloud platforms like iCloud, DropBox, Okeanos, Rackspace, and Amazon AWS for effective management of data collected form users.

Poenaru and Poenaru [11] mentioned a structural use case for remote patient monitoring (RPM) in IoT-based e-health monitoring system. A hierarchy was proposed that provide a reference path for any system by mentioning segment or group or sector or use case. RPM, timing-based services, tele-health consultation, personal healthcare data management, and location-based services are mainly highlighted in the proposed use cases.

An intelligent environment was built by Yang et al. [12] for observing the feedback system. This system collects real-time physical and environmental data of employees and transmits a warning message to minimize the accident. They worked on real-time data to analyze and to take an instant decision to provide an effective and beneficial environment.

Swiatek and Rucinsky [13] introduced a structural approach for combing e-health and IoT under a single service. They presented a general communication platform concept for the QoS delivery service. They also proposed two ways signalization for automatic configuration of different application modules and provide negotiation to any arbitrary group of atomic service according to application.

Fan et al. [14] proposed a rehabilitation system based on IoT. Ontology-based automating design methodology (ADM) was presented for smart rehabilitation systems in IoT. They highlighted various IoT-based technologies, multidisciplinary optimization methods, SOA methods, and ontology for disease diagnosis and to allocate resources.

A survey of IoT-based clinical environment was represented by López et al. [15]. The main highlighted field was to minimize the gap between the physical ecosystem and IoT ecosystem in terms of health care. Different clinical devices are implemented with new features such as observation of remotely located patients, warning analysis, and secured communication by the use of advanced technologies like Bluetooth Low Energy (BT-LE), 6LoWPAN/IEEE 802.15.4, and near-field communication (NFC). The focused areas are mainly e-health and m-health.

Trcek and Brodnik [16] focused on primitive members, identification medium (like RFIDs), and sensors for privacy issues of IoT-based health care. A strategy of continuous adjustment of protocols is considered for the implementation of wireless medical sensors body area networks (WMSBANs). This work will enforce privacy and quantifiably lightweight for the exchange of confidentially captured data. Security in terms of soft security provisioning and hard security is the key focused areas for computing devices.

Hu et al. [17] observed different areas to be covered on IoT-based health care like a remote observation of patients, analyzing collected data, diagnosis of disease, sharing of health-monitored data, generation of the warning message on time, generation of life saving action, and transfer of pharmaceutical things on real time.

A structured 6LoWPAN-based monitoring application was proposed by Le Moullec et al. [18]. IEEE 1588-2008/PTP was used for the effective synchronization of data collected from various nodes. The unified DSP modules were utilized to know the strength of different health parameters like ECG, SpO2, electrical bio-impedance, multi-axis acceleration, etc. These modules are combined with low power, short size 6LoWPAN controller for communication.

An android application was built by Mohammed et al. [19] for regular monitoring and visualizing the ECG waves and the collected data were to be transferred to a medical cloud platform for further diagnosis and analysis by the experts. On the basis of the healthcare domain, an infrastructure was presented that includes a secure and efficient transfer of large file, signal processing, communication protocols, the centralized cloud, database management system, and IOIO microcontroller.

Sebestyen et al. [20] highlighted the opportunities in the area of health care by the use of IoT and new technologies. Some real-life solutions are analyzed by applying some evaluation techniques. Healthcare applications based on IoT such as CardioNet can modify the idea of medical service.

Tahmasbi et al. [21] introduced an architecture for the improvement of healthcare applications on the general computing system. They proposed different solutions for qualitative features containing performance, interoperability, and availability.

A secured IoT framework was proposed by Choi et al. [22] to confirm a peer-to-peer encryption mechanism from application to IoT healthcare device under CoAP communication. This system encrypts vital data using symmetric encryption techniques and to reduce computation cost and for effective communication attribute-based encryption was used. IoT broker, application, and devices are involved in communication between nodes. CoAP and MQTT protocols are not concerned about security but they preferred security measures of DTLS.

Security on ECG signal transmission was the main focused area of Xu et al. [23] to protect a patient from various heart diseases. A dynamic encryption technique with biometric devices was used to gather information about frequency spectrums of ECG signals to confirm high classification rate and system energy efficiency. Additional spatial diversity gains are achieved by cooperative relay. Applying advantages of temporal and spatial diversities, transmission rate can be improved and the probability of data intercept and detection can be lowered by signal power capacity.

A new radio frequency identification authentication protocol based on elliptic curve cryptography (ECC) was introduced by Alamr et al. [24] to remove the vulnerabilities. Elliptic curve Diffie–Hellman (ECDH) key agreement protocol was used to encrypt the transmitted message by generating a short-term-shared key. Security features such as confidentiality, opposition to man-in-the-middle attack, opposition to impersonation attack, mutual authentication, forward security, opposition to replay attack, and anonymity are achieved by a new protocol in RFID system incorporating NXP Java smartcards (J3A040) and Omnikey smartcard reader (Omnikey 5421).

Ko and Song [25] introduced a secured system which contains unique identification of patient and vital information of health. A secured communication channel along with a hash function was implemented to resolve the security problem by creating a secure key. A dual hash function was used to create one-time password between the client and hospital to synchronize the updated data.

BSN-based modern healthcare system was highlighted by Gope et al. [4]. They introduced a security system using BSN to efficiently transmit the data.

Based on ciphertext policy and attribute-based encryption (CP-ABE), a cloud-based architecture using medical wireless sensor was suggested by Lounis et al. [26]. These resolve an access control problem to supports dynamic security policies in terms of efficiency and scalability.

A general review of WSN was given by Das et al. [27] in different fields of health monitoring applications such as remotely health monitoring of patient, power systems and health monitoring in automobiles. They also proposed an architecture to generate a automated warning message to convey geological hazards. This paper provides guidelines for WSN-based application on system monitoring, tracking, and surveillance.

12.2.1 IoT Application in the Field of Health Care

The concept of IoT health care may be introduced in the different area of applications which is shown in Fig. 12.2.

i. **Remote patient monitoring**: Through this application, the health condition of the rural patients can be easily monitored and provide a proper guideline by a doctor. Also for any bad situation, it sends a notification to the doctor and hence, death rate can be reduced by taking proper precautions.
ii. **Continues monitoring of glucose and calorie level**: This type of applications is very important for diabetes patients. In this type of application, glucose and calorie levels measured by sensor devices which are very closely attached with the human body and sent a signal/message to a smart device screen for any changes of base level and make a person fit.
iii. **Proper use of an inhaler for asthma patient**: Generally, we know asthma is not curable, but continues monitoring can be preventing the asthma attack. This continues monitoring is done by receiving data/signal through the IoT sensor device with the help of mobile apps and also suggests taking necessary action.
iv. **Continues monitoring of blood pressure**: The blood pressure(BP) of any patient can be up/down for any circumstance, so continues monitoring of BP is very important which is done by IoT healthcare application as why reduce the risk factor.

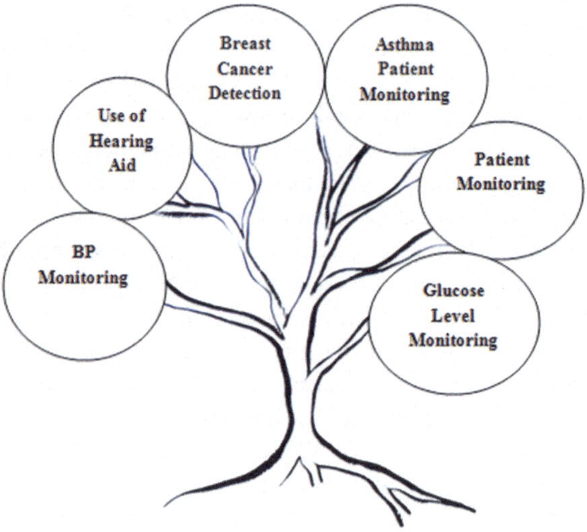

Fig. 12.2 Different types of application in the field of IoT health care

v. **IoT-enabled smartwatch for depression level measurement**: Nowadays, most of the peoples are suffering from depression and are taking the proper percussion to overcome these problems. Only the proper treatment can be possible when the root causes analysis will be perfect. So an innovative concept of IoT healthcare introduces a smartwatch, which measures the depression level. In these concept, applications continuously monitors the depression level with the help of sensor device and store the data in the cloud for further analysis.
vi. **Breast cancer detection**: The concept behind breast cancer detection is more powerful than other regular disease detection procedures. Here, sensor-enabled cloths detect the temperature changes from breast tissue.
vii. **IoT for hearing aid**: Today's daily life, million numbers of people suffering from their hearing loss problems. In this situation, IoT-enabled hearing aid becomes more popular because such type of application makes our daily life very easy. It is very useful for those people who have been suffering from hearing problems to listen the original sound from the noisy conversations.

12.2.2 Type of IoT Sensors Relates to Health Care

The activities of different sensing nodes play the primary role to accumulate a vareity of information from the human body. These body sensors do not work individually, i.e., it works as an integrated part of the entire healthcare system. The data sensing capability of different types of body sensors as mentioned in Table 12.1 may vary with respect to the applications.

Table 12.1 Types of sensor related to IoT healthcare application

Sensor type	Application
Blood pressure sensor	This type of sensor is used to measure the blood pressure of any person
Heart-rate monitoring sensor	This type of optical sensor detects and measures the heart or pulse rate
Air bubble detector	It is capable of checking the presence of air in a liquid flow like blood
Temperature sensor	It is responsible to monitor the body temperature at a regular time interval
Thermopile infrared (IR) sensors	This type of sensor is used in multiple applications in the medical sector which is used for non-contact temperature measurement
Photo optic sensors	It is responsible to calculate the oxygen level in blood
Humidity sensor	It is used to compute the humidity changes of the human body for various conditions
Ultrasonic sensor	This sensor is used as an integrated part of various medical equipment like as modern dialysis equipment

12.3 Vulnerabilities, Attacks, and Security Threats on Devices in IoT-Based Healthcare Network

In IoT healthcare platform, millions of heterogeneous data can route over a network with the help of big data concepts. Threats and attack these two are the major issues that directly relates to IoT security. These two facts may interrupt the personal private information of any individual. Also, these two are correlated to each other and accountable to hamper the original information.

12.3.1 IoT Threats

In this domain, any healthcare-related vital information can be theft during the routing over a network. This can be done due to the unavoidance interruption of any malicious person. Basically, threats create a pessimistic impact on the IoT security system. Nobody can prevent natural threats such as floods, hurricanes, etc., but we try to prevent different types of man-made threats by introducing a variety of protocols in IoT-layered architecture [28].

12.3.2 Different Attacks Related to IoT Health Care

Thousand of IoT devices are interconnected to each other for data communication over a network. In such situation, the possibility of data hacking also increases day by day. Some well-known attacks like denial-of-service attack, man-in-the-middle attack, replay attacks, etc., may hamper the original data during transmission or cloud storage which are briefly discussed in Table 12.2.

12.3.3 Challenges in IoT

IoT environment includes a variety of intelligent devices and application interface with the help of heterogeneous network structure where the scope and boundary may be limitless. In such situation, the security issue proportionally increases with the rapid development of IoT applications. Nowadays, unlimited uses of Internet make the network vulnerable and hence, the protection of data from cyber attacks is major challenges. In the world of digitization, users wish to acquire more digital services through the different IoT applications, which arises a big question of personal data fraudulent.

12.3.3.1 Speedy Development of Smart Devices

In the field of IoT health care, variety of new smart devices is introduced day by day to represent the growth of business development and fabricate a new market place. All these products amalgamate with new technology for the enlargement of

Table 12.2 Various types of major attack with respect to IoT healthcare are focused on different research area

Name of attacks	Description	Authors	Year of publication
Denial-of-service attack	This attack is based on traffic congestion of a network. The presences of this type of attack are suspected when the data access rate increases from the normal range. To overcome this attack, some adaptive techniques like packet dropping may be introduced to protect the server.	ul Sami et al. [35]	2018
Man in the middle attack	This is a very common attack where any suspicious person may interrupt between the sender and receiver and try to hack the valuable information. It may be used in a different technique where any malicious take over the proxy.	Cekerevac et al. [36]	2017
Sinkhole attack	Nowadays, different type of sinkhole attack may introduce in the field of IoT healthcare security where attacking node sent false information to original node through the routing process as an intruder and try to drop the packet on the basis of priority ranking.	Stephen and Arockiam [37]	2017

(continued)

Table 12.2 (continued)

Name of attacks	Description	Authors	Year of publication
Sybil attack	In the healthcare system, variety of sensors node collect the information from the environment and the human body. In this attack, any unknown person can provide fake identities to check the efficiency of a system that can hamper the original report of a normal user.	Chifor et al. [38]	2016
Replay attack	The attacker continuously monitors the data transmission of the source network as a spy and eavesdrops and decrypts original massage after some time later resent it by delaying the entire process in this attack.	Al Alkeem et al. [39]	2015

the market place to get up the business. Sometimes, these types of inventions launch some unknown challenges in the field of cybersecurity.

In IoT healthcare architecture, different body sensors object or node integrated with a large network via some small body sensor network and this type of integration rises the possibility of the information hacking and make the entire system vulnerable. In this environment, any vulnerable device may play the major role of a cyber attack in any situation. All the connected devices of an IoT network must respond to improve the service quality, but due to continues interruption of any malicious person the performance of the entire system degrades as well as deteriorates the facility to access vital sensitive information through some cyber attacks.

In recent days, a variety of applications is associated with our smart devices as an ornament which plays the major role of smartphone revolution. Some of them may be the causes of data hacking which act like malware, when users access their personal information. In twenty-first century research domain, it is a very flaming and burning issue to protect the entire system along with IoT healthcare devices from unauthorized access.

12.3.3.2 Data Privacy Issues

In the field of IoT health care, a huge amount of smart devices are responsible to deal with personal information of users such as BP, heart rate, body temperature, and amount of glucose. In such situations, most of the users do not reliable to share this type of sensitive information with the help of third-party applications due to lack of security. In healthcare system, a variety of heterogeneous data routes over a network to provide the service to different users which is very delicate. In such a situation, jumble and misplace of original data may rise another challenge of data security, so different types of encryption techniques and machine learning approaches may introduce for data privacy and to provide secure data transmission.

12.3.3.3 Utilization of Bandwidth

In IoT domain, millions of devices or nodes communicate to each other via a single server. In such situations, data can overflow due to congestion and the possibility of data missing may increase. This type of flooded situation can rise major difficulty for data security. In this circumstance, all the connected devices may utilize a dedicated communication link to solve such type of problems, but it is a very demanding issue in the field of IoT applications.

12.3.3.4 Cloud Security Issues

The idea of cloud computing creates a platform to monitor and control various IoT applications. Basically, cloud server is responsible to store all relevant data and provide efficient services for the users with the assistance of big data technologies. Various types of challenges relate with cloud security may be the major issues to degraded the overall performance of IoT services.

12.3.4 IoT Healthcare Vulnerabilities

IoT healthcare system incorporates some standard security mechanism at all level to protect healthcare-related information, although there exists some vulnerability which may hamper the entire process which is discussed below.

12.3.4.1 Hardware and Storage Vulnerability

In this IoT, physical device such as sensors and MCU node needs to be protected from both the attacks, natural or man-made. Some preventive methods may be introduced at physical layer to reduce the physical damage of IoT devices from environmental hazards. The valuable personal information may be stored at both local device and cloud storage. In such situation, sometimes, essential information may be lost due to bad security mechanism which may be the basic causes of hardware and storage vulnerability.

12.3.4.2 Network-Related Vulnerability

The network layer performs a major role in this type of applications because, here, heterogeneous information route as a packet over the network. A variety of network protocols is defined here to provide better service, but sometimes, vital data can be lost during different types of attacks such as unauthorized access, insider attacks, and replay attacks at this level. In IoT healthcare platform, different network infrastructures are associated with each other for better performance hence the characteristic of protocols also vary. So it makes the entire network system vulnerable.

12.3.4.3 Application-Related Vulnerability

This vulnerability happens at the application level. This vulnerability may arise due to poor application service of an un-trusted service provider or week encryption mechanism.

12.3.5 Techniques Applied to Resolve the Issues of IoT Healthcare Personal Data and Health Information

In the twenty-first century, the idea of different security mechanism and challenges focus on new research domain in the field of IoT health care. An efficient security mechanism ensures user to protect their privacy which is very challenging because millions of IoT devices are connected with heterogeneous network architecture.

12.3.6 IoT Security

Security is one of the major concerns for any network system. In this type of IoT application, data movement play an important role and hence security can be defined in various ways as here most of the data transmitted over an unguided medium termed as wireless sensor network (WSN). Encryption is the most popular term nowadays which is directly related to network security. In such situation, a congestion-free network provides the facility of reliable data transmission. The rapid development of different encryption algorithms is very helpful for safe data transmission over a network in the IoT healthcare system. This algorithm is also responsible to protect different types of attacks [29]. In IoT healthcare applications, all the personal data are very sensitive so it can be defined in many aspects as a whole.

i. **User Authentication**

It is the very basic requirement for any IoT-based system through which we can prevent any kind of unpredictable attacks. In IoT healthcare system, all the sensitive information passes from one node to another neighbor through proper coordination [30]. In such situation, proper user identification participates as a key role in authentication.

ii. **Data Confidentiality**

The term confidentiality relates to data security to represent the secrecy of personal information which route through an IoT network, i.e., all the information must be confidential when it sent via sensor network from any passive attack [9]. In this concept, a different type of encryption algorithm required for both physical storage along with transmission path.

iii. **Data Integrity**

In IoT healthcare domain, a large amount of data generated from a variety of body sensor node (BSN) at regular time intervals and hence, it is highly correlated with the security aspect. It ensures to prevent the insertion of any poisonous data into actual storage consequently the original information fully protected from any malicious attack.

iv. **Access Control**

It provides the authorization to access the service of the IoT system by getting the proper information. In this concept, Hussein et al. [31] define access control is a mechanism which provides the facility of ubiquitous access for users, services, devices, etc., at heterogeneous architectures of a different network. The idea of access control is based on security policies and privileges of different IoT users.

v. **Data Privacy**

Privacy is a major issue for IoT security. This is responsible to protect all relevant and vital information of a patient for both user and creator organization. Different types of attacks can degrade the performance of IoT application; hence, some of risk and challenges are introduced in the concept of IoT healthcare security. The strict security mechanism for data privacy in the field of IoT creates a new impact for the researchers and provides a space to overcome different types of challenges.

vi. **Data Encryption**

It is very powerful security mechanism to encode the original information, i.e., plain text and produce ciphertext hence the authorized user only can read the original information. In IoT healthcare domain, all the personal information is very sensitive and needs to protect the privacy of a patient. Here, popular encryption proposals are introduced in Table 12.3.

Table 12.3 Popular encryption methodology implemented for IoT healthcare data security

Encryption technique	Description	Authors	Year of publication
Data encryption standard	It is a very simple encryption mechanism that is sometimes unable to prevent any powerful attack. Basically, it is responsible to encrypt the data of block size 64 bit each, i.e., 64 bit plain text will be the input and produce 64 bit ciphertext as an output where the same key of size k is used for both encryption and decryption	Bhargavan et al. [40]	2016
Advanced encryption standard	Nowadays, AES is a more powerful and widely used symmetric key encryption technique that deals with the block size of 128 bit using a key size of 128/192/256 bit. It is faster than DES and very difficult to hack any original data through the implementation of AES	Elhoseny et al. [41, 42]	2018
RSA encryption	It is the most popular and secure asymmetric key cryptography algorithm which is based on public and private key concepts. Here, encryption technique based on the multiplication of two prime numbers m and n. Finally, this large multiplication value encrypt on the basis of some formulas	Vahdati et al. [43], Elhoseny et al. [42], Luo et al. [44]	2019 and 2018
Twofish encryption	Twofish based on blowfish algorithm where block size of 128 bit encrypted with the key size of 128/192/256 bits. This symmetric key encryption mechanism basically used for steganography and cryptography system. As per Rane [45], it should be responsible to encrypt every data of different sizes before outsourcing to the cloud server	Rane [45], Vijitha and Bhavani [46]	2016 and 2017

12.3.7 IoT Healthcare Framework Integrated with Cloud Computing

In this century, the application of IoT in the field of healthcare area becomes widely popular. This type of application is developed rapidly with the help of cloud computing. These two are highly correlated to each other where cloud computing enlarges its scope and provides different services for users with the help of distributed systems [32]. In IoT healthcare system, millions of IoT devices collect a variety of data from different objects of the human body and store all these things into a cloud server for further processing which plays a key role for personalized healthcare services [33]. Good cloud architecture provides quality and efficient service for medical diagnostic treatment. In these cases, data confidentiality built an assurance through medical data searing among authorized users or application providers.

Step-1 In this step, all the relevant medical data are gathered from the body sensors and all this information goes to the next step through a local area sensor network (LASN) by cover a short-distance transmission.

Step-2 The information of the previous step is routed to access network (AN) and transport network (TN) as packets based on some transmission technology.

Step-3 This step plays an important role because all the medical information is stored in a cloud server. This layer always interacts with a large dataset. Most of the security technique incorporates this layer to prevent different types of attacks. Here, another important feature is load distribution or balancing which required providing efficient service for users.

Step-4 In this step, doctor or any healthcare organization can retrieve necessary information about a patient as per requirement and provide required healthcare service

Sometimes, malicious attackers can hamper (delete, modify, leak, etc.) or hack the valuable information at any level of the above-mentioned architecture as to why enormous security mechanism may introduce in this framework. Figure 12.3 illustrated a multi-layered framework of IoT healthcare application [34].

12.3.8 Data Encryption and Decryption Techniques to Combat Security Concerns in IoT Health Care—A Case Study

We are going to implement a health monitoring system where any doctor can view or observe the health condition of the patient remotely through a Web application or any display unit and after that doctor can take action accordingly. But, the major concern in this system is security. At the time of data transmission from patient end to doctor end or doctor end to patient end, someone can attack that data and can change the information. So, our goal is to protect such important data using encryption–decryption techniques.

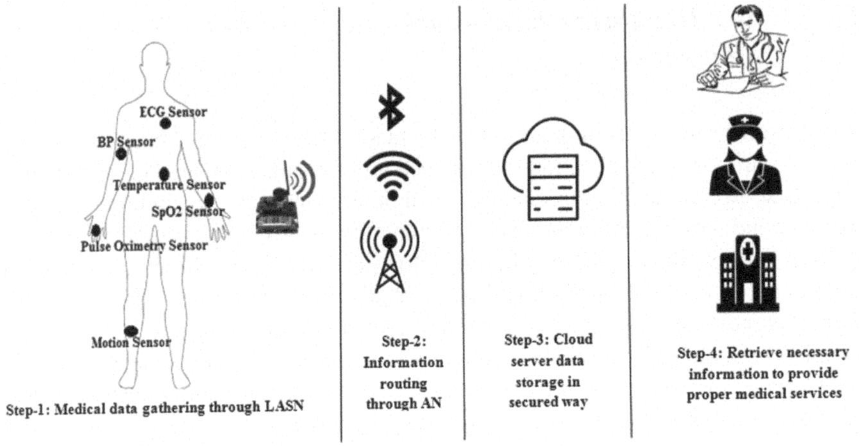

Fig. 12.3 IoT healthcare service based on cloud computing framework

12.3.9 System Overview of Health Monitoring System

In our health monitoring system prototype as shown in Fig. 12.4, we use two Nodemcu microcontrollers to send the data and receive the data. On the patient end, one microcontroller takes valuable data using heart-rate sensor and pulse oximeter IC for temperature and wearable health monitoring sensor using DS18B20 digital thermometer. After taking the raw data, we apply the encryption technique to prevent the cyber

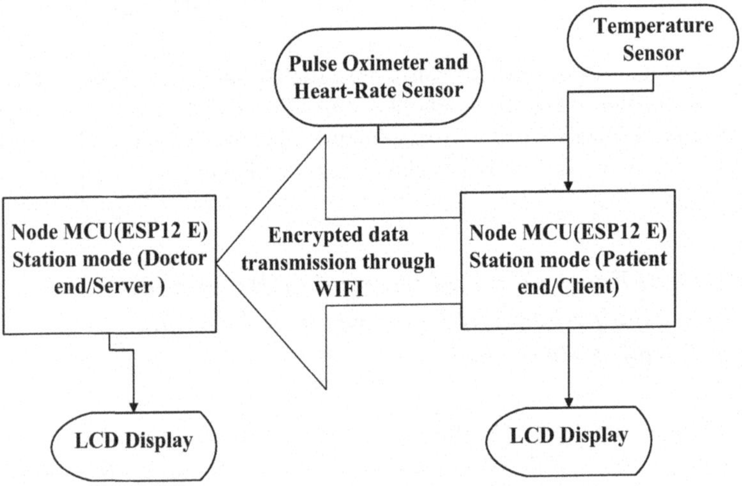

Fig. 12.4 Modular diagram of data communication between patient and doctor using encryption technique

attack and send the ciphertext through the wireless network to another microcontroller. On the other hand (doctor end), after receiving the ciphertext, it decrypts the ciphertext and shows the result in the output device. The microcontroller which takes and encrypts the sensor data is known as the client and the microcontroller which receives and decrypts the massage is known as the server. In this system, server and client talk to each other in a secret way.

12.3.10 Implementation of Encryption and Decryption Technique

In the above said heath monitoring system, we use the advanced encryption standard (AES) algorithm to encrypt/decrypt the data. In general, there are three types of AES used.

AES 128: It uses 128 bit secrete Key and the total round is 10 rounds.
AES 192: It uses 192 bit secrete Key and the total round is 12 rounds.
AES 256: It uses 256 bit secrete Key and the total round is 14 rounds.

Here, we use AES256 in health monitoring system. The AES encryption key is given below

aes_key[] = {0x30, 0x30, 0x30, 0x30, 0x30, 0x30, 0x30, 0x30, 0x30, 0x30, 0x30, 0x30, 0x30, 0x30, 0x30, 0x30};

12.3.10.1 AES Encryption Technique (Fig. 12.5)

The procedure of the AES encryption is mainly divided into three stages.

(a) The initial round
(b) The main rounds,
(c) The final round.

Above stages use the same sub-operations in separate combinations which are given below

- **Initial Round**
  - **Add Round Key**
- **Main Rounds**
  - **Sub Bytes**
  - **Shift Rows**
  - **Mix Columns**
  - **Add Round Key**

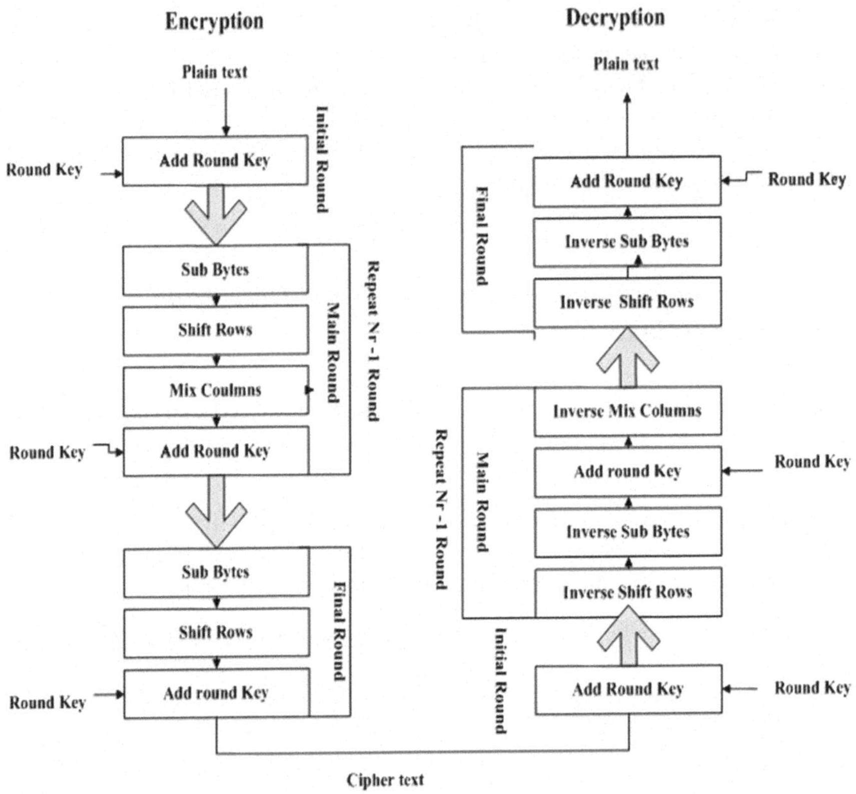

Fig. 12.5 Depicts the whole process of AES encryption and decryption techniques

- **Final Round**
  - **Sub Bytes**
  - **Shift Rows**
  - **Add Round Key.**

12.3.10.2 AES Decryption Technique (Fig. 12.5)

In AES technique, to decrypt the encrypted ciphertext, each stage followed during encryption process is reversed in which they are applied. The three stages of decryption are as follows:

(a) Inverse final round.
(b) Inverse main rounds.
(c) Inverse initial round.

Above stages use the same sub-operations in separate combinations which are given below

- **Final Round**
  - **Add Round Key**
  - **Inverse Shift Rows**
  - **Inverse Sub Bytes**
- **Main Rounds**
  - **Inverse Mix Columns**
  - **Add Round Key**
  - **Inverse Sub Bytes**
  - **Inverse Shift Rows**
- **Initial Round**
  - **Add Round Key**

12.3.11 Circuit Diagram

Figure 12.6 depicts how different devices are connected among themselves to collect the health-related information of a particular patient so that this information can be transmitted to the doctor or to the hospital for remote monitoring and prescribing medicines.

12.3.12 Workflow Diagram

In the IoT-based health monitoring system, information is collected from patient represented as station mode and that is transmitted to the doctor end represented as access mode. Before transmitting, original data are encrypted and then transmitted. Again received data are decrypted and converted to original data based on the key value. This system is represented by a flow diagram in Fig. 12.7 to remove the security issues. This vital information must be preserved from any fraud to restrict health hazards.

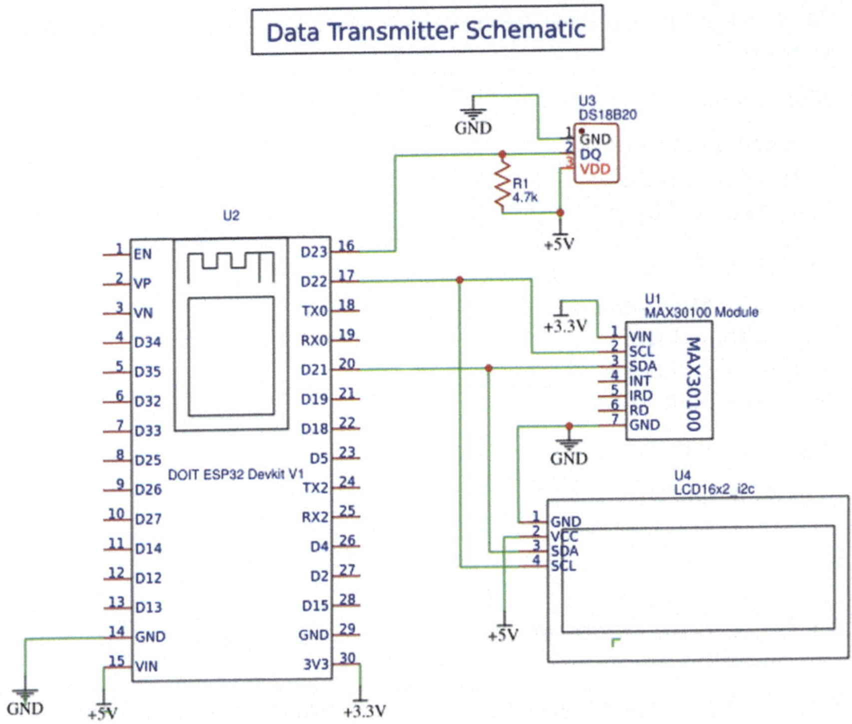

Fig. 12.6 Pin out diagram of the IoT devices connected to collect the health-related information

12.3.13 System Implementation

Figure 12.8 shows the original implementation of the application where blood pressure, oxygen percentage, and temperature of a patient are transmitting from one node to another. Here, data are encrypted before transmitted and decrypted at the access point. PHI is deployed in this system on the basis of PII. Main focused area in this system is to transmit both these information safely from station mode to access mode.

12.3.14 Result Analysis

Data collected at the patient end is shown in Fig. 12.9 and data accessed at the doctor end is shown in Fig. 12.10. This output depicts that a secure data transmission is possible between two nodes by implementing encryption and decryption techniques. Network security is the key feature implemented in this system to minimize the threats or attacks in the network.

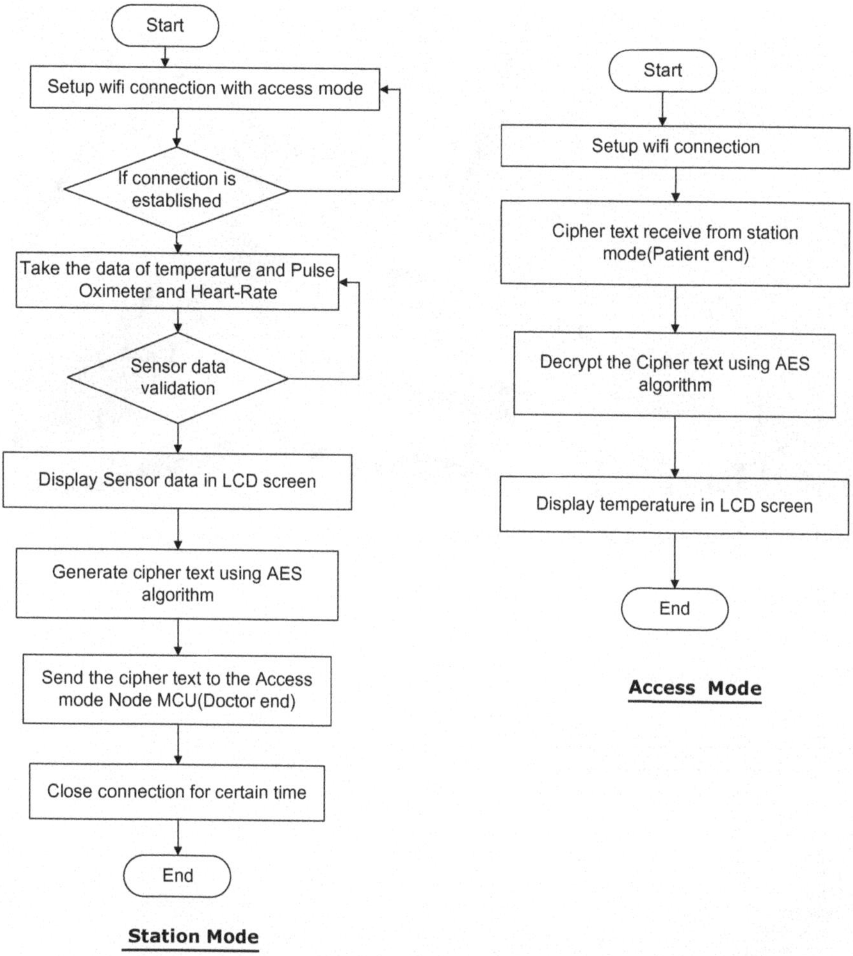

Fig. 12.7 Flow diagram of station mode and access mode of IoT-based health monitoring system

12.4 Conclusion and Future Scope

As the world is trending in the direction of utilizing IoT-based systems and applications in our daily health monitoring systems, the threats are equally increasing at the patients' end. The stakeholders connected with this system may illegally modify the information gathered from the devices (IoTs) that could have an adverse effect pertaining to patient care. Implementation of IoT security related to health care is the most important requirement in this century. This chapter mainly focused on problems in terms of security and highlighted the solutions to be implemented to enhance security mechanisms. Different cryptographic techniques can be used further to increase

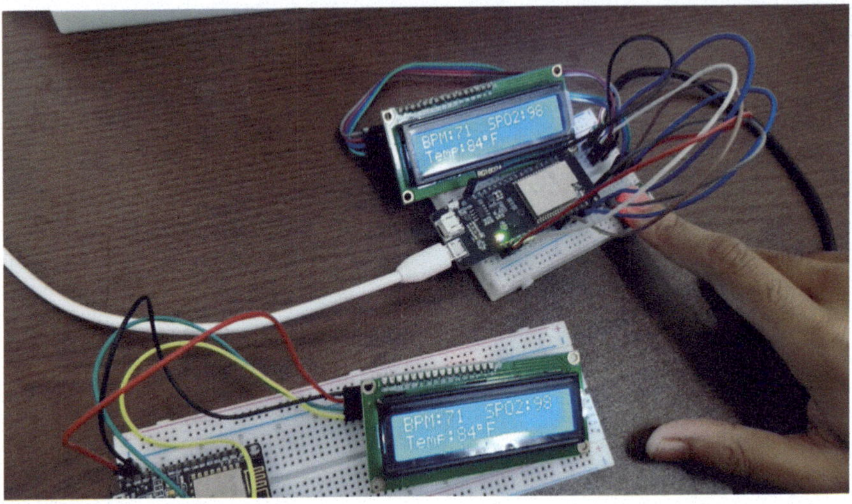

Fig. 12.8 Picture of health data transmission between station mode and access mode

At Patient End

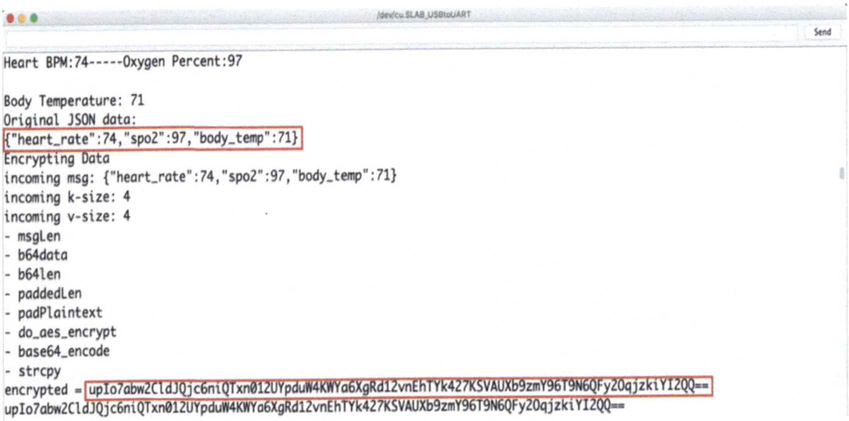

Fig. 12.9 Serial monitor output before transmission of original data

At Doctor's End:

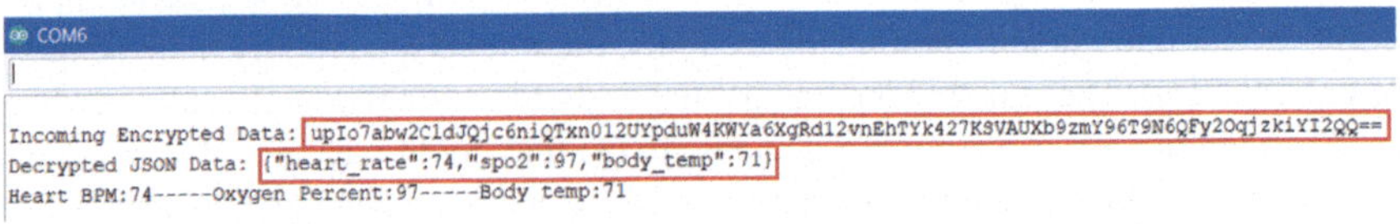

Fig. 12.10 Serial monitor output at the receiving end

the efficiency of vital data transmission. The illustrated case study represents a cryptographic technique to combat with network security issues. Optimization of security protocols leads to the high performance of the IoT healthcare systems. Development and current trends of IoT in the discipline of health care are the center of attention in this chapter for healthy and stable transmission of the important healthy reports. Further, more advanced techniques should be implemented that could detect the threats in IoT-based healthcare systems and could also change the modification in the applications.

References

1. Jing, Q., Vasilakos, A. V., Wan, J., Lu, J., & Qiu, D. (2014). Security of the Internet of Things: Perspectives and challenges. *Wireless Networks, 20*(8), 2481–2501.
2. Padhy, R. P., Patra, M. R., & Satapathy, S. C. (2012). Design and implementation of a cloud based rural healthcare information system model. *Universal Journal of Applied computer Science and Technology, 2*(1), 149–157.
3. Kakkar, A. (2019). An IoT equipped hospital model: A new approach for E-Governance Healthcare Framework. *IJMRHS, 8*(3), 36–42.
4. Gope, P., & Hwang, T. (2015). BSN-Care: A secure IoT-based modern healthcare system using body sensor network. *IEEE Sensors Journal, 16*(5), 1368–1376.
5. Alqahtani, F. H. (2018). The application of the Internet of Things in healthcare. *International Journal of Computers and Applications, 180*(18), 19–23.
6. Kumar, V. (2015). Ontology based public healthcare system in Internet of Things (IoT). *Procedia Computer Science, 50,* 99–102.
7. Yang, G., Xie, L., Mäntysalo, M., Zhou, X., Pang, Z., Da Xu, L., et al. (2014). A health-IoT platform based on the integration of intelligent packaging, unobtrusive bio-sensor, and intelligent medicine box. *IEEE Transactions on Industrial Informatics, 10*(4), 2180–2191.
8. Jara, A. J., Zamora-Izquierdo, M. A., & Skarmeta, A. F. (2013). Interconnection framework for mHealth and remote monitoring based on the internet of things. *IEEE Journal on Selected Areas in Communications, 31*(9), 47–65.
9. Castillejo, P., Martinez, J. F., Rodriguez-Molina, J., & Cuerva, A. (2013). Integration of wearable devices in a wireless sensor network for an E-health application. *IEEE Wireless Communications, 20*(4), 38–49.
10. Doukas, C., & Maglogiannis, I. (2012, July). Bringing IoT and cloud computing towards pervasive healthcare. In *2012 Sixth International Conference on Innovative Mobile and Internet Services in Ubiquitous Computing* (pp. 922–926). New York: IEEE.
11. Poenaru, E., & Poenaru, C. (2013, November). A structured approach of the Internet-of-Things eHealth use cases. In *2013 E-Health and Bioengineering Conference (EHB)* (pp. 1–4). New York: IEEE.
12. Yang, C. T., Liu, J. C., Liao, C. J., Wu, C. C., & Le, F. Y. (2013, December). On construction of an intelligent environmental monitoring system for healthcare. In *2013 International Conference on Parallel and Distributed Computing, Applications and Technologies* (pp. 246–253). New York: IEEE.
13. Świątek, P., & Rucinski, A. (2013, October). IoT as a service system for eHealth. In *2013 IEEE 15th International Conference on e-Health Networking, Applications and Services (Healthcom 2013)* (pp. 81–84). New York: IEEE.
14. Fan, Y. J., Yin, Y. H., Da Xu, L., Zeng, Y., & Wu, F. (2014). IoT-based smart rehabilitation system. *IEEE Transactions on Industrial Informatics, 10*(2), 1568–1577.

15. López, P., Fernández, D., Jara, A. J., & Skarmeta, A. F. (2013, March). Survey of internet of things technologies for clinical environments. In *2013 27th International Conference on Advanced Information Networking and Applications Workshops* (pp. 1349–1354). New York: IEEE.
16. Trcek, D., & Brodnik, A. (2013). Hard and soft security provisioning for computationally weak pervasive computing systems in e-health. *IEEE Wireless Communications, 20*(4), 22–29.
17. Hu, F., Xie, D., & Shen, S. (2013, August). On the application of the internet of things in the field of medical and healthcare. In *2013 IEEE International Conference on Green Computing and Communications and IEEE Internet of Things and IEEE Cyber, Physical and Social Computing* (pp. 2053–2058). New York: IEEE.
18. Le Moullec, Y., Lecat, Y., Annus, P., Land, R., Kuusik, A., Reidla, M.,. & Ruberg, P. (2014, December). A modular 6LoWPAN-based wireless sensor body area network for health-monitoring applications. In *Signal and Information Processing Association Annual Summit and Conference (APSIPA), 2014 Asia-Pacific* (pp. 1–4). New York: IEEE.
19. Mohammed, J., Lung, C. H., Ocneanu, A., Thakral, A., Jones, C., & Adler, A. (2014, September). Internet of things: Remote patient monitoring using web services and cloud computing. In *2014 IEEE International Conference on Internet of Things (iThings), and IEEE Green Computing and Communications (GreenCom) and IEEE Cyber, Physical and Social Computing (CPSCom)* (pp. 256–263). New York: IEEE.
20. Sebestyen, G., Hangan, A., Oniga, S., & Gál, Z. (2014, May). eHealth solutions in the context of Internet of Things. In *2014 IEEE International Conference on Automation, Quality and Testing, Robotics* (pp. 1–6). New York: IEEE.
21. Tahmasbi, A., Adabi, S., & Rezaee, A. (2016). Behavioral reference model for pervasive healthcare systems. *Journal of Medical Systems, 40*(12), 270.
22. Choi, J., In, Y., Park, C., Seok, S., Seo, H., & Kim, H. (2018). Secure IoT framework and 2D architecture for End-To-End security. *The Journal of Supercomputing, 74*(8), 3521–3535.
23. Xu, H., & Hua, K. (2016). Secured ECG signal transmission for human emotional stress classification in wireless body area networks. *EURASIP Journal on Information Security, 2016*(1), 5.
24. Alamr, A. A., Kausar, F., Kim, J., & Seo, C. (2018). A secure ECC-based RFID mutual authentication protocol for internet of things. *The Journal of Supercomputing, 74*(9), 4281–4294.
25. Ko, H., & Song, M. (2016). A study on the secure user profiling structure and procedure for home healthcare systems. *Journal of Medical Systems, 40*(1), 1.
26. Lounis, A., Hadjidj, A., Bouabdallah, A., & Challal, Y. (2016). Healing on the cloud: Secure cloud architecture for medical wireless sensor networks. *Future Generation Computer Systems, 55*, 266–277.
27. Das, A. T. A. N. U., & Bag, R. A. J. I. B. (2010). Wireless sensor network based monitoring systems: A review and state of art applications. *International Journal of Computer Applications in Engineering Technology and Sciences 3*, 1142.
28. Abomhara, M. (2015). Cyber security and the internet of things: Vulnerabilities, threats, intruders and attacks. *Journal of Cyber Security and Mobility, 4*(1), 65–88.
29. Dewangan, K., & Mishra, M. (2018). A review: security of IOT based healthcare system, vol. 3, 25–28.
30. Patel, S., Singh, N., & Pandya, S. (2017). IoT based smart hospital for secure healthcare system. *International Journal on Recent and Innovation Trends in Computing and Communication, 5*(5), 404–408.
31. Hussein, D., Bertin, E., & Frey, V. (2017, March). Access control in IoT: From requirements to a candidate vision. In *2017 20th Conference on Innovations in Clouds, Internet and Networks (ICIN)* (pp. 328–330). New York: IEEE.
32. Zhou, J., Leppanen, T., Harjula, E., Ylianttila, M., Ojala, T., Yu, C., et al. (2013, June). Cloudthings: A common architecture for integrating the internet of things with cloud computing. In *Proceedings of the 2013 IEEE 17th International Conference on Computer Supported Cooperative Work in Design (CSCWD)* (pp. 651–657). New York: IEEE.

33. Ida, I. B., Jemai, A., & Loukil, A. (2016, December). A survey on security of IoT in the context of eHealth and clouds. In *2016 11th International Design & Test Symposium (IDT)* (pp. 25–30). New YOrk: IEEE.
34. Ahmed, A., Latif, R., Latif, S., Abbas, H., & Khan, F. A. (2018). Malicious insiders attack in IoT based multi-cloud e-healthcare environment: A systematic literature review. *Multimedia Tools and Applications, 77*(17), 21947–21965.
35. ul Sami, I., Ahmad, M. B., Asif, M., & Ullah, R. (2018). DoS/DDoS detection for E-Healthcare in Internet of Things 9(1), 297–300.
36. Cekerevac, Z., Dvorak, Z., Prigoda, L., & Cekerevac, P. (2017). Internet of things and the man-in-the-middle attacks–security and economic risks. *MEST Journal, 5*(2), 15–25.
37. Stephen, R., & Arockiam, L. (2017). Intrusion detection system to detect sinkhole attack on RPL protocol in Internet of Things. *IJEECSE, 4*(4), 16–20.
38. Chifor, B. C., Bica, I., & Patriciu, V. V. (2017, June). Mitigating DoS attacks in publish-subscribe IoT networks. In *2017 9th International Conference on Electronics, Computers and Artificial Intelligence*, 1–6. New York: IEEE.
39. Al Alkeem, E., Yeun, C. Y., & Zemerly, M. J. (2015, December). Security and privacy framework for ubiquitous healthcare IoT devices. In *2015 10th International Conference for Internet Technology and Secured Transactions (ICITST)* (pp. 70–75). New York: IEEE.
40. Bhargavan, K., & Leurent, G. (2016, October). On the practical (in-) security of 64-bit block ciphers: Collision attacks on HTTP over TLS and OpenVPN. In *Proceedings of the 2016 ACM SIGSAC Conference on Computer and Communications Security* (pp. 456–467). ACM.
41. Elhoseny, M., Shankar, K., Lakshmanaprabu, S. K., Maseleno, A., & Arunkumar, N. (2018). Hybrid optimization with cryptography encryption for medical image security in Internet of Things. *Neural Computing and Applications*, 1–15.
42. Elhoseny, M., Ramírez-González, G., Abu-Elnasr, O. M., Shawkat, S. A., Arunkumar, N., & Farouk, A. (2018). Secure medical data transmission model for IoT-based healthcare systems. *IEEE Access, 6,* 20596–20608.
43. Vahdati, Z., Yasin, S. M., Ghasempour, A., & Salehi, M. (2019). Comparison of ECC and RSA algorithms in IoT devices. *Journal of Theoretical and Applied Information Technology, 97*(16).
44. Luo, E., Bhuiyan, M. Z. A., Wang, G., Rahman, M. A., Wu, J., & Atiquzzaman, M. (2018). Privacyprotector: Privacy-protected patient data collection in IoT-based healthcare systems. *IEEE Communications Magazine, 56*(2), 163–168.
45. Rane, D. D. (2016). Superiority of Twofish over Blowfish. *International Journal of Scientific Research and Management, 4*(11).
46. Vijitha, S., & Bhavani, S. (2017). WNTFLEP-worm node detection with two fish algorithm based secure routing and link expiry prediction. *International Journal of Pure and Applied Mathematics, 114*(7), 675–685.

Chapter 13
Applications of Internet of Things in Medical Area

Mamata Rath

Abstract In present-day, Internet of Things (IoT) has turned out to be industry-rationalist jargon to portray how innovation is presently being inserted in various fields and markets including healthcare and developing the manner by which commerce is led. The IoT has developed the manner in which interdisciplinary fields right now are associated with and will keep on streamlining the procedures engaged with forefront healthcare work. IoT in healthcare encourages ordinary yet significant assignments to improve patient results and furthermore takes a portion of the weight off of health professionals. Assignments like remote patient checking, treatment progress perception, and the lodging of immunizations are on the whole capacities of therapeutic gadgets with coordinated IoT. The current chapter describes applications of IoT in medical sector related developed systems.

Keywords Internet of Things · Healthcare · Sensor · Remote monitoring

13.1 Introduction

The IoT is portrayed as a system of physical gadgets that integrates devices and communicate intelligently to empower the direction of information. These gadgets are not really the unpredictable mechanical progressions. They do, be that as it may, streamline forms and empower healthcare laborers to finish undertakings in a convenient way. Organizations that spend significant time in healthcare or innovation will in general intensely put resources into IoT. In contemporary times, most tech gadgets accompany some category of the network, from bodily attached instruments, for example, health sensing instruments to scanning machines with Wi-Fi or Bluetooth. IoT-empowered therapeutic gadgets give basic information that helps health specialists play out their occupations [1].

M. Rath (✉)
School of Management (Information Technology), Birla Global University, Bhubaneswar, Odisha, India
e-mail: mamata.rath200@gmail.com

C. Chakraborty et al. (eds.), *Internet of Things for Healthcare Technologies*, Studies in Big Data 73, https://doi.org/10.1007/978-981-15-4112-4_13

One certified instance of the IoT being used in medicinal services is the Kinect HoloLens Assisted Rehabilitation Experience (KHARE) arrange, which was made by Microsoft Enterprise Services identified with the National Institute for Insurance Against Accidents at Work (INAIL) for reflecting neuron treatment. The KHARE arranges licenses ceaseless data supports that empower experts to make thorough and modified exercise-based recovery programs for patients paying little brain to their zone. The KHARE organize partners with Microsoft's Azure IoT Suite; through this, specialists can see data from a 30 min exercise-based recovery session. The KHARE organize is correct presently encountering a clinical report that is reserved to end in January 2020 [2].

Smart Fridge by Weka in an alternate model for antibodies, which tends to backbone issues in immunization the board, for example, putting away immunizations at a prescribed infection, the unwavering quality of electrical power, and stock mistakes prompting decay. The Weka Smart Fridge enables remote observing to guarantee antibodies are put away at the right temperature, and computerized stock administration administrations enable clinicians to feel calm and refreshed about putting away immunizations. The advantageous booth enables health professionals to sign on and indicate the immunization that is required, so, all things considered, the Shrewd Fridge gives admission to the solitary vial that was mentioned, leaving the remainder of the stock intact. Not exclusively does the Smart Fridge streamline the way toward interfacing with antibodies, it additionally takes into account information to be dissected and patterns to be bridled to make better immunization programs, particularly in high-chance provincial territories [3].

Not exclusively are simply the IoT gadgets significant, the part of breaking down information is an auxiliary advantage that they offer. In this way, IoT information investigation stages, for example, Kaa (KaaIoT Technologies), MindSphere (Siemens), and Azure (Microsoft) enable information to be examined from IoT gadgets to draw important significant patterns. IoT has made considerable progress as of late and is all-around coordinated inside various businesses, including the healthcare space. The proceeded with execution of IoT inside healthcare will prompt an exceptional increment in efficiency and investigation of information. Headways in innovation as to therapeutic gadgets will improve patient results with better examination, and Global Data accepts the IoT will speed up this procedure [4].

Essential healthcare would get unfriendly to the gigantic majority, an enormous area of society would go inefficient logical to mature age and individuals would be progressively inclined to incessant malady. Is it harmless to say that it isn't the catastrophe we disbelieved? Whatever IoT submission advancement is at your salvage. While innovation can't prevent the populace from maturing or annihilate incessant infections on the double, it can, at any rate, make healthcare simpler on a pocket and in terms of openness [5].

Remedial symptomatic eats up a tremendous bit of crisis center bills. Development can move the calendars of restorative checks from a center (crisis facility headed) to the patient's (home-driven). The right finding will in like manner reduce the need for hospitalization. Another perspective, known as the Internet of Things (IoT), has a wide relevance in different zones, including healthcare. The full use of this perspective in human services zone is a mutual desire since it empowers remedial concentrations to work even more ability and patients to procure better treatment. With the use of this advancement-based medicinal services technique, there are unequaled points of interest that could improve the quality and capability of drugs and in like way improve the wellbeing of the patients [6].

13.2 Advantages in Medical Sector Due to IoT

Synchronous itemizing and watching—Constant checking by methods for related contraptions can save lives in event of a wellbeing-related emergency like cardiovascular breakdown, diabetes, asthma attacks, etc. With steady seeing of the condition set up by strategies for a quick therapeutic device related to a mobile phone application, related contraptions can accumulate helpful and other required wellbeing data and use the data relationship of the PDA to move assembled information to a specialist. Focal point of Connected Health Policy coordinated an examination that shows that there was a half diminishing in 30-day readmission rate in perspective on remote patient keeping an eye on cardiovascular breakdown patients. The IoT device accumulates and moves wellbeing data: circulatory strain, oxygen, and glucose levels, weight, and ECGs. These data are taken care of in the cloud and can be conferred to an affirmed person, who could be a specialist, your protection organization, a taking an intrigue wellbeing firm or an external pro, to empower them to look at the assembled data paying little brain to their place, time, or gadget [7].

IoT can modernize tolerant consideration work process with the help of social insurance adaptability course of action and other new progressions, and bleeding-edge medicinal services workplaces. IoT in medicinal services enables interoperability, machine-to-machine correspondence, information exchange, and data improvement that makes social insurance organization movement convincing. Accessibility shows: Bluetooth LE, Wi-Fi, Z-wave, ZigBee, and other current shows, human services work power can change the way where they spot affliction and infections in patients and can moreover improve dynamic techniques for treatment. In this manner, a development driven course of action chops down the cost, by cleaving down pointless visits, utilizing better quality resources, and improving the assignment and arranging [8].

Data assortment and assessment—Tremendous proportion of data that a social insurance device sends in a brief time span inferable from their steady application is hard to store and supervise if the passage to cloud is difficult to reach. In any occasion, for medicinal services providers to verify data starting from different contraptions and sources and inspect it truly is an outrageous bet. IoT contraptions can assemble, report, and examine the data consistently and cut the need to store the rough data. This all can happen overcloud with the providers simply picking up permission to convincing reports with diagrams. Likewise, medicinal services exercises empower relationship to get basic social insurance examination and data-driven bits of information which quicken essential administration and is less disposed to mistakes [9].

13.3 Remotely Taking Care of Health

On-time alert is fundamental in the event of dangerous conditions. Remedial IoT devices amass basic data and move that data to masters for consistent after, while simultaneously dropping alerts to people about fundamental parts through versatile applications and other associated devices. Reports and alerts give a firm decision about a patient's condition, autonomous of spot and time. It in like manner empowers choose to learned decisions and give on-time treatment. Along these lines, IoT enables continuous advised, after, and watching, which licenses hands-on prescriptions, better precision, appropriate intervention by masters and improve absolute patient consideration transport results [9].

a. Remote remedial assistance

In the event of an emergency, patients can contact a master who is various kilometers away with splendid compact applications. With conveyability game plans in medicinal services, the specialists can instantly check the patients and recognize the distresses in a rush. Moreover, different medicinal services transport grapples that are evaluating to manufacture machines that can fitting drugs dependent on patient's cure and torment related data available by methods for associated devices. IoT will improve the patient's consideration in medicinal center. This along these lines will cut on people's expansiveness on human services [10].

b. Research on IoT in medical sector

IoT for healthcare can likewise be utilized to inquire about purposes. This is on the grounds that IoT empowers us to gather an enormous measure of information about the patient's disease which would have taken numerous years in the event that we gathered it physically. This information accordingly gathered can be utilized for measurable investigation that would bolster the medicinal research. Along these lines, IoT doesn't just spare time yet in addition our cash which would go in the exploration. Along these lines, IoT has an incredible effect in the field of therapeutic research. It empowers the presentation of greater and better restorative medicines. IoT is utilized in an assortment of gadgets that improve the nature of the healthcare administrations got by the patients. Indeed, even the current gadgets are presently being refreshed by IoT by essentially utilizing implanting chips of brilliant gadgets. This chip improves the help and cares that a patient requires [11].

13.4 Contests in Implementing IoT in Healthcare

One of the most basic threats that IoT presents is data security and insurance. IoT contraptions get and transmit data constantly. Regardless, most by far of the IoT contraptions need data shows and benchmarks. Despite that, there is a basic vulnerability regarding data ownership rule. All of these components make the data significantly defenseless against cybercriminals who can hack into the structure and deal Personal Health Information (PHI) of the two patients similarly as masters. Cybercriminals can manhandle patient's data to make fake IDs to buy meds and therapeutic equipment which they can sell later. Software engineers can in like manner record a bogus insurance ensure in patient's name [12].

IoT and Medical sector: different gadgets and conventions—Joining of different gadgets additionally cause impediment in the execution of IoT in the healthcare division. The explanation behind this deterrent is that gadget producers haven't arrived at an accord with respect to correspondence conventions and standards. In this way, regardless of whether the assortment of gadgets is associated; the distinction in their correspondence convention entangles and thwarts the procedure of information conglomeration. This non-consistency of the associated gadget's conventions hinders the entire procedure and lessens the extent of the versatility of IoT in healthcare [13].

13.5 Information Over-Burden and Accuracy

As examined before, information conglomeration is troublesome because of the utilization of various correspondence conventions and benchmarks. Be that as it may, IoT gadgets still record a huge amount of information. The information gathered by IoT gadgets is used to increase essential bits of knowledge. Notwithstanding, the measure of information is huge to such an extent that getting bits of knowledge from it is getting very hard for specialists which, at last influences the nature of basic leadership. In addition, these challenges are ascending as more gadgets are associated which record an ever-increasing number of information [14].

Cost—Amazed to see cost thoughts in the test portions? I know most of you would be; yet the primary concern is: IoT has not made the medicinal services urges sensible to the fundamental man yet. The impact on the healthcare costs is focusing on a sign for everybody especially the made countries. The situation is to such a degree, that it offered rise to "Helpful Tourism" in which patients with essential conditions find a workable pace of the making nations which costs them as less as one-tenth. IoT in human services as a thought is a charming and promising idea. Regardless, it hasn't fathomed the cost considerations beginning at now. To viably execute IoT application progression and to choose up its all improvement the partners must make it monetarily exquisite else it will reliably avoid everyone's degree besides the people from the high class [15].

The present decade may well watch a rebellion in the treatment and finish of disorder. The Internet of Things (IoT) has opened up a vast expanse of possible results in drug: when related with the Internet, standard helpful devices can accumulate precious additional data, give extra information into reactions and examples, engage remote consideration, and all-around give patients more control over their lives and treatment. Here are a couple of cases of IoT in human services that show what drug is getting fit for appreciation to innovation [16].

13.5.1 Ailment Treatment

In June 2018, data was presented at the ASCO Annual Meeting from a randomized clinical primer of 357 patients getting treatment for head and neck dangerous development. The starter used a Bluetooth-enabled weight scale and circulatory strain sleeve, together with a sign after application, to send updates to patients' primary care physicians on indications and responses to treatment each weekday [17].

The patients who used this exquisite checking system, known as CYCORE, experienced less outrageous symptoms related to both the harmful development and its treatment when stood out from a benchmark gathering of patients who proceeded with typical step by step specialist visits (with no extra watching). Bruce E. Johnson, President of ASCO (the American Society of Clinical Oncology), said that the splendid advancement "revamped care for the two patients and their consideration providers by engaging creating responses to be recognized and tended to quickly and viably to encourage the heaviness of treatment". The examination displays the potential focal points of sharp development concerning improving patient contact with specialists, and seeing of patients' conditions, to such an extent that causes irrelevant check with their consistently lives. As Richard Cooper, Head of Digital at AXA PPP Healthcare, educated Econsultancy in a gathering concerning the destiny of wellbeing tech, "A bit of the enhancement we see have stopped people being connected to their home, or kept them from being reliably in the restorative clinic" [18].

13.5.2 Intense Consistent Glucose Checking (CGM) and Insulin Taking Devices

Diabetes has shown to be a ready ground for the headway of splendid contraptions, as a condition that impacts around one of each ten adults, and one that requires perpetual watching and association of treatment. A Continuous Glucose Monitor (CGM) is a device that makes diabetics reliably screen their blood glucose levels for a couple of days in a steady progression, by taking readings at customary between times. The first CGM structure was supported by the US Food and Drug Administration

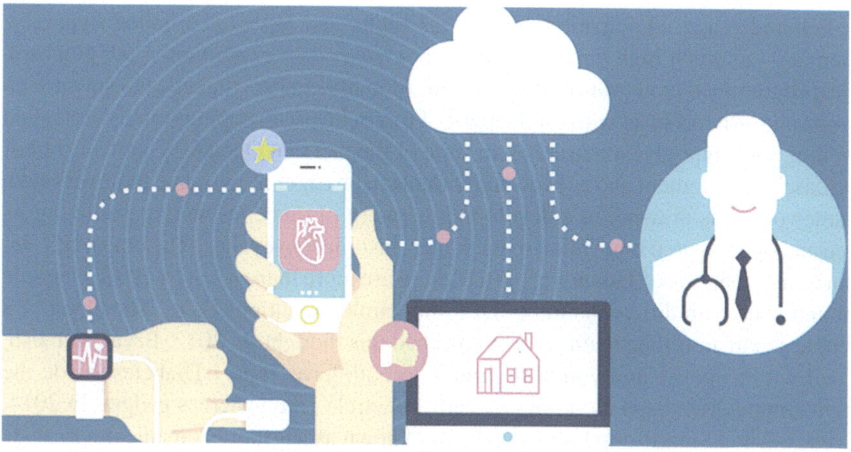

Fig. 13.1 Smart continuous glucose monitoring (CGM) device

(FDA) in 1999, and of late, different wise CGMs have hit the market [19]. Rich CGMs like Eversense and Freestyle Libre send data on blood glucose levels to an application on iPhone, Android or Apple Watch, empowering the wearer to easily check their information and recognize designs. The FreeStyle LibreLink application furthermore mulls over remote watching by means of parental figures, which could consolidate the watchmen of diabetic youths or the relatives of old patients. These devices are in any occasion, starting to get open on the NHS: on World Diabetes Day 2018 (fourteenth November), the NHS proclaimed that it would make the FreeStyle Libre adroit CGM available on answer for Type 1 Diabetes sufferers. It evaluated this would grow the degree of diabetes patients who approach sharp CGM contraptions in England from 3–5% to 20–25% [20] (Fig. 13.1).

Another important gadget as of now improving the lives of diabetes patients is the elegant insulin pen. Savvy insulin pens—or pen tops—like Gocap, InPen, and Esysta can naturally record the time, sum and sort of insulin infused in a portion, and suggest the right kind of insulin infusion at the opportune time. The gadgets communicate with a cell phone application that can store long haul information, help diabetes patients ascertain their insulin portion, and even (on account of the Gocap) enable patients to record their suppers and glucose levels, to perceive how their nourishment and insulin admission are influencing their glucose [21].

13.5.3 Automatic Delivery of Insulin in Patient Body

By observing a person's blood glucose levels and consequently modifying the measure of insulin conveyed into their framework, the APS keeps blood glucose inside a sheltered range, anticipating outrageous highs and lows (also called hyperglycaemia—too much high glucose—and hypoglycaemia—exorbitantly low glucose). The programmed conveyance of insulin additionally enables diabetics to stay asleep from sundown to sunset without the peril of their glucose dropping (otherwise called evening time hypoglycaemia) [23]. In spite of the fact that OpenAPS isn't an "out of the case" arrangement and expects individuals to be eager to fabricate their very own framework, it is drawing in a developing network of diabetics who are utilizing its free and open-source innovation to hack their insulin conveyance. The OpenAPS site announces that "As of January 15, 2018, there are more than $(n = 1) * 1078 +$ people far and wide with different sorts of DIY shut circle executions" [24]. The OpenAPS people group aren't the main ones to have had this thought. In 2013, Bryan Mazlish, a dad with a spouse and youthful child who both have Type 1 Diabetes, made the main computerized and cloud-associated shut circle fake pancreas gadget. In 2014, he established SmartLoop Labs—presently known as Bigfoot Biomedical—to scale and popularize the advancement of a mechanized insulin conveyance framework dependent on his development. The organization is at present planning for a significant preliminary of its answer, subtleties of which are expected to be reported in "late 2018 or mid-2019". Bigfoot as of now foresees that its robotized framework will be propelled financially in 2020, pending FDA audit and endorsement [25].

13.5.4 Associated Respiratory Inhalers

Asthma is another disease like diabetes where the condition is that affects the lives of a huge number of individuals over the world. Keen innovation is starting to give them expanded understanding into and command over their side effects and treatment, on account of associated inhalers. The greatest maker of shrewd inhaler innovation is Propeller Health. As opposed to delivering whole inhalers, Propeller has made a sensor that appends to an inhaler or blue tooth spirometer. It interfaces up to an application and helps individuals with asthma and COPD (Chronic Obstructive Pulmonary Disease, which incorporates emphysema and incessant bronchitis) comprehend what may be causing their side effects, track employments of salvage medicine, and furthermore gives allergen estimates [26]. The association was built up in 2010, and in 2014 got FDA opportunity for two sensors proposed to work with inhalers from critical pharma associations: GlaxoSmithKline's Diskus inhaler, and the Respimat inhaler from Boehringer Ingelheim. Starting now and into the foreseeable future, Propeller has continued collaborating with different noteworthy producers of inhalers, and now says that its sensor "works with most inhalers and driving bluetooth spirometers" [27]. One of the benefits of using a related inhaler is improved adherence—by the day's end, the prescription is taken even more dependably and even more as often as possible. The Propeller sensor produces gives insights about inhaler use that can be granted to a patient's essential consideration doctor, and show whether they are using it as often as possible as is suggested. For patients, this gives motivation and moreover clearness, exhibiting how the use of their inhaler is authentically improving their condition [28].

13.5.5 Digital Sensor Treatment

Proteus Digital Health and its ingestible sensors are another instances of how sharp prescriptions can screen adherence. As demonstrated by an assessment by the World Health Organization in 2003, half of the drugs are not taken as facilitated. Proteus' system is one effort to decrease this figure: the association has made pills that separate in the stomach and produce a little sign that is gotten by a sensor worn on the body. The data is then moved to a wireless application, confirming that the patient has acknowledged their solution as facilitated [29].

Proteus has so far trialed the system with pills for treating uncontrolled hypertension and Type 2 Diabetes, and antipsychotic solution. In late 2017, ABILIFY MYCITE—an antipsychotic drug made by Proteus and Otsuka Pharmaceutical Co.—transformed into the vital FDA-confirmed cure with an electronic after framework [30].

Also as with related inhalers, ingestible sensors can follow and improve how typically patients take their medication, similarly empowering them to have a dynamically instructed trade with their PCP about treatment. While taking pills with a sensor may give off an impression of being meddling, the system is pick in as for patients, and they can end sharing a couple of sorts of information, or quit the program all things considered, at whatever point.

13.5.6 Related Contact Lens

Remedial more intelligent contact focal point is a forceful use of the Internet of Things in a human services setting. While the thought has a great deal of potential, as of recently, the science hasn't commonly made sense of how to fulfill trust. In 2014, Google Life Sciences (by and by known as Verily, a helper of Google's parent association Alphabet) detailed it would develop an astute contact point of convergence that could measure tear glucose and give an early advised system to diabetics to caution them when their blood glucose levels had dropped or climbed past a particular breaking point. It joined together with Alcon, the eyecare division of pharmaceutical association Novartis, for the undertaking [31].

In any case, the endeavor pulled in a ton of doubt from experts who acknowledged that evaluating blood glucose levels by methods for tears wasn't deductively steady—and finally, they were exhibited right. After an extensive stretch with no certified news about errand headways, in November 2018 Verily asserted that the endeavor was being racked [32].

In any case, other restorative applications for sharp contact central focuses may show dynamically productive. Verily is up 'til now working on two keen points of convergence programs with Alcon, which intend to treat presbyopia (long-sightedness realized by lost adaptability in the point of convergence of an eye) and cascade medicinal method recovery. Swiss association Sensimed has also developed a noninvasive quick contact point of convergence called Triggerfish, which normally records changes in eye estimations that can incite glaucoma. First made in 2010, Triggerfish is by and by CE-checked and FDA-supported, which implies it is confirmed for exhibiting and arrangement in Europe and the U.S. and was embraced accessible to be obtained in Japan in September 2018 [33].

13.5.7 "Watch" as Solution—Apple Watch Application that Screens Misery

Wearable advancement doesn't, for the most part, should be organized considering a helpful use to have medicinal services benefits. Takeda Pharmaceuticals U.S.A. moreover, Cognition Kit Limited, a phase for assessing abstract wellbeing, collaborated in 2017 to research the use of an Apple Watch application for checking and assessing patients with Major Depressive Disorder (MDD). The results from the exploratory examination were presented in November 2017 at the pharma and biotech gathering CNS Summit [34].

The examination found a raised degree of consistence with the application, which individuals used each day to screen their attitude and acumen. The application's step by step assessments were furthermore found to relate with target acumen tests and patient-uncovered outcomes, showing that scholarly tests passed on by methods for an application can at present be lively and dependable [35]. While the assessment was only an exploratory pilot, it has displayed the potential for wearable tech to be used to assess the effects of distress dynamically. Like other adroit helpful devices that aggregate data, the Apple Watch application could in like manner give patients and human services specialists more information into their condition, and enable progressively taught conversations about consideration.

13.5.8 Coagulation Testing

In 2016, Roche propelled a Bluetooth-empowered coagulation framework that enables patients to check how rapidly their blood coagulates. This is the primary gadget of its sort for anticoagulated patients, with self-testing appeared to assist patients with remaining inside their restorative range and lower the danger of stroke or dying. Having the option to transmit results to healthcare suppliers implies less visits to the center. The gadget likewise enables patients to add remarks to their outcomes, reminds them to test, and banners the outcomes in connection to the objective range.

13.5.9 Apple's ResearchKit and Parkinson's Disease

In 2018, Apple included another "Development Disorder API" to its open-source Research Kit API, which permits Apple Watches to screen Parkinson's Disease manifestations. Regularly side effects are checked by a doctor at a center by means of physical indicative tests, and patients are urged to maintain a journal in control to give a more extensive knowledge into manifestations after some time. The API intends to make that procedure programmed and constant. An application on an associated iPhone can show the information in a chart, giving day by day and hourly breakdowns, just as moment by-minute indication variance. Apple's ResearchKit has likewise been utilized in various diverse health thinks about, including a joint inflammation study completed in association with GSK, and an epilepsy study that pre-owned sensors in the Apple Watch to identify the beginning and length of seizures.

Apple is quick to tout the potential for its applications to help with medicinal research and care, and keeping that in mind, in 2017 it propelled CareKit, an open-source system intended to assist engineers with creating applications for overseeing ailments. Not at all like HealthKit, which is pointed more at general wellness and prosperity, CareKit can be utilized to structure applications with a particular therapeutic reason—so watch this space for increasingly restorative developments that utilize iPhone and Apple Watch innovation.

13.5.10 Asthma Monitoring Using Technology

The gadget was initially expected to accomplish FDA freedom and be discharged for shoppers toward the finish of 2017, yet hasn't yet been cleared, demonstrating that these gadgets can now and then set aside a long effort to come to advertise even once created. Be that as it may, an examination on patient health checking stages that consolidate IoT gadgets distributed in July 2018 notices that ADAMM is "relied upon to get FDA freedom soon".

There are clear worries of defenselessness associated with associated healthcare, which alongside the meticulousness of medication improvement might be easing back the advancement of new computerized meds. Be that as it may, it's unmistakable what direction the breeze is blowing. From adherence to analysis, the applications are complex. Specifically, lifelogging (which conceded is regularly an instance of versatile health, not carefully IoT) appears to be still to be an influential thought, changing how patients collaborate with their center. This is especially the situation for estimating emotional information for those experiencing uneasiness or wretchedness. At last, one can perceive any reason why Apple is getting into this space with HealthKit, ResearchKit, and CareKit, and Google with GoogleFit and backups like Verily. It's not hard to envision a future in which iOS or Android applications communicate with a lot of our drugs. As a greater amount of these gadgets are brought to advertise and even become accessible as physician recommended prescription, for instance on the NHS, advanced healthcare will begin to turn into the standard as opposed to the special case.

13.6 IoMT [Internet of Medical Things]

It is difficult to overestimate the spot of IoT in healthcare nowadays. Brilliant gadgets, wearables, and the general degree of network and advancements in current restorative hardware have changed the business for eternity. Also, unquestionably to improve things. In this piece, you'll locate an exhaustive response to most of the inquiries you can have about the territory of IoT in healthcare in 2019 [1].

13.7 Prominence of IoT in Healthcare

To state that advanced prescription is endeavoring would be a moderate articulation. The advancement quickens each day "with no regret", changing all known therapeutic practices. Worldwide healthcare develops dependent on the most recent accomplishments of the planet's most prominent personalities and astonishing possibilities of independent, self-learning tech arrangements. Alongside such quick advancement, in any case, comes a severe need to stay aware of the pace. Interestingly, all medicinal fields are either looking to or as of now go connected at the hip with trend-setting innovations—from diagnostics to therapeutics, from pediatrics to complex medical procedures.

Innovations are various—man-made brainpower, AI—and so on. In any case, what specific tech idea or a mix of ideas can give adequate observing and overseeing forces such an evergrowing, worldwide specialty requires? The appropriate response might be found on the Internet of Things or IoT. In spite of the idea's generally youthful age, it's as of now gotten firmly snared with healthcare. So much that it is regularly begat as the Internet of Medical Things. Broad centralization and interconnection limits the IoT tech gives are hard to overestimate. It brings health checking, remote treatment, medical clinic physical, and advanced framework association to an unheard-of level. However, how about we consider on IoT controls in healthcare in more fine-grained detail. IoT-Based centralized network of interconnected devices which indicates that the innovation has an assorted field of application in medication. Well, we investigate some significant executions.

13.8 IoT Use Cases in Healthcare

a. Remote Patient Monitoring

In 2018, NHS England—an "official nondepartmental open body of the Department of Health and Social Care" declared that it will bolster a remote diabetes treatment arrangement. The announcement was made on World Diabetes Day 2018. The arrangement is a Continuous Glucose Monitor (CGM). A gadget that is the size of a penny that screens blood glucose level relentlessly after it's embedded in a patient's arm.

The checking information can be effectively gotten to by means of your Android or iOS gadget. Mass-showcase occasions of such items are Freestyle Libre and Eversense. Such savvy health observing gadgets carry tremendous incentive to the examination and treatment of diabetics. The Eversense persistent glucose checking sensor can be embedded in the patient's arm and keeps going as long as 90 days. What's more, in numerous different cases, remote abilities (additionally called telehealth) may make the need to visit your neighborhood emergency clinic for all intents and purposes out of date [37]. Going further into the remote subject, the IoT system can interface and track essentially any sensor embedded into a human body for therapeutic purposes. This will help forestall heart failures (MoMe Kardia from InfoBionic), a wide range of seizures, and give medicinal assistance to basic patients without a moment to spare. InfoBionic's wearable cardinal tracker streams ECG and movement information to the specialist continuously.

The World Health Organization led an examination in 2003 to discover that around 50% of endorsed prescriptions aren't taken the correct way or totally disregarded. An unmistakable case of settling this issue is the ingestible sensors arrangement created by Proteus. These little sensors happen of a solution and send a sign an accepting gadget upon disintegration in the stomach. An astounding propelled creation, Proteus' "brilliant pills" will without a doubt help lessen the paces of erroneous, silly utilization of profoundly significant medicinal remedies. Presently, this is the thing that one can call a really propelled medication the board. While being a propelled bit of medicinal innovation, Porteus Smart Pills have a similar little size as the genuine pills. There are additionally brilliant pills that element small cameras, which permit helpfully imagining within the condition of one's life form. PillCam from Medtronic is one model.

13.9 Health Care in Mobility Condition

Likewise called mHealth, it's the method for watching and dealing with one's health through portable can be a genuine lifeline for current patients, basically, every one of whom uses cell phones normally. Versatile health is a rising field that contributes vigorously to both basic medicinal circumstances and ordinary treatment examples.

As we've just referenced in the "Remote patient observing" segment, portable applications can fill in as the administration implies for health GPS beacons. There are a few new companies who are attempting to pick up a piece of the overall industry with their portable application. Such applications can be utilized as your all-out healthcare center where you can get to significant restorative data, break down your life form conduct patterns, oversee other body-embedded IoT sensors, and contact your primary care physician with a solitary tap.

This is a particularly significant answer for immature nations of the reality where individuals can't bear the cost of ordinary visits to medical clinics yet, most likely, have cell phones. What's more, governments, thusly, get an ability to perceive how the populace is getting along as far as health, collecting monstrous insights. There are numerous applications effectively accessible available, running in usefulness and reason:

- Medication the board applications
- Fitness applications
- Body, movement, and rest following applications
- Pregnancy observing applications
- Individual health recording applications.

13.10 Beaming Hospitals

The disappointment with defective, hard to oversee medical clinic foundations is a typical issue of a greater part of the globe's nations (even the created ones). Enormous heaps of desk work, long and baffling lines, and employed over-burden most medical caretakers and specialists experience—this is the place the issue stalks. Basically, all these circumstances can be turned around with a mix of IoT arrangements. Immense, bulky research can be supplanted with a computerized, brought together a database, which can be furthermore upgraded as far as dependability with blockchain and brilliant agreements; a solitary administration framework can get entries, help ideally control lines, and track staff individuals by means of their cell phones; all the hardware can likewise be remotely observed and overseen (e.g., shut down in exceptional cases). Such developments can help incredibly lessen in-house costs for clinics, safeguard backwoods, and make the two patients' and therapeutic staff's lives simpler. The general profitability will likewise increment because of the computerized savvy arrangements' ability to quickly perceive health issues which would somehow or another take a long time of live specialist diagnostics.

With IoT-controlled wearables, sensors, information investigation, and portable chances, fighting interminable sicknesses become progressively proficient and available. The thing is, repeating health issues must be checked and dissected over extensive stretches of time. That way, slants in the sickness variances can be characterized and compared so as to be most productively treated. All that tech permits doing only that, with numerous extra abilities gave by the mix of blockchain and AI what's more. This is significant with regards to health issues as hard to comprehend and underexplored as the constant ones.

13.11 IoT-Related Challenges in Healthcare

As much as the Internet of Medical Things is by all accounts progressive and profoundly effective, there are still some significant difficulties of IoT in healthcare this tech idea must defeat not far off. With huge, game-changing incorporations, for example, this one, there goes along a horde of specialized troubles and adjustment issues. The fundamental include:

- Underdeveloped activities. Numerous IoMT activities coordinated at doing combating interminable maladies or different issues still need time to develop and create. This mechanical specialty, in general, should grow a ton so as to begin giving standard upgrade results.
- Possible absence of accessible memory. IoT sensors and gadgets can general enormous measures of information, which is all significant and should be broken down. This offers a conversation starter of gigantic information stores that must hold every one of those volumes of data for inconclusive terms.
- Difficulties with customary updates. With such a significant number of equipment, arrangements come as a lot of programming for controlling and overseeing everything. This product must be conveniently refreshed so as to run easily and remain at its most recent rendition.
- Personal delicate information security. An IoT-controlled drug is an equipment sponsored framework.
- Global healthcare guidelines. The IoMT still must be endorsed by worldwide healthcare administrative bodies around the world. This will require some serious energy and may keep numerous advancements under control as a result of certain conventions.

Compensation and Disadvantages of IoT in Healthcare—Considering the previously mentioned difficulties of IoT in healthcare, there are, surely, drawbacks just as advantages with regards to the restorative IoT.

Role of IoT in Healthcare

The "all-expending" association of health gadgets and information centralization carries numerous critical advantages to the table, for example, all-around mechanical upgrade. Rendering clinic visits superfluous, latently collecting and profoundly investigating significant health information, and so on. We've just considered on all these propelled tech limits aplenty enough. The IoMT gives space to fabulous long haul advancements. Table 13.1 concludes the research with recent and prominent contributions in this magnificent field.

Cost investment funds. Probably the best bit of leeway of IoT in healthcare is that effective self-sufficient frameworks will cost less to oversee and "utilize" over the

Table 13.1 Prominent contributions in this magnificent field

Contributor details	Details of contribution
Rath et al. [2]	Technological Development in health care
Lomotey et al. [3]	Wearable IoT data stream in DHIS (Distributed health Information System)
Farahani et al. [6]	Fog-driven IoT in e-health care
Riazul Islam et al. [7]	IoT Health prescription assistant
Djedi et al. [8]	Flexible design of wireless body sensor network for health care
Adame et al. [9]	RFID-WSN hybrid smart health care system
Lloret et al. [10]	5G based protocol for smart and continuous e-health monitoring system
Zachariae et al. [11]	Cloud-based personalized system for cancer patients
Olayinka et al. [12]	Big data information in global health education
Knoppers et al. [13]	Ethics and big data in Health Sector

long haul. Things are far and away superior with regards to patient cost reserve funds because of less emergency clinic travels just as quickened diagnostics and treatment.

Accessibility—Specialists can see all the fundamental information on the direction and check ongoing patient conditions without leaving their office.

13.12 Drawbacks of IoT in Healthcare

A few drawbacks that join the huge usage of the IoT in healthcare include:

- Privacy can be conceivably undermined. As we've just referenced, frameworks get hacked. Heaps of consideration should be centered around information security, which requires critical extra spendings.
- Unauthorized access to centralization. Quite possibly untrustworthy intruders may get to concentrated frameworks and understand some coldblooded aims.
- Global healthcare guidelines. Universal health organizations are now giving rules that must be carefully trailed by legislative medicinal foundations incorporating the IoT in their work process. These may limit potential abilities somewhat.

13.13 IoT Trends in Healthcare

In 2019, there can be characterized a few IoMT patterns executed by larger parts of new businesses around the world.

- Wearables keep on fixing the market. Significant versatile innovation suppliers like Apple and Android are improving and refreshing their real wearables, including them with more health following highlights. What's more, the remainder of the world isn't bashful to pursue the propensity, bringing forth various different reasons smaller than expected gadgets.
- Surgical mechanical technology becomes a typical reality. Artificial intelligence fueled, automated careful methods show to be more exact than genuine specialists over and over. There are still confinements and dangers included, yet the innovation is certainly in the spotlight and is hoping to turn out to be increasing across the board in the closest future.
- Integration of other unmistakable advancements with the IoT grows the skyline. Man-made intelligence, AR, Machine Learning, Big Data, blockchain, and savvy contracts—the entirety of that fuel up and grows the IoT controls significantly further. Artificial intelligence is as of now better and unquestionably progressively exact in anticipating, for one occurrence, ladies' cancer disease.

13.14 Prospect of Future IoT in Healthcare

Out and out keen emergency clinics by 2020, mHealth as a standard, normal thing on a worldwide scale, and decreased physical visits to medical clinics—this is just an inexact image of the IoMT achievement [36]. All things considered, as youthful as the idea seems to be, it isn't generally respected to be that novel by dynamic clinics of the now. The vast majority of them are either actualizing major IoT methods or capacities or as of now have upgraded parts that are in their adjustment arrange. It is assessed that the introduce base of IoT gadgets in healthcare will be in excess of 161 million units before the finish of 2020. As indicated by some autonomous forecasts, very nearly 90% of healthcare foundations and association worldwide will utilize the IoT as a normal in-house apparatus before the finish of 2019. Along these lines, the "now" of the healthcare IoT is truly distinctive, with its future looking much more brilliant.

13.15 Conclusion

Let us stress again that the IoT can be out and out an upset in the field as significant on the worldwide scale as healthcare. There are as yet numerous troubles, characteristics, and innovative obstructions to survive. What's more, despite the fact that there are, at present, drawbacks just as points of interest to the idea, things appear to go very well for this mechanical advancement. We are really sure that on the off chance that you get some information about their supposition regarding the matter, they will say that full IoMT reconciliation and adjustment is the main legitimate method for improvement for cutting edge prescription of things to come.

References

1. https://dzone.com/articles/iot-in-healthcare-use-cases-trends-advantages-and. Last accessed on 31st Dec, 2019.
2. Rath, M., & Pattanayak, B. (2019). Technological improvement in modern medical sector applications using IoT and proposal of novel medical sector approach. *International Journal of Human Rights in Medical sector, Emerald Group Publishing, 12*(2), 148–162.
3. Lomotey, R. K., Pry, J., & Sriramoju, S. (2017). Wearable IoT data stream traceability in a distributed health information system. *Pervasive and Mobile Computing, 40*, 692–707. ISSN 1574-1192.
4. Qiu, H. J. F., Ho, I. W. H., Tse, C. K., & Xie, Y. (2015). A methodology for studying 802.11p VANET broadcasting performance with practical vehicle distribution. *IEEE Transactions on Vehicular Technology, 64*(10), 4756–4769.
5. Sun, E., Zhang, X., & Li, Z. (2012). The Internet of Things (IOT) and cloud computing (CC) based tailings dam monitoring and pre-alarm system in mines. *Safety Science, 50*, 811–815.
6. Farahani, B., Firouzi, F., Chang, V., Badaroglu, M., Constant, N., & Mankodiya, K. (2018). Towards fog-driven IoT eHealth: Promises and challenges of IoT in medicine and healthcare. *Future Generation Computer Systems, 78*(Part 2), 659–676. ISSN 0167-739X.
7. Hossain, M., Riazul Islam, S. M., Ali, F., Kwak, K.-S., & Hasan, R. (2017). An Internet of Things-based health prescription assistant and its security system design. *Future Generation Computer Systems*. https://doi.org/10.1016/j.future.2017.11.020. Available online 2 December 2017. ISSN 0167-739X.
8. Harbouche, A., Djedi, N., Erradi, M., Ben-Othman, J., & Kobbane, A. (2017). Model driven flexible design of a wireless body sensor network for health monitoring. *Computer Networks, 129*(Part 2), 548–571. https://doi.org/10.1016/j.comnet.2017.06.014. ISSN 1389-1286. http://www.sciencedirect.com/science/article/pii/S138912861730258X.
9. Adame, T., Bel, A., Carreras, A., Melià-Seguí, J., Oliver, M., & Pous, R. (2018). CUIDATS: An RFID–WSN hybrid monitoring system for smart medical sector environments. *Future Generation Computer Systems, 78*(Part 2), 602–615. ISSN 0167-739X.
10. Lloret, J., Parra, L., Taha, M., & Tomás, J. (2017). An architecture and protocol for smart continuous eHealth monitoring using 5G. *Computer Networks, 129*(Part 2), 340–351. https://doi.org/10.1016/j.comnet.2017.05.018. ISSN 1389-1286.
11. Kyriazakos, S., Valentini, V., Cesario, A., & Zachariae, R. (2017). FORECAST—A cloud-based personalized intelligent virtual coaching platform for the well-being of cancer patients. *Clinical and Translational Radiation Oncology*. ISSN 2405-6308.
12. Olayinka, O., Kekeh, M., Sheth-Chandra, M., & Akpinar-Elci, M. (2017). Big data knowledge in global health education. *Annals of Global Health*. ISSN 2214-9996.
13. Knoppers, B. M., & Thorogood, A. M. (2017). Ethics and Big Data in health. *Current Opinion in Systems Biology, 4*, 53–57. https://doi.org/10.1016/j.coisb.2017.07.001. ISSN 2452-3100.
14. Pramanik, M. I., Lau, R. Y. K., Demirkan, H., & Azad, M. A. K. (2017). Smart health: Big data enabled health paradigm within smart cities. *Expert Systems with Applications, 87*, 370–383. https://doi.org/10.1016/j.eswa.2017.06.027. ISSN 0957-4174.
15. Wang, Y., Kung, L. A., Wang, W. Y. C., & Cegielski, C. G. (2017). An integrated big data analytics-enabled transformation model: Application to medical sector. *Information & Management*. https://doi.org/10.1016/j.im.2017.04.001. ISSN 0378-7206.
16. Carney, T. J., & Kong, A. Y. (2017). Leveraging health informatics to foster a smart systems response to health disparities and health equity challenges. *Journal of Biomedical Informatics, 68*, 184–189. ISSN 1532-0464.

17. Hussain, A., Wenbi, R., da Silva, A. L., Nadher, M., & Mudhish, M. (2015). Health and emergency-care platform for the elderly and disabled people in the Smart City. *Journal of Systems and Software, 110*, 253–263. ISSN 0164-1212.
18. Finlay, D. (2016). Chapter Seven—Connected health approaches to wound monitoring. In J. Davis, A. McLister, J. Cundell & D. Finlay (Eds.), *Smart bandage technologies* (pp. 229–244). Cambridge: Academic. ISBN 9780128037621.
19. Rogers, W. A., & Mitzner, T. L. (2017). Envisioning the future for older adults: Autonomy, health, well-being, and social connectedness with technology support. *Futures, 87*, 133–139. https://doi.org/10.1016/j.futures.2016.07.002. ISSN 0016-3287.
20. Jeste, D. V., Blazer, D. G., Buckwalter, K. C., Keri-Leigh, K. C., Fishman, L., Gwyther, L. P., et al. (2016). Age-friendly communities initiative: Public health approach to promoting successful aging. *The American Journal of Geriatric Psychiatry, 24*(12), 1158–1170. https://doi.org/10.1016/j.jagp.2016.07.021. ISSN 1064-7481.
21. Shamim Hossain, M., Rahman, M. A., & Muhammad, G. (2017). Towards energy-aware cloud-oriented cyber-physical therapy system. *Future Generation Computer Systems*. https://doi.org/10.1016/j.future.2017.08.045. ISSN 0167-739X.
22. Au, M. H., Yuen, T. H., Liu, J. K., Susilo, W., Huang, X., Xiang, Y., et al. (2017). A general framework for secure sharing of personal health records in cloud system. *Journal of Computer and System Sciences, 90*, 46–62. ISSN 0022-0000.
23. Neethirajan, S., Tuteja, S. K., Huang, S.-T., & Kelton, D. (2017). Recent advancement in biosensors technology for animal and livestock health management. *Biosensors and Bioelectronics, 98*, 398–407. ISSN 0956-5663.
24. Archenaa, J., & Mary Anita, E. A. (2015). A survey of big data analytics in healthcare and government. *Procedia Computer Science, 50*, 408–413. https://doi.org/10.1016/j.procs.2015.04.021. ISSN 1877-0509.
25. Khalifa, M., & Zabani, I. (2016). Utilizing health analytics in improving the performance of healthcare services: A case study on a tertiary care hospital. *Journal of Infection and Public Health, 9*(6), 757–765. ISSN 1876-0341.
26. Fotopoulou, E., et al. (2016). Linked data analytics in interdisciplinary studies: The health impact of air pollution in urban areas. *IEEE Access, 4*, 149–164.
27. Lepeule, J., Laden, F., Dockery, D., & Schwartz, J. (2012). Chronic exposure to fine particles and mortality: An extended follow-up of the Harvard six cities study from 1974 to 2009. *Environmental Health Perspectives, 120*(7), 965–970.
28. Samoli, E. (2014). Which specific causes of death are associated with short term exposure to fine and coarse particles in Southern Europe? Results from the MED-PARTICLES project. *Environment International, 67*, 54–61.
29. Kiesewetter, G., Schoepp, W., Heyes, C., & Amann, M. (2015). Modelling $PM_{2.5}$ impact indicators in Europe: Health effects and legal compliance. *Environmental Modelling & Software, 74*, 201–211.
30. Vippalapalli, V., & Ananthula, S. (2016). Internet of things (IoT) based smart medical sector system. In *2016 International Conference on Signal Processing, Communication, Power and Embedded System (SCOPES), Paralakhemundi*, pp. 1229–1233.
31. Satheesh, S. R., Sangeetha, D., & Vaidehi, V. (2013). EPSSHIC-enabling privacy and security of smart medical sector system in cloud. In *2013 International Conference on Recent Trends in Information Technology (ICRTIT), Chennai*, pp. 79–83.
32. Wu, H.-T., & Horng, G.-J. (2017). Establishing an intelligent transportation system with a network security mechanism in an internet of vehicle environment. *IEEE Access*, 2169–3536 (c) 2017 IEEE. Translations and content mining, https://doi.org/10.1109/access.2017.2752420.
33. https://www.asianhhm.com/information-technology/smart-health. Last Accessed on 10th Dec, 2017.
34. Shah, T., et al. (2016). Remote medical sector cyber-physical system: Quality of service (QoS) challenges and opportunities. *IET Cyber-Physical Systems: Theory & Applications, 1*(1), 40–48. https://doi.org/10.1049/iet-cps.2016.0023.

35. Patel, P., Intizar Ali, M., & Sheth, A. (2017, September/October). On using the intelligent edge for IoT analytics. *IEEE Intelligent Systems, 32*(5), 64–69.
36. Scarfò, A. (2018). Chapter 3—The cyber security challenges in the IoT era. In M. Ficco & F. Palmieri (Eds.), *Security and resilience in intelligent data-centric systems and communication networks*. Intelligent data-centric systems (pp. 53–76). Academic. ISBN 9780128113738.
37. Chakraborty C. (2019). Mobile Health (m-Health) for tele-wound monitoring. *IGI: Mobile Health Applications for Quality Healthcare Delivery* (Ch. 5, pp. 98–116).
38. Chakraborty, C., Gupta, B., & Ghosh, S. K. (2013). A review on telemedicine-based WBAN framework for patient monitoring. *International Journal of Telemedicine and e-Health, 19*(8), 619–626.

Chapter 14
Bigdata in the Management of Diabetes Mellitus Treatment

Dhanaraj Rajesh Kumar, K. Rajkumar, K. Lalitha, and V. Dhanakoti

Abstract Due to technological advancement and digitalization within the medical field, there is tremendous growth in the medical data on a daily basis. The data includes but not limited to, personal data of patients and other frequent clinical data generated through health centers, government and private hospitals, etc. This data is represented in the form of electronic health records, registers, and patient wearable sensors and stored in a secure cloud. Eventually, the storage will have heterogeneous data. A large amount of information stored on cloud space is required to extract the data by applying the efficient big data analytic techniques, to assemble and handle the analysis. The various applications of big data analytics tools and techniques are growing quickly in the domain of management of diabetes mellitus treatment as it is considered one of the most common deficiencies of the current era. Applying machine learning and deep learning techniques to produce a prediction of disease risk and collect the various hospital's performance related to diabetes. It provides a large number of benefits such as available treatments, costs of treatment, outbreaks prediction of epidemics, and to recommend the best health care system. In this chapter, we are going to discuss the various types of diabetes and its management, sustainable healthcare systems, and health care information exchanges using big data, decrease medical errors and supporting collaboration, etc. Also, the big data technology plays vital role to manage the diabetic mellitus treatment in the trustworthy and security. The identification of fraud in medical information and misuse of medical resources

D. Rajesh Kumar
School of Computing Science and Engineering, Galgotias University, Greater Noida, India

K. Rajkumar
Department of Information Technology, Galgotias College of Engineering and Technology, Greater Noida, India

K. Lalitha (✉)
Department of Information Technology, Kongu Engineering College, Erode, Tamil Nadu, India
e-mail: klalitha.it@kongu.edu

V. Dhanakoti
Department of Computer Science and Engineering, SRM Valliammai Engineering College, Chennai, Tamil Nadu 603203, India

C. Chakraborty et al. (eds.), *Internet of Things for Healthcare Technologies*, Studies in Big Data 73, https://doi.org/10.1007/978-981-15-4112-4_14

are discussed briefly in this chapter. A deep study is carried out on key issues and the actual use of big data analytics in diabetes healthcare.

Keywords Diabetes mellitus treatment · Big data analytics · Predictive models · Machine learning · Deep learning

14.1 Introduction

Diabetes mellitus (DM), typically referred to as diabetic issues, diabetes mellitus is actually a variety of illnesses recognized by huge amounts of glucose within the blood caused by defects in deep insulin generation (insulin deficiency), insulin actions (insulin resistance), or perhaps the two. Insulin is actually a hormone created by the pancreas. When consumed, food items transform into a sugar type known as glucose, which enters the bloodstream. Insulin is actually necessary to go glucose directly into the entire body cells in which it's utilized for power, as well as excesses are actually kept in body fat cells and the liver. Inadequate quantities of dealing insulin lead to blood sugar level quantities to increase as well as huge amounts of glucose are actually excreted within the urine. Regularly, tall amounts of glucose within the bloodstream injure the nervous feelings as well as blood vessels and may result in center disorders, stroke, high blood pressure levels, loss of sight, kidney disorders, amputations, as well as dentistry disease [1, 2].

14.1.1 Diagnosis As Well As Classification of Diabetes

Diabetic issues are usually categorized straight into these basic groups [3, 4]:

1. Type one diabetes (due to autoimmune β-cell devastation, typically bringing about complete insulin deficiency)
2. Type two diabetes (due to a progressive loss in β-cell insulin secretion often on the track record of insulin resistance)
3. Gestational diabetic issues mellitus (GDM) (diabetic issues identified during the third or second trimester of pregnancy, which wasn't overt diabetic issues just before gestation)
4. Specific types of diabetic issues because of various other reasons, e.g., monogenic diabetic issues syndromes (such as neonatal diabetic issues as well as maturity-onset diabetic issues of younger [MODY]), illnesses of this exocrine pancreas (such as cystic fibrosis as well as pancreatitis), as well as chemical-induced or drug-diabetic issues (such much like glucocorticoid make use of, inside the therapy of HIV/AIDS, or even subsequent to body organ transplantation).

14.1.2 Type 1 Diabetes

Type 1 diabetic issue is actually a persistent illness recognized through the body's failure to create insulin as a result of the autoimmune damage of these beta cells within the pancreas. Even though beginning often arises within the youth, the illness may also build around grownups [4]. The symptoms of type I diabetic issue are listed below

Polyuria—creation of abnormally big volumes of dilute urine,

Polydipsia—abnormally amazing desire as a warning sign of an ailment (such as mental disturbance or diabetes),

Polyphagia—too much diet or maybe urge for food, particularly as a warning sign of this illness Unexplained weight reduction, Other signs can include fatigue, serious exhaustion caused by physical or mental effort or maybe an illness, nausea a sensation of sickness having a tendency to vomit, as well as blurry eyesight. Examination of type one diabetes consists of all of the following [5]:

- A fasting plasma glucose (FPG) amount ≥126 mg/DL (7.0 mmol/L), or A 2-h plasma glucose amount ≥200 mg/DL (11.1 mmol/L) while in a 75 g dental glucose tolerance check (OGTT), or
- An arbitrary plasma glucose ≥200 mg/DL (11.1 mmol/L) inside an individual with traditional signs of hypoglycemic crisis or even hyperglycemia.

14.1.3 Type 2 Diabetes

Diabetic issues are a difficulty with the body of yours which brings about blood glucose (sugar) that amounts to increase above regular. This is additionally known as hyperglycemia. Type two diabetic issues are probably the most typical type of diabetic issues. In case you've type two diabetes, the entire body of yours doesn't make use of insulin correctly. This is known as insulin opposition. In the beginning, the pancreas of people help to make additional insulin to compensate for it. Nevertheless, with time, it is not in a position to continue as well as cannot earn plenty of insulin to keep the blood glucose of peoples at giving amounts that are typical. Type two diabetic issues once were recognized as adult-onset diabetic issues, but these days additional kids are now being identified as having the condition, most likely as a result of the increase in youth being overweight. There is no remedy for these type two diabetes, but weight loss, consuming food properly and regular exercise will help control the illness. When diet plan and also exercising are not adequate to handle your blood sugar levels properly, you may even need to eat diabetic issues medicines or maybe insulin treatment. Regular symptoms of type one diabetic issues are elevated desire, frequent urination, increased food cravings, unintended weight reduction, fatigue, blurred eyesight, slow-healing sores, frequent infections, aspects of darkened epidermis, typically within the armpits as well as neck. Type two diabetic issues is generally identified utilizing the following:

- ***Glycated hemoglobin (A1C) check***: This blood check signifies your typical blood glucose amount within the last 2–3 weeks. Amounts that are typical are actually under 5.7%, along with a consequence in between 5.7 along with 6.4% is recognized as prediabetes. An A1C degree of 6.5% or even greater on two distinct assessments indicates you've diabetic issues.
- ***Random blood sugar levels test***: Blood sugar level values are actually conveyed around milligrams a deciliter (millimoles or mg/DL) a liter (mmol/L). Irrespective of whenever you survive consumed, a blood sample indicating that the blood sugar level of yours is actually 200 mg/DL (11.1 mmol/L) or even greater hints diabetic issues, particularly in case additionally you have clues and clues of diabetic issues, for example, excessive desire and regular urination.
- ***Fasting blood sugar levels test***: A blood sample will be tested promptly. A reading through a bit less compared to a hundred mg/DL (5.6 mmol/L) is actually typical. An amount through a hundred to 125 mg/DL (5.6–6.9 mmol/L) is recognized as prediabetes.

In case you are fasting, blood sugar levels are actually 126 mg/DL (7 mmol/L) or even greater on two distinct assessments, you've diabetic issues.

- ***Oral glucose tolerance check***: This examine is much less widely used as opposed to the others, besides throughout pregnancy. The person will get increased sugary fluid level in overnight, the blood sugar level amounts are analyzed occasionally for that coming 2 several hours.

Blood sugar level amounts under 140 mg/DL (7.8 mmol/L) is actually typical. Reading through in between 140 along with 199 mg/DL (7.8 mmol/L as well as 11.0 mmol/L) suggests prediabetes. A reading of 200 mg/DL (11.1 mmol/L) or even greater when to several hours indicates diabetic issues.

14.1.4 Gestational Diabetes Mellitus

Gestational diabetic issues are build up throughout pregnancy (gestation). Just like the remaining types of diabetic issues, gestational diabetes issues have an effect on the way your cells make use of high sugar (glucose). Gestational diabetic issues sources higher blood glucose, which may change the pregnancy of women as well as your baby's overall health. Almost any pregnancy problem is worried, but there is news that is good. Expectant females are able to aid manage gestational diabetic issues by eating ingredients that are healthy, working out as well as, if needed, using drugs. Managing blood sugar levels is able to stop a hard birth as well as prevent the patient and the infant in good health. For gestational diabetic issues, blood sugar levels typically return to usual immediately after shipping. In this case, you may have gestational diabetes issues with type two diabetes. You will do work together with your medical treatment staff to keep track of, as well as controls the blood sugar levels of yours. Indications of gestational diabetes, women with gestational diabetes ordinarily have absolutely no signs and symptoms. Most people master they have it throughout regular pregnancy screening assessments. Hardly ever, particularly, when the gestational diabetic issues are actually from command, you could possibly notice: Feeling a lot thirstier, feeling more often starved as well as consuming more, a requirement to pee.

Gestational diabetes analysis generally takes place within the second one half of pregnancy. The physician of yours may test to find out if you've gestational diabetic issues last few days and the result may be analyzed shortly. To check for gestational diabetic issues, you will rapidly consume a sugary beverage. This can increase blood sugar quantities of yours. One hour later on, you will have a blood examination to find out the way your entire body managed all of that high sugar. When the outcomes indicate that the blood glucose of yours is actually greater when compared to a particular cutoff (anywhere through 130 mg/dL or maybe greater), you are going to need a lot more assessments. This simply means evaluating the blood sugar levels of yours while fasting as well as an extended glucose check of more than 3 h [6].

If the outcome of yours are actually regular though they have an excessive chance of receiving gestational diabetic issues, it might have to be followed–up and checked later on in the pregnancy of yours to ensure you will still not get it. In order to deal with the gestational diabetes of yours, the doctor of yours is going to ask you to look at your blood sugar levels amounts four or maybe a lot more occasions in one day, do urine assessments which look for ketones that implies that the diabetes of yours isn't in check, eat a nutritious diet that is consistent with your physician's suggestions, make physical exercise a practice. The physician of doctors is going to track just how much fat you gain and also allow to find out should to have another medication or insulin for the gestational diabetic issues. Problems of gestational diabetes due to some reasons such as infant birth with high mass, quick birth, respiratory distress syndrome, low blood sugar levels, Mom with hypertension etc. In order to avoid gestational diabetes or upcoming diabetes, obtain, subjected to testing, reports for diabetic issues six to twelve days after giving birth as well as every 1–3years [5–7].

14.1.5 Specific Types of Diabetes Due to Other Causes

Certain varieties of diabetic issues because of various other reasons include things like monogenic diabetic issues syndromes, for example, neonatal diabetic issues or maybe maturity-onset diabetic issues of younger (MODY); illnesses of this exocrine pancreas, for example, serious pancreatitis; cystic fibrosis; endocrinopathies; chemical-induced diabetes or drug, for example, inside the therapy of HIV/AIDS or even subsequent to body organ transplantation; infections; unusual types of immune-mediated diabetic issues; along with other hereditary syndromes which are actually related to diabetic issues. Neonatal diabetic issues are actually identified within the very first six weeks of living as well as isn't normal autoimmune style one diabetes. It can easily be permanent or transient. MODY is actually recognized by impaired insulin secretion without any defects or maybe merely nominal defects in deep insulin excitement. It's passed down within an autosomal dominant pattern. So long as a kid is actually identified as having diabetic issues within the very first six weeks of daily life, has a solid household historical past of diabetic issues (with no common style two diabetes features), has bad autoantibodies, doesn't have indications of insulin opposition, isn't heavy and also displays just moderate hyperglycemia, subsequently, an examination of monogenic diabetic issues must be thought about. Cystic fibrosis related diabetic issues is typical only in cystic fibrosis individuals (20% of adolescents as well as 40, 50% of adults). It worsens health conditions, as well as plays a role in worse inflammatory lung illness as well as increased mortality, though the latter has been enhanced by making use of intense insulin treatment.

14.1.6 Management of Diabetes Mellitus Treatment

Controlling Diabetes: There's absolutely no remedy for diabetic issues, though it may be handled as well as managed. The objectives of dealing with diabetic issues are keeping the blood glucose amounts of yours as close to usual as you can by controlling food items ingestion with actions as well as drugs.

Maintain the blood cholesterol of yours as well as triglyceride (lipid) amounts as close to the standard ranges as practical. Control the blood pressure levels of yours. The blood pressure levels of yours shouldn't go more than 140/90. You can control the diabetic issues of your by observing a healthy supper program, working out, routinely shooting drugs in case recommended, along with strongly adopting the recommendations on when and how to do checking the blood glucose of yours as well as blood pressure levels amounts at home [6].

14.2 Introduction to Big Data and Its Role in the Health Care System

Data: Symbols, characters, or the quantities where businesses are actually done by your personal computer, that might be saved as well as transmitted within the type of electric indicators as well as captured on magnetic, optical, or maybe physical recording media [8]. *Large Data*: Large data details information sets come to be extremely huge which they're hard to thing to do utilizing just data source managing equipment or maybe conventional info managing equipment. Large data additionally identifies every one of the services, infrastructures, and the technologies which allow it to be easy to gather, grocery as well as evaluate information gathered as well as manufactured in boosting numbers, making use of automated synthetic intelligence

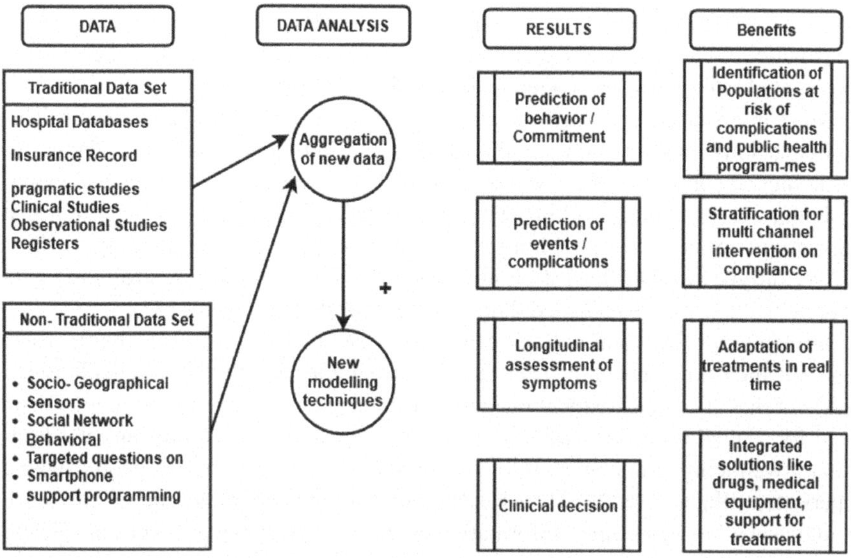

Fig. 14.1 Comparing traditional and non-traditional data

and processing activity systems [9]. It is regular process the '4Vs' which characterized in big data: an explosion of this volume on the information, velocity of the info as well as simultaneous processing velocity, as well as the great represented by the information because of the entity or even person. Diabetic issues as well as heart problems are actually two of the essentially priciest as well as common persistent circumstances impacting individuals within India, reputable the health care business to invest enormous amounts each year for treating as well as control the conditions.

As treatment shipping continues to evolve against reactive illness therapy to hands-on preventive attention, a lot more businesses actually want to complex systems such as man-made intelligence plus printer learning to help with inhaling actionable conclusions coming from the large details of their resources, see in Fig. 14.1 [10].

Large data entails the aggregation as well as merging of large and heterogeneous datasets while training analytics to embrace an examination of patterns to come down with academic process or maybe overall performance within aggregate or single detail sets. Health treatment suppliers nowadays have to become knowledgeable on the managing of powerful and complex characteristics of big data and analytics to guarantee expert informative applications are actually responsible for those applications operated as well as designed. Even though utilizing digital engineering has typically produced a few small amounts of on the happenings whereby these were used as well as the way they had been used to these activities. Large data exploits several details of energy as well as hints that the majority of huge information that may be employed in overall health treatment provider training analysis the majority of probable weren't found for training reasons. For instance, the information which may be gathered by using numerous institutions as well as merged along with other details, which includes the following: public demographics or maybe wellness results information, to determine broader patterns of conduct and the effect of it compared to potential making use of academic details alone [8, 11].

Most information types are usually examined working with large details. This particular info consists of these types of details as important symptoms, diagnoses, medicines, recommended, as well as countless types of noted illnesses and symptoms may be examined working with large details. Scientists have found out that an examination associated with a sexual or maybe gender condition amplified the danger of type two DM by 130%; practically the identical price as struggling with hypertension, a well-established threat element for diabetic issues [12].

Implementing big data analytics can lead to sizable expense, cost savings and also the same measurements of the keep (LOS) for diabetics additionally, on readmission fees. For diabetics that are mentioned to a medical center, there's a tremendous basic need for diabetic inpatient training just before discharge. It requires an interdisciplinary wellbeing treatment staff to offer products for a big public of people having a persistent illness like DM [13]. Health information has a multitude of info, each digital as well as newspaper. Information could be the following: Electronic Health Reports (EHR) of sufferer's information, clinical accounts, crisis treatment information, physician's doctor prescribed, analysis accounts, health-related photographs, drugstore info, wellness insurance-related details, every other clinical details through the Computerized Patient Order Entry (CPOE) process, information coming from social networking (including Twitter feeds (so-called tweets), logs, condition revisions on other operating system and Facebook, as well as net pages); as well as much less patient-specific info like media feeds, as well as posts to come down with health-related or maybe nursing journals. Information that is raw also could be examined more for glucose dimensions, blood pressure levels readings, as well as other dimensions or even readings [14, 15].

14.3 Comparative Study on Various Big Data Analytic Methods in the Health Care System

Though essentially, the most recently available ten years, at this time there continues to be a quick digitalization across the business organizations. A therapeutic system works with Electronic Medical Records (EMRs); Healthcare Information Systems as well as handheld, wearable outstanding devices. Thus, a huge amount as well as assortment of health connected info nowadays is within the sophisticated framework that incorporates' comic's info, socio socioeconomic info as well as safety assertions info divided against clinical info. This phenomenal interpersonal insurance info provides possible motivation for improving proper care conveyance, nonetheless, it's even now "seen as a consequence of man solutions conveyance, rather than a focal learning resource hotspot for top hands" [9] Since the electric health info stays to an excellent level underutilized also hence squandered, there's a necessity for switching during crude info in significant and important details info contained wellness treatment expertise is actually spread as well as dispersed, originating by using various energy sources as well as owning styles and buildings various, we can see in Table 14.1 [16].

The conceptual framework for a huge information analytics task in deep healthcare is actually akin to this of a regular health and fitness informatics or maybe analytics task. The crucial distinction is based on the way processing is actually performed. Within a typical health and fitness analytics task, the evaluation could be done having a company intelligence application set up for a standalone phone system, like a desktop computer or even laptop computer. Since great details are actually by characterization big, processing is actually divided as well as carried out throughout several nodes. The idea of sent out processing has been around for many years. What's fairly brand-new is the usage place of it within examining huge info sets as health care suppliers begin to take advantage of their big detail's repositories attain awareness to make better-informed health-related choices. In addition, receptive supply operates the system, for example, Hadoop/MapReduce, on the cloud, has urged the use of serious details analytics in deep overall health therapy.

Even though the algorithms as well as clothes airers are actually very similar, the end-user interfaces of standard analytics equipment as well as all those employed for great details are completely different; conventional health and fitness analytics equipment are becoming extremely individual warm and friendly as well as transparent. Large details analytics equipment, however, are incredibly intricate, programming extensive, as well as need the use of an assortment of abilities. They've emerged within an advertisement hoc manner largely as open source growth equipment and also data set, consequently they are lacking the help and user-friendliness which vendor-driven proprietary resources have. As Fig. 14.2 suggests that the intricacy takes place using the information itself [17] (Table 14.2).

14.4 Machine Learning Approaches in Diabetes Mellitus Treatment

Machine learning techniques that can check out the 200 variables rather than 5 or maybe 6 variables, there is an extremely considerable jump of phrases of accuracy. Researchers will even make use of printer learning how to enhance persistent illness managing as well as therapy protocols for the circumstances. Present therapy protocols usually use a one-size-fits-all strategy, evaluating the point of illness instead of the unique affected person. With printer mastering algorithms, nonetheless, suppliers are able to structure personalized interventions for every affected person, out of improved checking of altered therapy programs. These customized attempts are able to assist them to intervene ahead of when a person's problem gets to a crucial stage, leading to reduced proper care expenses as well as enhanced overall health results.

Table 14.1 Various sources we collecting health care data

S. No.	Category	Source of health care data	Description	Sources
1	Diabetics clinical data	Electronic Medical Records (EMRs)	Thorough patient-related info (physician prescriptions, medicines, healthcare history)	Clinics and hospitals
		Diagnostic	Analysis results (imaging benefits, lab reports)	Laboratories, radiology departments
		Molecular characteristic	Molecular {datal details linfo} (genomic, proteomic, transcript to mic, meta bolomic)	Analysis companies
		Administrative data	Administrative details (admission, discharge, monetary data and transfer) (claims)	Clinics and clinics data clustering
2	Diabetics healthcare-claims	Medical claims	Healthcare reimbursement information (procedures, medical center keeps, insurance policy details)	Data clustering
		Prescription claims	Doctor prescribed reimbursement information (drugs, serving, duration)	Data clustering
3	Diabetics clinical test	Clinical trails	Style details (compound, sizing, conclusion points)	Pharma companies, medical journals
4	Patient generated data	Social media, wearable, and sensors	Town considerations, wellness, and way of life information (smartphones, health and fitness monitors)	Net health portals social networking websites, device data systems

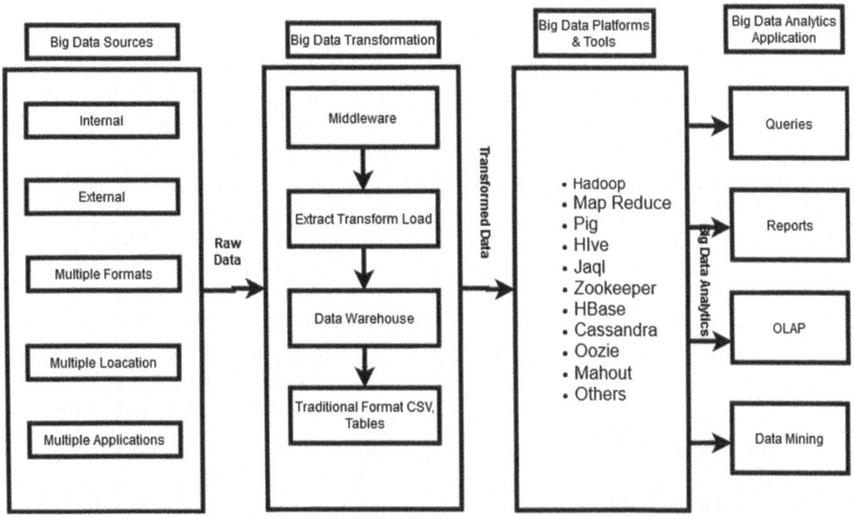

Fig. 14.2 The intricacy takes place using the information itself

> If you take a look within the present status of healthcare found India, we're really proficient at dealing with factors whenever they show up, and once the circumstances start to be considerable adequate to warrant focus in the wellbeing treatment program. Nevertheless, I do not believe we're very great only in phrases of stopping the conditions,
>
> Using printer learning how to think of personalized predictions as well as suggestions will considerably reinforce avoidance attempts. Far better avoidance cannot merely enhance results for people, but additionally significantly bring down wellness treatment spending.

In order to obtain the aim, nonetheless, printer mastering equipment should be rooted, accurate, and trustworthy within details that are dependable. A particular likely possibility of utilizing printer learning would be that the information might be incorrect. When we're teaching algorithms, which are generating predictions on incorrect details, there's a threat that any of us could possibly achieve a bad conclusion. We've checked out diabetic issues and heart problems, these staying maybe the two most prominent persistent sicknesses which impact probably the most individuals. Diabetes mellitus might be a persistent sickness recognized by signs. It must cause a lot of problems. In the Earth, the diabetic people will be increased to 642 zillions before 2040. Later on, is actually laid minimal with the polygenic condition. There is very little doubting this forbidding figure would like excellent interest using the fast advancement of printer learning, printer learning has been put on to a number of areas of healthcare health and wellbeing.

A far more comprehensive as well as official meaning of printer learning is actually provided by Mitchel [18, 19]: A pc plan is actually believed learning through expertise *E* related to several category of projects *T* and also general performance degree *P*, in case the performance of its of projects within *T*, as assessed by *P*, gets better with expertise *E*. Acquisition of expertise is actually a vital necessity of treatments

Table 14.2 Big data techniques in diabetics health care system

S. No.	Big data analytics techniques	Healthcare application
1	Machine learning	Prediction of illness danger, assessment of this medical center efficiency, determination of epidemics, etc.
2	Natural Language Processing (NLP)	Enhancement of performance of attention and managing expenses, providing treatments, consultation, and training, identification of high-risk elements, extraction of info out of clinical paperwork, reducing the chance of mortality and morbidity
3	Neural networks	Examination of persistent illnesses, prediction of patients' long-term illness
4	Pattern recognition	Enhancement of public health and wellbeing surveillance
5	Spatial analysis	Removing significant population-level insights through the use of advanced, spatial, and visual analytics
6	Cluster analysis	Dedication of morbid obesity clusters for determining high-risk organizations, determination of public clusters with certain wellbeing determinants for therapy of persistent diseases
7	Data mining	Bio-signal keeping track of for health-related irregularities, determination of epidemics, inductive thought as well as exploratory details evaluation inside healthcare
8	Graph analytics	Evaluation of medical center overall performance throughout a variety of quality measures

meant to display smart actions. Given that mastering is a good method to expose some awareness, the majority of synthetic intelligence research thus far has used mastering strategies. The main goal of studying under expertise is allowing pcs to educate yourself instantly with no man treatment or even guidance. This method may entail some technique which contains a few inductive parts, which range from a fairly easy Kalman filtration system to an elaborate convolution neural community. Absolutely no technique is inherently superior to any type or other; each is much more or maybe much less good suited to various scenarios, e.g., a much softer mastering curve, quicker delivery, or perhaps much more adaptable fixes. In addition, the show of different techniques are directly connected with the quality and also volume of information: when a bit more info is actually gathered, as well as a lesser amount of racket is actually contained in the information, more effective remedies could be received. The most crucial households of methods are pointed out below (Fig. 14.3).

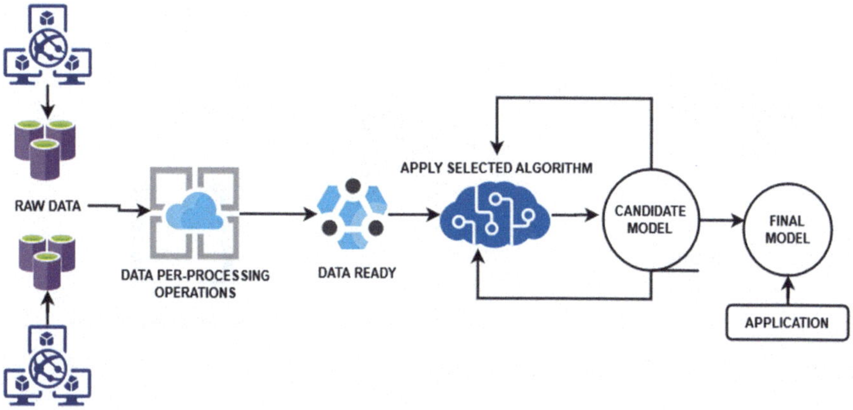

Fig. 14.3 General diagram for machine learning algorithm process

Machine Learning is classified into three board categories [20], which are given as follows:

I. ***Supervised Learning***—whereby the device infers a characteristic out of marked instruction information, you've entered variables (a result and x) adjustable (Y) and also you drive an algorithm to master the mapping feature in the feedback to the result. $Y = f(X)$, at this time there are actually two types of mastering job to begin with a single classification and also regression. Distinction clothes airers make an effort to anticipate unique instructional classes, for instance, like blood organizations, hemoglobin amount, and so on. Within the regression version, it is going to predict numerical values. Several of the typical methods within supervised discovering are actually decision tree (DT), rule learning (RL), as well as instance based learning (IBL), artificial neural network (ANN), as well as support vector machines (SVM).

II. ***Unsupervised Learning***—may be the instruction of a synthetic intelligence (AI) algorithm utilizing info that's neither categorized neither marked as well as making it possible for the algorithm to act on this info with no direction. The objective of unsupervised learning is commonly to bunch the information into characteristically various organizations. Unsupervised piece of equipment mastering tends to be more complicated compared to supervised mastering because of the lack of product labels. Exact same details could be clustered directly into organizations that are various based on how clustering is completed (Fig. 14.4).

Unsupervised mastering has two types, at this time there are actually: Clustering: Clustering is actually utilized for examining as well as grouping information and that doesn't incorporate pre-labeled category or maybe category characteristics. Clustering types are actually Hierarchical clustering, K-means clustering, KNN (k nearest neighbors), Principal Component Analysis, Singular Value Decomposition, Independent Component Analysis. Association:

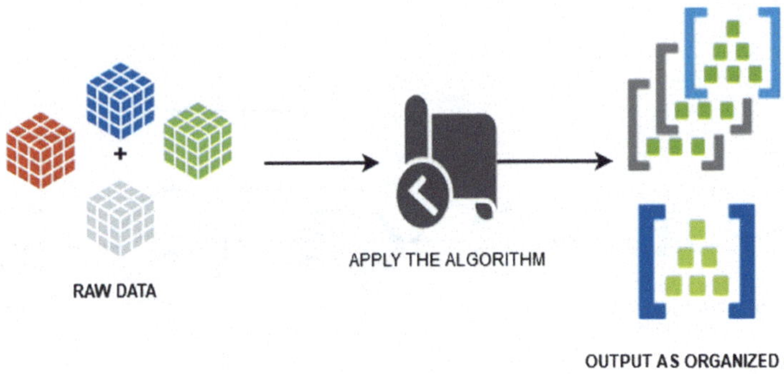

Fig. 14.4 Diagrammatic representation of unsupervised learning

Association discovers the likelihood of this co-occurrence of products inside a set.

III. ***Reinforcement Learning***—Reinforcement learning will be the instruction of printer mastering clothes airers to create a sequence of choices. The agent learns to attain an objective within an unsure, likely complicated setting. Inside reinforcement learning, synthetic intelligence faces a game-like circumstance. The hp EliteBook 8740w mobile workstation engages error and trial to think of a means to fix the issue. In order to have the printer to complete what the coder desires, synthetic intelligence will get possibly penalties or incentives for all the activities it works. The objective of it is maximizing the entire incentive. Even though custom sets the incentive policy that is actually the guidelines of a game he provides the product absolutely no tips or maybe ideas for how you can resolve the game. It is as much as the design to discover how you can do the job to optimize the incentive, beginning out of completely arbitrary trials as well as completing with superhuman abilities and advanced techniques. By using the strength of many trials and the search engines, reinforcement learning is presently the most reliable method to hint the machine's imagination. In comparison to man, synthetic intelligence is able to collect practical experience coming from a large number of parallel gameplays when a reinforcement mastering algorithm is actually operated on completely impressive computer system infrastructure (Tables 14.3 and 14.4).

14.5 Deep Learning Approach in Diabetes Mellitus Treatment

Full mastering contained overall health treatment that helps you to present the physicians, the evaluation of manual and disease them in dealing with a certain illness within a far better method. Thus, the health conclusions produced by the medical

Table 14.3 Diabetes mellitus with comparing various machine learning techniques

Publication details	Machine learning technique	Type of DM	Source of healthcare data	Validation method	Accuracy level (%)
Diabetes prediction using artificial neural network [21]	Neural networks	Type 1	The dataset for the diagnoses of diabetes was gathered from the documentation of the Association of diabetic's city of Urmia which contains 1004 samples with nine attributes	Cross-validation	87.3
End-to-end data science example: predicting diabetes with logistic regression [22]	Logistic regression	Type 1 and Type 2	The information had been collected and also created ideal by "National Institute of Diabetes as well as Digestive as well as Kidney Diseases" together with the Pima Indians Diabetes Database. The information established is made up of a history of 767 individuals to come down with total	Cross-validation	78
An accurate diabetes prediction system based on K-means clustering and proposed classification approach [23]	K-mean clustering	Type 1 and Type 2	The information had been collected and also created ideal by "National Institute of Diabetes as well as Digestive as well as Kidney Diseases" together with the Pima Indians Diabetes Database. The information establish is made up of history of 767 individuals to come down with total	Cross-validation	98.7

Table 14.4 Comparison results of the different system

Used method	Accuracy (%)
Naïve Bayes	79.56
SVM	78
SVM + modified k-means	96.71
LDA − MWSVM	89.74
SVM + fuzzy C-means clustering	94.30
K-means clustering	98.7

professionals could be done much more sensitive and therefore are getting better around criteria. Rich mastering is actually a type of printer learning. In contrast to contained printer learning, function extraction as well as distinction isn't explicitly completed in serious mastering networks. The concealed levels of full mastering networking do this implicitly inside itself while not including the outside researcher. A brief explanation of rich mastering networks is actually provided beneath.

14.5.1 Recurrent Neural Network

Recurrent neural community (RNN) is capable of doing removing powerful temporal actions coming from a type in time period sequence. Fundamental RNNs is actually networking of nodes emulating neurons, each one having a directed (one way) link with each and every alternative node. Each and every node includes a time-varying real-valued activation. Every hookup (synapse) includes a real-valued industry that could be altered in each and every iteration. Nodes are sometimes entering nodes to get information at the exterior of this networking or maybe paper nodes which produce scans, or maybe concealed nodes that alter the information and that goes by via them through the course of theirs at type into result. The distinction through the conventional feedforward neural networks is actually RNN is capable of doing utilizing the inner status of it, normally referred to as mind, to thing to do sequences of inputs (Fig. 14.5).

14.5.2 Long-Short-Term Memory

Lengthy short-term remembering (LSTM) devices are actually a specific type of creating devices for RNN. It is able to evaluate, classify as well as foresee temporal details sequences of precious time lags of every dimension. A common LSTM networking consists of mind, feedback, result, and also does not remember gates. The remembering contained LSTM can easily recall values more than arbitrary period times. Every one of the three gates are actually a type of the neuron (which computes an activation perform associated with a weighted sum). A lot more than this, the

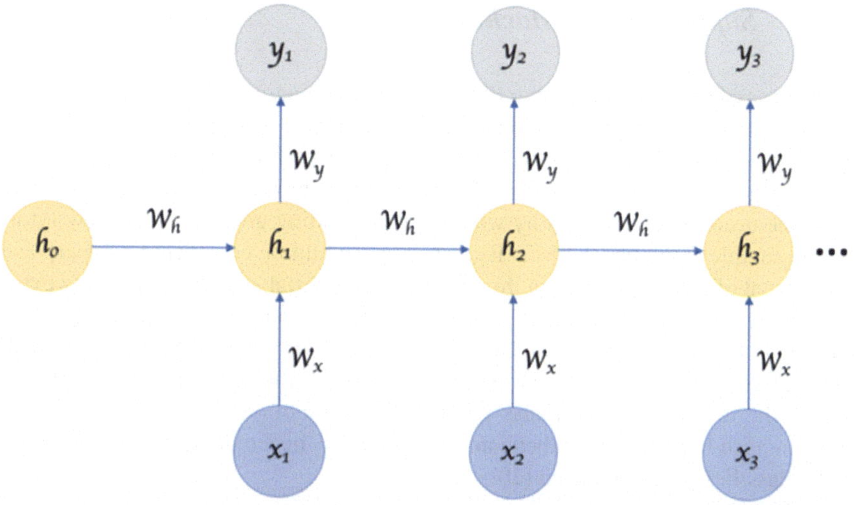

Fig. 14.5 A recurrent neural network, with a hidden state that is meant to carry pertinent information from one input item in the series to others

gates limit the passage of values within LSTM layers; hence these specific neurons are actually called gates. By lengthy short-term, the reality underlined is the fact that LSTM's mind is able to keep going for a big period length. LSTM discusses the problem of exploding as well as disappearing gradient issues that is a crucial problem while instruction conventional RNNs.

14.5.3 Convolutional Neural Network

Convolutional neural community (CNN) is actually an improvised version of a multilayer perceptron. CNN is frequently comprised of feedback, a paper level, and lots of concealed levels. The concealed levels of a CNN usually are comprised of convolutional, pooling, moreover completely connected levels.

14.5.4 Hybrid Networks

Inside crossbreed networks, the original component is actually CNN comprising of max pooling levels as well as convolution just. The maxpooling1D layer's paper is actually given to the type in the level of subsequent rich mastering structure as LSTM or RNN utilized.

14.5.5 Support Vector Machine

Inside the assistance vector printer (SVM), every information sample is actually represented like a place inside the room. It's guaranteed that a large splitting up prevails for samples of various groups. Whenever a brand-new information sample comes, mapping to area very first occurs. The grouping of brand-new sample is actually made the decision determined by what edge of dividing gap; the brand-new information sample stage lies. SVM's distinction gap could be considered a hyperplane in the event of binary distinction. In case over two martial arts classes actually exist, subsequently, the dividing gap is usually considered a pair of hyperplanes put into a substantial dimensional room. The perfect hyperplane is actually selected in such a fashion that there's an optimum probable distance through the closest sample per edge to the sorting out hyperplane. From the situation of ours, distinction is simply to distinguish between the diabetic and normal HRV, hence the fundamental binary SVM classifier is actually used [20].

14.5.6 Diabetes Mellitus with Comparing Various Deep Learning Techniques

14.5.6.1 Using Convolution Neural Networks

See Table 14.5.

14.5.6.2 Using Recurrent Neural Networks

Dataset: The data sets considered for this project were obtained from the online Machine Learning UCI repository. The links of the data sets are given [24].

Attributes	Glucose	Insulin	BMI	Pregnancies	D.P.F	B.P	S.T	Age
Assigned weight	0.8	0.7	0.7	0.615	0.61	0.59	0.55	0.47

		Predicted classes	
		0 (diabetic)	1 (non-diabetic)
Actual classes	0 (diabetic)	421	79
	1 (Non-diabetic)	67	201

Table 14.5 Diabetes mellitus with comparing various deep learning management system

Publication details	Source of healthcare data	Compared algorithms	Validation method	Accuracy level
Diabetes detection using deep learning algorithms Swapna G., Vinayakumar R., Soman K. P.	DIARETDB0 dataset which is publicly available has been used	CNN 1 with SVM	5-fold cross-validation	0.648
		CNN 2 with SVM		0.755
		CNN 3 with SVM		0.887
		CNN 4 with SVM		0.913
		CNN 5 with SVM		0.939
		CNN 1. LSTM with SVM		0.743
		CNN 2. LSTM with SVM		0.764
		CNN 3. LSTM with SVM		0.853
		CNN 4. LSTM with SVM		0.937
		CNN 5. LSTM with SVM		0.957

	Deep learning (type 1 diabetes mellitus)	Deep learning (Pima Indians' diabetes)
Precision for non-diabetic i.e. 0	0.8064	0.75
Precision for diabetic i.e. 1	0.7777	0.842
Recall for non-diabetic i.e. 0	0.9259	0.9066
Recall for diabetic i.e. 1	0.53846	0.55138
Error rate	0.20	0.145

14.5.6.3 Using SVM (Support Vector Machine)

Dataset:
The Pima Indian diabetic issues dataset, donated by Vincent Sigillito, is actually a set of health-related analysis accounts coming from 768 documents of female individuals a minimum of twenty-one years of age of Pima Indian historical past, a public residing close to Phoenix, Arizona, USA [25, 26] (Table 14.6).

14.6 Security and Trustworthy of the Health Management System

Privacy is actually considered a vital governing concept of patient–physician relationship. Patients are needed in order to discuss info with the doctors of theirs to facilitate analysis that is accurate as well as therapy, and also to stay away from negative drug interactions. Nevertheless, people might reveal info that is crucial to situations of health issues such as for instance psychiatric conduct as well as HIV, as the disclosure of theirs could result in public stigma as well as discrimination. With time, a person's healthcare history accumulates considerable private info such as identification, record of healthcare analysis, digital renderings of health-related pictures, treatment options, prescribed medication past, dietary behavior, sexual preference, hereditary info, mental bookmark profiles, work past, cash flow and physicians' very subjective assessments of mental state and character.

Table 14.6 Classification accuracy using SVM

Data set	Samples	Training data	Testing data	Attributes	No. of classes	Using SVM (with RBF Kernel)
Diabetes	460	200	260	8	2	0.755

14.6.1 The Threat to Information Privacy

Even though overall health info privacy continues to be commonly talked about within the interpersonal science as well as small business media, the academic literature doesn't have a systematic investigation to determine as well as classify a variety of energy sources of threats to info privacy as well as security. Recent policy-based scientific studies broadly categories privacy threats, or maybe method to obtain info safety measures, directly into two areas:

1. Organizational threats which crop up against inappropriate gain access to of affected person information by possibly inner elements mistreating the privileges of theirs or maybe outside elements exploiting a vulnerability of this info systems
2. Systemic threats that crop up as a result of an agent within the info flow chain exploiting the disclosed information over and above the planned make use of its.

14.6.2 Privacy Concerns Among Healthcare Consumers

With rising reliance on web-based systems for dealing with the deployment and health info of individual health and wellbeing banks, privacy issues of health care customers came to the cutting edge. Recently, available analysis in this region has usually centered on limited pc user bases, like pupils. Long-term research should check out the variance of privacy tastes within the context of on the internet systems among a broader assortment of owners, which includes the normal functioning public as well as senior citizens. A greater comprehension of the elements influencing health care consumers' willingness to disclose private info will allow much better policymaking and enhance the adoption of e-health.

14.6.3 Providers' Perspective of Regulatory Compliance

Regulatory mandates, like HIPAA, are usually criticized for not enough lucidity. Present minimal amounts of total compliance among hospitals involve focus on the analysis group to look at compliance relate disuse on a number of fronts. For instance, scientists can examine: the variance in employee protection hygiene as well as very best methods used by executives to advertise regulatory compliance; the impact of regulatory compliance initiatives on assistance quality; the economics of obtaining and sustaining regulatory compliance; the problems of managing regulatory compliance throughout states with diverging demands; or maybe the outcome of regulatory demands on the digital methods of businesses as well as the partners of theirs.

14.6.4 Information Access Control

Recent exploration of info gain access has mainly focused don' technological fixes. You will discover not many economic scientific studies that provide deeper insights on cost effectively coping with information access command. Healthcare organizations should commit in numerous info protection procedures, like gain access to control systems, intrusion detection methods, policies, and also personnel. Malfunction of those information security methods might interrupt company continuity as well as diminish running effectiveness. Provider groups using movable systems providing ubiquitous access to affected person info might recognize advantages that are considerable within phrases of decreased mistake and increased client satisfaction.

Modeled info governance making use of the game concept to learn the effect of incentives as well as auditing on gain access , revising and establishing gain access to management policies in hospital locations owing to a large number of roles, interdependent information systems, as well as powerful dynamics of function task is actually a pricey Endeavor. Long-term area analysis which accounts for your peculiarities of health care groups (e.g., overriding behavior) is actually necessary in order to look at healthcare's complicated governance problems and also to discover the best methods. From the feedback of ours, we discover just one empirical analysis reporting on real use as well as access privilege provision. In addition, noting the intricacy of process networks within healthcare, fruitful investigation guidance might be developing an understanding of interdependency in between company procedures empowered by info methods, and then how such networks may be unduly impacted by info protection problems.

14.6.5 Data Interoperability and Information Security

The fundamental idea of information interoperability is to facilitate seamless and accurate details exchange in just as well as in between groups to support regular healthcare. Recently available initiatives, like Security and Privacy Solutions to Promote Interoperable Health Information Exchange, have facilitated advancement towards the development of HIEs, enactment of state-level privacy as well as protection legislation, and development of shared privacy and protection treatments (AHRQ, 2007c). Through the policy perspective, long-term analysis is required to a number of places such as for instance the effect of legislative efforts on variants within privacy and protection investments by stakeholders within the states that participate as part of overall health info exchange as well as the improvement of typical data elements for consent to allow the flow of affected person medical-related info across organizations.

14.6.6 Information Security Issues of E-Health

During the previous 5 years, the health care industry has experienced considerable progress within the usage of movable equipment as well as web-based applications. Contemporaneously, info protection studies have focused entirely on the improvement of frameworks as well as protocols to deal with protection problems to come down with e-health.

Inside a recently available examination of privacy as well as protection problems of e-health sites, a number of strategies such as the pseudonymization of metadata, anonymous authentication and multiple identities, obfuscation to counterattacks on patients' privacy especially through what can be viewed as insiders (e.g., insurance companies).

Long-term analysis is actually necessary to look at the usefulness of these privacy-enhancing frameworks and protocols on the operational effectiveness of consumer satisfaction and health care suppliers. An additional potential fertile stream of investigation would be the analysis of personal health bank account diffusion vis-à-vis info protection consequences and also the effect on patients 'privacy, the impact on organizational protection policies, as well as need on info security management online resources.

14.6.7 Information Security Risks in Authorized Data Disclosure

In past times, research has devoted to creating theoretical ways for protected details disclosure. However, healthcare suppliers might not constantly deploy state-of-the-art know-how to disclose data for secondary uses. A field-level comprehension of the operational strength of data disclosure engineering will assist the administrator's perfect disclosure policies as well as choose appropriate information disclosure strategies.

14.6.8 Information Integrity in Deep Healthcare

Past exploration evaluating the effect of investment in wellness IT on healthcare mistakes has been restricted to just one instantiation of system deployment. Long-term analysis is actually necessary to span a number of CPOE installations, each at giving national and is gonial fitness level, to characterize the effect of this type of device on health mistakes and information integrity. This type of scientific studies could possibly think about the impact of a number of factors such as medical center attributes, drug security alert overriding conduct, phony alerts due to the inadequacy of expertise platform (clinical decision support system), incomplete or erroneous affected person history, as well workflow interruptions or even waiting times.

14.6.9 Financial Risk

With developing digitization of overall health captures, healthcare identity theft has turned into a bigger looming problem, being individuals and payers. Facts protection problems may also result in financial losses to different stakeholders such as payers, providers, and patients arising from fraudulent attention as well as drug costs by put-together crooks, the selling of medical identities to unlawful immigrants, as well as fraudulent billing for services hardly ever got bringing about incorrect overall health captures as well as prospective injury to individuals. Besides these anecdotal proofs, organized research of fiscal danger is actually to guide info protection policy growth as well as inform overall health maintenance organizations because they shift towards broader adoption of EHRs methods [7].

14.6.10 Regulatory Implications for Healthcare Practice

As we highlighted previously, at this time there are several avenues for long-term exploration of regulatory compliance problems in the providers' perspective. Nevertheless, the health care industry consists of a number of other players including payers (insurance), companies, wellness info switches, personal health banks in addition to medical scientists. Laws, like HIPAA, are promulgated to guarantee patients' privacy and keep protection through health care networking. Coming from a public policy perspective, we imagine which macroeconomic scientific studies are actually required to calculate the outcome of these laws.

14.6.11 Information Security Risk Management

Recent exploration of info protection chance control in deep healthcare is actually confined to anecdotal proof of profitable setup of frameworks as OCTAVE. Keeping in your mind that an individual dimension doesn't fit in each, long-term study needs to check out exactly how these frameworks are now being applied by diverse businesses as well as look at the economics of modification. This particular investigation might possibly inform providers on the greatest methods for applying OCTAVE like frameworks.

In addition, several of the outside threats which might interrupt businesses call for company continuity preparation. The study is actually necessary to guide health care groups on continuity preparation. We believe in this assessment plus proposed succeeding paths will promote additional study that should provide useful insights to decision-makers within the part of health care info privacy as well as security [27].

14.7 Issues and challenges in Management of Diabetes Mellitus Treatment

14.7.1 Type 2

The improved comprehension of this pathophysiology of sort two diabetes (T2D) has resulted in the improvement of different drug courses with novel systems of motion, for instance, these based upon incretin stress hormones. In spite of the breakthroughs to come down with healthcare treatment, the first-line therapy for many T2D individuals is actually metformin, a dental antihyperglycemic medicine that grew to be commercially accessible. As T2D is actually progressive, nearly all people are going to require therapy intensification to attain suggested glycemic (HbA1c) quantities. This usually includes mixture treatment of two or maybe a lot of more dental drugs or maybe escalation to injectable treatments (insulin or maybe GLP 1 receptor agonists). Two combination treatments or maybe move to GLP 1 receptor agonists or maybe insulin is able to bring in brand-new unwanted side effects, like diarrhea or vomiting within the situation of GLP 1 receptor agonists or perhaps hypoglycemia as well as fat gain as well as the situation with insulin.

While we have seen outstanding developments recently, at this time there remain to become deficits within T2D treatments. An optimum therapy would meaningfully bring down HbA1c, reduce diligent adherence as an aspect contained therapy effectiveness, and also have little complications. If it had been attained, the usage of health care methods—such as the quantity of period in which health care suppliers invest in T2D managing—might be substantially decreased while enhancing the lives of countless individuals.

These actions can help keep the blood sugar levels amount closer to usual, which may hold off and/or protect against problems.

14.7.1.1 Weight Loss

Slimming down is able to reduce the blood sugar quantities in the human body. Shedding simply 5–10% of the weight is able to generate a positive change, though a sustained fat loss of 7% plus of the original weight appears to be best. This means somebody who weighs in at 180 excess weight (22 kg) will have to shed a bit under 13 excess weight (5.9 kg) to produce an influence on blood sugar levels quantities. Managing meal portions as well as consuming foods that are healthy are easy solutions to begin having the fat off.

14.7.1.2 Healthy Eating

In contrast to the famous notion, there is absolutely no certain diabetic issues diet plan. Nevertheless, it is essential to century our diet plan around:

- Fewer calories
- Fewer enhanced carbs, particularly sweets
- Fewer ingredients that contain saturated fats
- Fruits as well as veggies
- More food with fibre.

A registered dietitian is able to make it easier to develop a supper strategy which suits the health objectives of people, foods tastes, as well as way of life. She or he is able to likewise educate on exactly how to keep an eye on the carbohydrate consumption and also allow them to be familiar with just how a lot of carbs they have to consume together with their snack, foods, and dishes to maintain their blood sugar levels quantities much steadier.

14.7.1.3 Physical Activity

Every person requires frequent cardiovascular physical exercise, as well as individuals that have type two diabetic issues, aren't any different. Get the physician's OK before beginning a workout plan. Pick things people like, walks, going swimming, as well as biking, such they are able to cause them to become a part of the daily program [23, 28].

Goal for a minimum of 30–60 min on average (or 15–30 min of vigorous) of cardiovascular physical exercise on the majority of the days or weeks of this week. A mix of routines—cardiovascular workouts, like going for walks or maybe dancing on many days or weeks, put together with opposition training courses, like weightlifting or even yoga exercises two times every week—provides additional advantages compared to whichever exercise type on its own.

Keep in mind that strenuous activity reduces blood sugar levels. Check the blood sugar levels amount of yours just before virtually any exercise. You may have to consume a bite just before physical exercise to help you stop very low blood sugar levels in case you are taking diabetic issues drugs which bring down the blood sugar of yours. It's also important to reduce the amount of time you spend on inactive activities, such as watching TV. Try to move around a bit every 30 min.

14.7.1.4 Monitoring Your Blood Sugar

Based on the therapy program of yours, you might have to test as well as capture your blood sugar levels amount then and now or even, in case you are on insulin, many times one day. Question the doctor of yours how frequently he or maybe she needs one to examine the blood sugar levels of yours. Thorough keeping track of is definitely the best way to ensure that the blood glucose amount of yours continues to be inside the goal span of yours.

14.7.1.5 Diabetes Medications and Insulin Therapy

A number of individuals who have type two diabetes are able to attain their goal of blood glucose amounts with exercise and diet, but several likewise need diabetic issues medicines or maybe insulin treatment. Their decision regarding what medicines are perfect depends upon elements that are a lot of, such as the blood glucose amount of them and some other health conditions. The physician may blend medicines coming from various instructional classes to support and control the blood sugar levels within a number of distinct ways [29, 30].

14.7.2 Type 1

The occurrence of T1DM is actually overlooked as approximately 5–15% of adult style two diabetes mellitus (T2DM) instances may be T1DM. The important distinguisher in between T2DM and T1DM could be the detection of autoantibodies from islet beta-cell antigens at giving illness business presentation. About 85–90% of T1DM patients showed ≥1 of these autoantibodies: those reactive to insulin (IAA), glutamic acid decarboxylase 65 (GAD65), insulinoma-associated autoantigen 2 (IA2A), zinc transporter 8 (ZnT8A), and tyrosine phosphatase IA-2β and IA-2β antibodies. Correct examination of T1DM is vital for giving adequate attention and stopping problems.

There's absolutely no certain remedy for T1DM, as well as insulin treatment is actually needed for lifestyle. The main objective is actually maintaining normoglycemia, reduce hypoglycemia, as well as minimize the danger of problems. A common plan for treatment consists of regular keeping track of glucose quantities as well as an individualized insulin program.

Self-monitoring of blood glucose (SMBG) is able to guide appropriate insulin dosing as well as meal/snack make up. SMBG have a glucose meter to keep track of glycemia patterns to counteract hypoglycemia. A glucose sensor used on the epidermis top comes with an insertable probe which continuously monitors glucose amounts within the cell's interstitial solution. Such a real-time constant glucose overseeing (rt CGM) Hojo motor magnetic generator enables individuals to have fast precautionary measures for keeping normoglycemia. It's additionally helpful for individuals with recurrent asymptomatic hypoglycemia (i.e., hypoglycemia unawareness).

Throughout 14 randomized, controlled clinical trials, rt CGM has resulted in a much better decrease in smaller durations and A1C of all hypoglycemia as well as hyperglycemia when in contrast with SMBG with a glucose meter. There is actually some lag (up to 7 min) in between interstitial substance glucose and plasma, as well as individuals have to regularly adjust the rt CGM unit with capillary blood glucose samples for end result confirmation. Precision of rt CGM gadget isn't regarded as sufficient with the FDA to change the traditional glucose meters for point-of-care tests of hospitalized patients. Anybody who has type one diabetic issues must have long-term insulin treatment.

Types of insulin are numerous and also include: short-acting (regular) insulin, rapid-acting insulin, intermediate-acting (NPH) insulin, and long-acting insulin instances of short-acting (regular) insulin consist of Humulin R, as well as Novolin R. Rapid-acting insulin instances, are actually insulin glulisine (Apidra), insulin lispro (Humalog) and also insulin Aspart (Novolog). Long-acting insulins consist of insulin glargine (Lantus, Toujeo Solostar), insulin detemir (Levemir) and also insulin degludec (Tresiba). Intermediate-acting insulins consist of insulin NPH (Novolin N, Humulin N).

14.7.2.1 Insulin Administration

Insulin cannot be used orally to reduced blood sugar levels due to the fact belly enzymes will fail the insulin, stopping the motion of its. Patients will have to obtain it often by way of injection therapy or maybe an insulin pump.

14.7.2.2 Injections

To utilize a good needle as well as a syringe or maybe an insulin dog pen to inject insulin below the epidermis of yours. Insulin pens appear much like printer ink pens and therefore are made only in refillable or disposable variations.

If injection therapy is chosen by doctors, and they will probably have a combination of insulin types that can be used during the day as well as evening. Several days injection therapy which includes a mix of long-acting insulin coupled with rapid-acting insulin much more strongly imitate the body's regular utilization of insulin compared to do more aged insulin regimens which just needed just one or maybe 2 photos one day. A program of three or maybe a lot more insulin injection therapy one day has been found to enhance blood sugar levels quantities.

14.7.2.3 Artificial Pancreas

The Food and Drug Administration authorized the very first synthetic pancreas for individuals with type one diabetes that are age range 14 as well as more mature. It is likewise known as closed-loop insulin shipping. The implanted Hojo motor magnetic generator links a consistent glucose computer monitor, and that determines blood sugar levels amounts every 5 min, to an insulin pump. The unit instantly provides the right quantity of insulin whenever the computer monitor signifies it is required.

There will find much more synthetic pancreas (closed-loop) methods already for clinical trials [30, 31].

14.8 Future Work

Profitable Diabetes Treatment needs data, discussion on the utilization of man-made intelligence (AI health and) particularly is ubiquitous within the lay and medical media reflecting the notion that it's an opportunity that is overwhelming to minimize the global and personal concern of numerous long-range health conditions. Presently, diabetic issues seem to be the poster kid of the use of AI found overall health takes care of a selection of reasons. All over the world, the selection of grownups plus kids acquiring diabetic issues carries on to increase around parallel with worldwide entry to smartphone solutions. During an everyday foundation, private details of individuals coping with diabetic issues are continually produced as well as logging. Though the key variable of fascination is sugar, using the increase in customer monitoring solutions, sugar information is now being supplemented with extra info relevant to nourishment, exercise, and then rest. With all the growing options of extra sensor solutions for biological keeping track of, as well as sensible insulin pens, social networking, and also documents of online searches, the diabetic issues information swimming pool will proceed to grow. Moreover, additional data generating comorbidities (e.g., cardiac arrhythmias and high blood pressure) in addition to info via screening assessments for problems (e.g., retinopathy) will also be contributing to this particular "big data" useful resource.

14.9 Conclusion

Diabetic mellitus issues are actually an ailment that may cause numerous problems. Tips on how to really anticipate as well as identify the condition by utilizing printer learning may be worth learning. Printer mastering techniques are now being progressively developed as appropriate for using wearing clinical day procedure, and also because of the self-management of diabetic issues. For that reason, the options offer highly effective resources for boosting patients' quality of living.

Within the literature, smart algorithms are commonly used within data-driven techniques to allow for superior analytics and supply personalized healthcare tools. There's additionally proof that an escalating variety of overall health treatment businesses are putting on the strategies. Short-term prospects suggest they're more likely to have a lot of results within the clinical process. The primary factors for the development consist of the intense rise in the quantity of information that is available, together with the much better functionality of smart methodologies able to deal with and process this particular info, each of that contain resulted in the improvement of equipment plus programs which could improve the real managing of complex illnesses, which includes cancer and diabetic issues rich knowing could additionally be worn within healthcare distinction, segmentation, registration, as well as other tasks. Deep learning is actually utilized around aspects of medication such as retinal, pulmonary, digital pathology, neural and so on. Rich mastering is a continuously building pattern within the area of information evaluation. Rich mastering is actually a development of man-made neural networks that be made up of even more levels from greater amounts of abstraction.

There's an enhancement within the predictions in the information created utilizing heavy mastering algorithms. Full mastering is actually appearing as an extremely crucial printer mastering instrument for imaging, convolutional neural networks, personal computer domains eyesight, etc. It learns the key associations in the information of yours as well as documents the info regarding previous customers that can be worn an upcoming guide for your individuals with indications that are quite similar or even illnesses. It permits us to produce a model based on no matter what method to obtain information out there once you need a threat score after administration apart from discharge. Serious mastering gives timely and accurate threat scores that allow the self-confidence as well as a rough allocation of online resources. It approaches result in reduced expenses and supplies much better outcomes. When the full mastering algorithms connect to the instruction information, they start to be far more exact as well as correct enabling people to attain unprecedented insights directly into proper care procedures, variability, as well as diagnostics.

References

1. Baynes, H. W. (2015). Classification, pathophysiology, diagnosis, and management of diabetes mellitus. *Journal of Diabetes and Metabolism, 6*(5). https://doi.org/10.4172/2155-6156.1000541.
2. Punthakee, Z., Goldenberg, R., & Katz, P. (2018). Definition, classification and diagnosis of diabetes, prediabetes and metabolic syndrome. *Canadian Journal of Diabetes, 42*, S10–S15.
3. American Diabetes Association. (2014). Diagnosis and classification of diabetes mellitus. *Diabetes Care, 37*, S81–S90.
4. American Diabetes Association. (2010, January). Diagnosis and classification of diabetes mellitus. *Diabetes Care, 33*(Suppl. 1), S62–S69.
5. Metzger, B. E., & Coustan, D. R. (Eds.). (1998). *Proceedings of the Fourth International Workshop–Conference on Gestational Diabetes Mellitus. Diabetes Care, 21*(Suppl. 2), B1–B167.
6. American Diabetes Association. (2003, January). Gestational diabetes mellitus. *Diabetes Care, 26*(Suppl. 1), s103–s105. https://doi.org/10.2337/diacare.26.2007.S103.
7. Udhayakumar, H. (2019). Safety measures for EHR systems. In *Security and privacy of electronic healthcare records: Concepts, paradigms and solutions* (pp. 272–289). London: Institution of Engineering and Technology. https://doi.org/10.1049/PBHE020E_ch10.
8. Wullianallur, R., & Raghupathi, V. (2014). Big data analytics in healthcare: Promise and potential. *Health Information Science and Systems, 2014,* 2–3. https://doi.org/10.1186/2047-2501-2-3.
9. Murdoch, T. B., & Detsky, A. S. (2016). The inevitable application of big data to health care. *JAMA, 309*, 1351–1352.

10. Zimmet, P., Alberti, K. G., & Shaw, J. (2001, December 13). Global and societal implications of the diabetes epidemic. *Nature, 414*(6865), 782–787.
11. Saravana Kumar, N. M., Eswari, T., Sampath, P., & Lavanya, S. (2015). Predictive methodology for diabetic data analysis in big data. *Procedia Computer Science, 50*, 203–208.
12. Ramesh, S., Caytiles, R. D., Iyengar, N. Ch. S. N. (2017). *A deep learning approach to identify diabetes*. UCI Repository of Bioinformatics Databases. Website: http://www.ics.uci.edu/~mlearn/MLRepository.html.
13. Anuja Kumari, V., & Chitra, R. (2013, March–April). Classification of diabetes disease using support vector machine. *International Journal of Engineering Research and Applications (IJERA), 3*(2), 1797–1801.
14. Raghupathi, W., & Raghupathi, V. (2014). *Health Information Science and Systems, 2*, 3. https://doi.org/10.1186/2047-2501-2-3.
15. El-Jerjawi, N. S., & Abu-Naser, S. (2018). Diabetes prediction using artificial neural network. *Journal of Advanced Science, 124*, 1–10.
16. Rouse, W. B., & Serban, N., (2014). *Understanding and managing the complexity of healthcare*. Cambridge, MA: The MIT Press.
17. Amit, B., Chinmay, C., Anand, K., & Debabrata, B. (2019). Emerging trends in IoT and big data analytics for biomedical and health care technologies. *Handbook of data science approaches for biomedical engineering* (Ch. 5, pp. 121–152). Amsterdam: Elsevier. ISBN: 9780128183182.
18. Han, J., Kamber, M., & Pei, J. (2011). *Data mining: Concepts and techniques (The Morgan Kaufmann series in data management systems)* (3rd ed.).
19. Alpaydin, E. (2004). *Introduction to machine learning*. Cambridge, MA: The MIT Press.
20. Swapna, G., Vinayakumar, R., & Soman, K. P. (2018). Diabetes detection using deep learning algorithms. *ICT Express, 4*, 243–246.
21. Akash, G., Chinmay, C., & Bharat, G. (2019). Sensing and monitoring of epileptical seizure under IoT platform. In *Smart medical data sensing and IoT systems design in healthcare* (pp. 201–223). IGI. https://doi.org/10.4018/978-1-7998-0261-7.ch009.
22. Chakraborty, C., Gupta, B., & Ghosh, S. K. (2013). A review on telemedicine-based WBAN framework for patient monitoring. *International Journal of Telemedicine and e-Health, 19*(8), 619–626. ISSN: 1530-5627.
23. Hardee, S. G., Osborne, K. C., Njuguna, N., Allis, D., Brewington, D., Patil, S. P., … Tanenberg, R. J. (2015). Interdisciplinary diabetes care: A new model for inpatient diabetes education. *Diabetes Spectrum, 28*(4), 276–282. https://doi.org/10.2337/diaspect.28.4.276.
24. Dhandhania, K. (2018). *Towards data science*. https://towardsdatascience.com/end-to-end-data-science-example-predicting-diabetes-with-logistic-regression-db9bc88b4d16.
25. Kadhm, M. S., Ghindawi, I. W., Mhawi, D. E. (2018). An accurate diabetes prediction system based on K-means clustering and proposed classification approach. *International Journal of Applied Engineering Research*. https://technostacks.com/blog/deep-learning-in-healthcare/.
26. Chakraborty, C. (2019). Mobile health (m-Health) for tele-wound monitoring. *Mobile health applications for quality healthcare delivery* (Ch. 5, pp. 98–116). IGI. https://doi.org/10.4018/978-1-5225-8021-8.ch005. ISBN: 9781522580218.
27. Appari, A., & Eric Johnson, M. (2010). Information security and privacy in healthcare: Current state of research. *International Journal of Internet and Enterprise Management, 6*(4), 279–314.
28. Ellaway, R. H., Pusic, M. V., Galbraith, R. M., & Cameron, T. (2014). Developing the role of big data and analytics in health professional education. *Medical Teacher, 36*(3), 216–222. https://doi.org/10.3109/0142159X.2014.874553.
29. Chu, T. (2016). Current challenges in the management of diabetes, meta cure Type 1 diabetes mellitus: Management challenges. *US Pharmacist, 41*(6), 21–26. Venkatachalam, M. (2019). *Recurrent neural network: Towards data science*. mayoclinic.org.
30. Wang, L., & Alexander, C. A. (2016). Big data analytics as applied to diabetes management. *European Journal of Clinical and Biomedical Sciences, 2*(5), 29–38. https://doi.org/10.11648/j.ejcbs.20160205.11.
31. Contreras, I., & Vehi, J. (2018). Artificial intelligence for diabetes management and decision support: Literature review. *Journal of Medical Internet Research, 20*, e10775. Introduction to BIG DATA: What is, types, characteristics & example. guru99.com.

32. Anderson, A. E., Kerr, W. T., Thames, A., Li, T., Xiao, J., & Cohen, M. S. (2016). Electronic health record phenotyping improves detection and screening of type 2 diabetes in the general United States population: A cross-sectional, unselected retrospective study. *Journal of Biomedical Informatics, 54,* 162–168. https://doi.org/10.1016/j.jbi.2015.12.006.

The manufacturer's authorised representative in the EU is Springer Nature Customer Service Centre GmbH, Europaplatz 3, 69115 Heidelberg, Germany. If you have any concerns regarding our products, please contact ProductSafety@springernature.com

Printed and bound by CPI Group (UK) Ltd, Croydon, CR0 4YY
05/10/2026
02228126-0009